New Methods in Language Processing

Studies in Computational Linguistics

Series Editor
Harold Somers

Further titles in the series

A course in Generalized Phrase Structure Grammar Paul Bennett

Abduction, beliefs and context: studies in computational pragmatics
William J. Black & Harry Bunt (eds)

Linguistic and computational techniques in Machine Translation system design
Peter Whitelock & †Kieran Kilby

Analogical Natural Language Processing Daniel Jones

New Methods in Language Processing

Edited by

D. B. Jones & H. L. Somers

Published in association with
the Centre for Computational Linguistics

UCL PRESS

First published in 1997 by UCL Press
Published in association with the Centre for Computational Linguistics

UCL Press Limited
1 Gunpowder Square
London
EC4A 3DE

and

1900 Frost Road, Suite 101
Bristol
Pennsylvania 19007-1598

British Library Cataloguing-in-Publication Data
A catalogue record for this book is available from the British Library.

Library of Congress Cataloging-in-Publication Data are available

ISBN: 1-85728-711-8

This book has been typeset, proofed and passed for press by the editors.
Typeset in Times Roman and Helvetica.
Printed in Great Britain by T. J. International Ltd, Padstow, Cornwall.

Contents

List of contributors

Melina Alexa Universität Darmstadt
Maria Aretoulaki Universität Erlangen-Nürnberg
Roberto Basili Università Roma II
Dominique Béroule LIMSI-CNRS, Orsay, France
William J. Black UMIST, Manchester
Derek Bridge University of York
Norbert Bröker Universität Freiburg
John D. Burger The MITRE Corporation, Bedford, Mass.
Marie-Hélène Candito Université Paris VII
Alex Collier University of Liverpool
Dennis Connolly Ameritech, Inc., Hoffman Estates, Ill.
Matthew Crocker University of Edinburgh
Hamish Cunningham University of Sheffield
Walter Daelemans Katholieke Universiteit Brabant, Tilburg, The Netherlands
David S. Day The MITRE Corporation, Bedford, Mass.
Gert Durieux Universitaire Instelling Antwerpen, Belgium
David Elworthy Canon Research Centre Europe Ltd, Guildford, Surrey
Jim Entwisle The Flinders University of South Australia, Adelaide
Stefano Federici Par.O.La. Sas, Pisa
Andrew Fordham Price Waterhouse, London
Mike Freeman UMIST, Manchester
Roberto Garigliano University of Durham
Éric Gaussier Université Paris VII
Steven Gillis Universitaire Instelling Antwerpen, Belgium
Michael Groves The Flinders University of South Australia, Adelaide
Gregory Guthrie Maharishi University of Management, Fairfield, Iowa
Udo Hahn Universität Freiburg
Satoru Ikehara Tottori University, Japan
Daniel Jones UMIST, Manchester
Patrick Juola Oxford University
Nenad Koncar Imperial College, London
Jean-Marc Langé IBM, Paris
Michael McTear University of Ulster at Jordanstown, Newtownabbey, Co. Antrim
Yoshihiro Matsuo NTT Communication Science Laboratories, Yokosuka, Japan
Ruslan Mitkov University of Wolverhampton
Hermann Moisl University of Newcastle upon Tyne
Simonetta Montemagni Par.O.La. Sas, Pisa
David J. Nettleton University of Durham

Yoshihiko Nitta Hitachi Ltd, Saitama, Japan
Tadashi Nomoto Hitachi Ltd, Saitama, Japan
Piyush Ojha University of Ulster at Jordanstown, Newtownabbey, Co. Antrim
Miles Osborne University of York
Maria Teresa Pazienza Università di Roma II
Vito Pirrelli ILC-CNR, Pisa
Martine Roques Ecole d'Architecture, Paris-Tolbiac
Susanne Schacht Universität Freiburg
Gabriele Scheler Technische Universität München, Munich
Helmut Schmid Universität Stuttgart
Satoshi Sekine New York University
Satoshi Shirai NTT Communication Science Laboratories, Yokosuka, Japan
Khalil Sima'an Rijksuniversiteit Utrecht
Michael Strube Universität Freiburg
Paola Velardi Università di Ancona, Italy
Per Westerlund Kungliga Tekniska Högskolan, Stockholm
Xinyu Wu University of Ulster at Jordanstown, Newtownabbey, Co. Antrim
Akio Yokoo NTT Communication Science Laboratories, Yokosuka, Japan

Preface

The contributions to this collection are a selection of some of the papers which were presented at NeMLaP, an International Conference on New Methods in Language Processing, held at UMIST, Manchester, in September 1994. Most of the papers have been substantially revised since then to allow, for example, for the incorporation of more recent experimental results, where appropriate.

We were motivated to host NeMLaP by the steadily increasing interest in theories and methodologies in natural language processing (NLP) which could be seen as alternatives to the mainstream techniques of symbolic computational linguistics. NeMLaP aimed to provide a forum for researchers in the broad area of new methods in NLP, i.e. symbolic and non-symbolic techniques of analogy-based, statistical, and connectionist processing, to present their most recent research and to discuss its implications. Although focusing on the processing of *written* language, it was hoped that topics of interest would include

- example- and memory-based machine translation
- corpus-based NLP
- bootstrapping techniques
- analogy-based NLP
- connectionist NLP
- statistical machine translation/NLP
- theoretical issues of sub-symbolic vs symbolic NLP
- hybrid approaches

The high quality of the papers, and the interest that has been expressed in the results of the conference persuaded us to produce this anthology of representative contributions.

Faced with contributions on a wide variety of topics, it is always difficult for the editors to decide how to arrange them. The papers contained in this collection cover a wide variety of topics, from a wide variety of approaches. We decided to group them according to the latter: Part I contains three papers on analogy-based methods, Part II looks at connectionism, Part III the use of corpora, Part IV example-based machine translation, Part V statistical approaches, Part VI hybrid approaches, with a discussion of methodological issues by Cunningham et al. making up Part VII. But we might equally have arranged the work so that papers addressing similar topics were grouped, perhaps as follows.

The biggest section would have covered – not surprisingly – **parsing** and **disambiguation**. Montemagni et al. present an analogy-based approach to the difficult problem of recognizing grammatical relations in a relatively free-word-order language like Italian. Moisl and Wu et al. both take a Simple Recurrent Network approach to parsing. The former compares neural networks and traditional finite-state automata, arguing against the widely held reservations about FSA parsing, and proposes a general SRN approach. The latter concentrates on disambiguation of semantic roles. Basili et al. take a probability-based approach to PP-disambiguation, whereas Entwisle & Groves take a purely algebraic approach to parsing, using constraint-based reasoning rather than probability calculations, exploiting inflections and closed-class word sequences. Westerlund et al. tackle the problem of parsing natural speech using a Guided Propagation Network. Message passing is the technique adopted by Bröker et al., who adapt it to a fully lexicalized, head-driven, dependency-oriented approach. Government–Binding theory is the framework in which Fordham & Crocker discuss the unification of specifications of syntax based on psychologically plausible hypotheses about language learning and the use of probabilistic information in principle-based grammars and parsers. Osborne & Bridge show how a unification-based grammar can be acquired using a hybrid of model-based and data-driven learning. Sima'an works in the framework of Stochastic Tree Substitution Grammars, and presents algorithms for computing the probability of a parse and the probability of an input sentence and its most probable derivation.

Related to parsing is the problem of **tagging**, a discipline that has certainly undergone a renaissance with the increased use of non-symbolic methods and the increased availability of large corpora. Schmid addresses the problems that taggers based on the Markov Model face when they have to estimate transition probabilities from sparse data by the use of a decision tree. Elworthy describes a technique for detecting errors made by Hidden Markov Model taggers, based on comparing observable values of the tagging process with a threshold.

Discourse is the topic of four papers. Mitkov presents a method for identifying the focus (or "center") in a discourse segment by recalculating probabilities using Bayes's formula. Nomoto & Nitta describe experiments in discovering coherence in unconstrained text using quantitative techniques from information retrieval: their technique makes use of their theory of discourse segments for Japanese, and the experiments show an analysis of newspaper editorials. Connolly et al. describe the application of machine learning to the resolution of anaphoric reference, in particular casting anaphoric reference as a classification problem, and comparing various classification techniques. Nettleton & Garigliano describe the use of evolutionary algorithms inspired by research in biology in the task of optimizing dialogues.

Papers looking at **translation** can be divided between those presenting an overall model of translation and those focusing on particular inherent problems. The former category is represented by Koncar & Guthrie's neural network approach to English–Serbo-Croatian translation, and Juola's use of the Marker Hypothesis from language-learning research in an English–Urdu system based on simulated annealing. Papers looking at individual problems include Scheler's experiments with supervised learning using standard back-propagation to generate Russian aspect from English interlingual representations, and Jones & Alexa's attempts at aligning German compounds with English multi-word groups using *n*-gram associations. Matsuo et al. present a proposal to do English–Japanese transfer by pattern-matching parse trees as an alternative to writing transfer rules. Related to translation is the question of bilingual terminology, which is addressed by Gaussier & Langé, who evaluate a number of statistics-based approaches to the task.

Other branches of language processing are represented by one paper each. Daelemans et al. use the example, from **phonology**, of learning stress patterns in Dutch to illustrate their comparison of two approaches to modelling. Federici & Pirrelli take an analogical approach to **morphology**, considering a number of problems from English, Italian, Turkish and Rotuman. The use of neural networks to generate **abstracts** is described by Aretoulaki; Collier discusses the use of statistical measures of lexical collocation in order to facilitate the extraction of relevant information from **concordances**; and Sekine considers the problem of identifying **sublangauges**, and presents some experiments based on statistical measures of lexical appearance.

Natural language proceessing is a wide-ranging topic, and the emergence of so many new techniques makes this an exciting time to be involved in this field. As this collection of papers goes to press, the second NeMLaP conference is taking place at Bilkent University in Ankara, Turkey, and a third NeMLaP conference is planned in Australia in January 1998. At some point in the future, of course, the methods and techniques described in this collection, and at subsequent NeMLaP conferences, will cease to be "new" – perhaps they will even become "mainstream". Until that time, however, it is with great enjoyment that we continue our efforts at the cutting edge of language processing technology.

Daniel B. Jones and Harold L. Somers
Manchester

Part I
Analogy-based methods

1 Skousen's analogical modelling algorithm: a comparison with lazy learning

WALTER DAELEMANS,
STEVEN GILLIS AND GERT DURIEUX

1.1 Introduction

Machine learning techniques may help in solving knowledge acquisition bottlenecks in natural language processing. Instead of hand-crafting linguistic knowledge bases like rule bases and lexicons almost from scratch for each new domain, language, application, and theoretical formalism, we can apply machine learning algorithms to a corpus of examples, and automatically induce the required knowledge.

This paper explores one such class of algorithms, "lazy learning" (LL), for which there has been an increased interest in machine learning recently. In this type of similarity-based learning, classifiers keep in memory a selection of examples without creating abstractions in the form of rules or decision trees. Generalization to a new (previously unseen) input pattern is achieved by retrieving the most similar memory items according to some distance metric, and extrapolating the category of these items to the new input pattern. Instances of this form of "nearest-neighbour method" include instance-based learning (Aha et al. 1991), exemplar-based learning (Salzberg 1991; Cost & Salzberg 1993), and memory-based reasoning (Stanfill & Waltz 1986).

The approach has been applied to a wide range of problems using not only numeric and binary values (for which nearest-neighbour methods are traditionally used), but also using symbolic, unordered features. Advantages of the approach include an often surprisingly high classification accuracy, the capacity to learn polymorphous concepts, high speed of learning, and perspicuity of algorithm and classification (Cost & Salzberg 1993). Aha et al. (1991) have shown that the basic instance-based learning algorithm can theoretically learn any concept whose boundary is a union of a finite number of closed hyper-curves of finite size (a class of concepts similar to that which decision-tree induction algorithms and neural networks trained by back-propagation can learn). Training speed is extremely fast (it consists basically of storing patterns), and classification speed, while relatively slow on serial machines, can be considerably reduced by using indexing mechanisms on serial machines (Friedman et al. 1977), massively parallel machines (Stanfill & Waltz 1986), or wafer-scale integration (Kitano 1993).

In natural language processing, LL techniques are currently being applied by various Japanese groups to parsing and machine translation under the names "exemplar-based translation" or "memory-based translation and parsing" (Kitano 1993). In work by Cardie (1993) and by the present authors (Daelemans 1995; Daelemans et al. 1994), variants of LL are applied to disambiguation tasks at different levels of linguistic representation (from phonology to semantics).

One LL variant, "analogical modelling" (AM) (Skousen 1989) was explicitly developed as a linguistic model. On the one hand, despite its interesting claims and properties, it seems to have escaped the attention of the computational linguistics and machine learning communities, while on the other hand, the AM literature seems to be largely oblivious of the very similar LL and nearest-neighbour techniques. In this paper we provide a qualitative and empirical comparison of AM to the more mainstream variants of LL.

In the next section the concept of LL is elaborated further and a basic lazy learner is described. A number of improvements to that basic scheme will be discussed. Next, AM is presented in considerable detail. We will then turn to the main theme of this paper: a comparison of the basic lazy learner and AM. This comparison will mainly focus on two aspects: (a) the global performance of both algorithms on a selected linguistic task, and (b) the algorithms' resistance to noise: the performance of the algorithms is monitored in conditions in which the learning material contains progressively more "noise".

1.2 Variants of LL

LL is a form of "supervised learning". Examples are represented as a vector of feature values with an associated category label. Features define a pattern space, in which similar examples occupy regions that are associated with the same category (note that with symbolic, unordered feature values, this geometric interpretation does not make sense). Several regions can be associated with the same category, allowing polymorphous concepts to be represented and learned.

During training, a set of examples (the training set) is presented in an incremental fashion to the classifier, and added to memory. During testing, a set of previously unseen feature–value patterns (the test set) is presented to the system. For each test pattern, its distance to each example in memory is computed, and the category of the least distant instance is used as the predicted category for the test pattern.

In LL, performance depends crucially on the distance metric used. The most straightforward distance metric would be the one in (1), where X and Y are the patterns to be compared, and $\delta(x_i,y_i)$ is the distance between the values of the ith feature in a pattern with n features.

(1) $$\Delta(X,Y) = \sum_{i=1}^{n} \delta(x_i, y_i)$$

Distance between two values is measured using (2) for numeric features (using scaling to make the effect of numeric features with different lower and upper bounds comparable), and (3), an overlap metric, for symbolic features.

(2) $$\delta(x_i, y_i) = \frac{|x_i - y_i|}{\max_i - \min_i}$$

(3) $$\delta(x_i, y_i) = 0 \text{ if } x_i = y_i, \text{ else } 1$$

1.2.1 Feature weighting

In the distance metric described above, all features describing an example are interpreted as being equally important in solving the classification problem, but this is not necessarily the case. Elsewhere (Daelemans & van den Bosch 1992) we introduced into LL the concept of "information gain", which is also used in decision tree learning (Quinlan 1986, 1993), to weigh the importance of different features in a domain-independent way. Many other methods to weigh the relative importance of features have been designed, both in statistical pattern recognition and in machine learning (Aha (1990) and Kira & Rendell (1992) are examples), but the one we used will suffice as a baseline for the purpose of this paper.

The main idea of "information gain weighting" is to interpret the training set as an information source capable of generating a number of messages (the different category labels) with a certain probability. The information entropy of such an information source can be compared in turn for each feature to the average information entropy of the information source when the value of that feature is known.

Database information entropy is equal to the number of bits of information needed to know the category, given a pattern. It is computed by (4), where p_i (the probability of category i) is estimated by its relative frequency in the training set.

$$H(D) = \sum p_i \log_2 p_i \tag{4}$$

For each feature, the information gain from knowing its value is now computed. To do this, we compute the average information entropy for this feature and subtract it from the information entropy of the database. To compute the average information entropy for a feature (5), we take the average information entropy of the database restricted to each possible value for the feature. The expression $D_{[f=v_i]}$ refers to those patterns in the database that have value v_i for feature f; V is the set of possible values for feature f. Finally, $|D|$ is the number of patterns in a (sub)database.

$$H\left(D_{[f]}\right) = \sum_{v_i \in V} H\left(D_{[f=v_i]}\right) \frac{\left|D_{[f=v_i]}\right|}{|D|} \tag{5}$$

Information gain is then obtained by (6), and scaled for use as a weight for the feature during distance computation.

$$G(f) = H(D) - H\left(D_{[f]}\right) \tag{6}$$

Finally, the distance metric in (1) is modified to take into account the information gain weight associated with each feature (7).

$$\Delta(X,Y) = \sum_{i=1}^{n} G(f_i)\delta(x_i, y_i) \tag{7}$$

1.2.2 Symbolic features

A second problem confronting the basic LL approach concerns the overlap metric (3) for symbolic, unordered feature values. When using this metric, all values of a feature are interpreted as equally distant from each other. This may lead to insufficient discriminatory power between patterns. It also makes impossible the well-understood "Euclidean distance in pattern space" interpretation of the distance metric. Stanfill & Waltz (1986) proposed a "value difference metric" (VDM) which takes into account the overall similarity of classification of all examples for each value of each feature. Recently, Cost & Salzberg (1993) modified this metric by making it symmetric. In their approach, for each feature, a matrix is computed with the differences (represented as real values) between each value using (8), where V_1 and V_2 are two possible values for feature *f*, the distance is the sum over all *n* categories, C_{1i} is the total number of times value V_1 was classified as category *i*, and C_1 is the total number of times V_1 occurred.

(8)
$$\delta(V_1, V_2) = \sum_{i=1}^{n} \left| \frac{C_{1i}}{C_1} - \frac{C_{2i}}{C_2} \right|$$

The value difference matrices, computed for each feature, are used to compute the distance between two patterns with symbolic values, so that the distance metric in (2) can be used instead of (3), thereby safeguarding the "Euclidean distance in pattern space" concept. Cost & Salzberg report excellent classification accuracy on a number of tasks with symbolic, unordered features with this modified Stanfill–Waltz VDM (MVDM).

1.2.3 Variants not considered

Apart from weighting the relative importance of different features, and computing the numeric distance between symbolic feature values, several other improvements and modifications to the basic LL scheme have been proposed: weighting the examples themselves based on typicality of performance, minimizing storage by keeping only a selection of examples, etc. These variations will not concern us here. We will compare the AM approach to be discussed shortly to (a) the basic LL scheme, (b) LL with information-gain weighting of features, and (c) LL using the MVDM. We will consider both normal circumstances and the presence of noise.

1.3 The AM algorithm

1.3.1 Background

AM has been proposed as a model of language usage, as an alternative to current rule-based linguistic descriptions. The main assumption underlying this approach is that many aspects of speaker performance are better accounted for in terms of "analogy", i.e. the identification of similarities or differences with forms in memory (the lexicon), than by referring to explicit but inaccessible rules. See Derwing & Skousen (1989) and Chandler (1993) for psycholinguistic research supporting this assumption. As in LL, the notion of "analogy" is given an operational definition in terms of a matching process between an input pattern and a database of stored exemplars. The result of this matching process is a collection of examples called the "analogical set", and classification of the input pattern is achieved through extrapolation from this set. AM thus shares some important characteristics with LL: the main source of knowledge in both approaches is a database of stored exemplars. These exemplars themselves are used to classify new items, without intermediate abstractions in the form of rules. In order to achieve this, an exhaustive database search is needed, and during this search, less relevant examples need to be discarded.

The main difference between the two approaches lies in the way this selection is made. In LL with feature selection, the different features are assigned a relative importance, which is used during matching to filter out the influence of irrelevant features. In AM, essentially the same effect is achieved without precomputing the relative importance of individual features. Instead, all features are equally important initially, and serve to partition the database into several disjoint classes of examples. Filtering out irrelevant exemplars is done by considering properties of these classes rather than by inspecting individual features that their members may share with the input pattern. To explain how this works, we will describe the matching procedure in more detail.[1]

1.3.2 The algorithm

The first stage in the matching process is the construction of "subcontexts": these are sets of examples, and they are obtained by matching the input pattern, feature by feature, to each item in the database, on an equal/not-equal basis, and classifying the database exemplars accordingly. Taking an input pattern **ABC** as an example, eight ($=2^3$) different subcontexts would be constructed: ABC, $\bar{A}BC$, $A\bar{B}C$, $AB\bar{C}$, $\bar{A}\bar{B}C$, $\bar{A}B\bar{C}$, $A\bar{B}\bar{C}$ and $\bar{A}\bar{B}\bar{C}$, where the macron denotes complementation. Thus, exemplars in the class ABC share all their features with the input pattern, whereas for those in $\bar{A}\bar{B}C$ only the value for the third feature is shared. In general, n features yield 2^n mutually disjoint subcontexts. Subcontexts can be either "deterministic", which means that their members all have the same associated category, or "non-deterministic", when several categories occur.

In the following stage, "supracontexts" are constructed by generalising over specific feature values. This is done by systematically discarding features from the input pattern, and taking the union of the subcontexts that are subsumed by this new pattern. Supracontexts can be ordered with respect to generality, so that the most specific supracontext contains examples that share all n features with the input pattern, less specific supracontexts contain items that share at least $n-1$ features, and the most general supracontext contains all database exemplars, whether or not they have any features in common with the input pattern. In Table 1.1, the supracontexts for our previous example are displayed, together with the subcontexts they subsume.

An important notion with respect to supracontexts is "homogeneity". A supracontext is called "homogeneous" when any of the following conditions holds:

- The supracontext contains nothing but empty subcontexts.

1. Our description of the algorithm is based on the PASCAL code in Skousen (1989).

Table 1.1 Supracontexts and subcontexts.

Supracontext	Subcontexts
A B C	ABC
A B -	ABC, $AB\bar{C}$
A - C	ABC, $A\bar{B}C$
- B C	ABC, $\bar{A}BC$
A - -	ABC, $A\bar{B}C$, $AB\bar{C}$, $A\bar{B}\bar{C}$
- B -	ABC, $\bar{A}BC$, $AB\bar{C}$, $\bar{A}B\bar{C}$
- - C	ABC, $\bar{A}BC$, $A\bar{B}C$, $\bar{A}\bar{B}C$
- - -	ABC, $\bar{A}BC$, $A\bar{B}C$, $AB\bar{C}$, $\bar{A}\bar{B}C$, $\bar{A}B\bar{C}$, $A\bar{B}\bar{C}$, $\bar{A}\bar{B}\bar{C}$

- The supracontext contains only deterministic subcontexts with the same category.
- The supracontext contains a single non-empty, non-deterministic subcontext.

Heterogeneous supracontexts are obtained by combining deterministic and non-deterministic subcontexts. Going from least to most general, this means that as soon as a supracontext is heterogeneous, any more general supracontext will be heterogeneous too.

In the final stage, the analogical set is constructed. This set contains all of the exemplars from each of the homogeneous supracontexts. Two remarks are in order here. First, since some exemplars will occur in more than one supracontext, each exemplar is weighted according to its distribution across different supracontexts. This is accomplished by maintaining a score for each exemplar. This score is simply the summed cardinality of each of the supracontexts in which the exemplar occurs. The intent of this scoring mechanism is to favour frequent patterns over less frequent ones, and patterns closer to the input pattern over more distant patterns, since the former will surface in more than one supracontext. Second, banning heterogeneous supracontexts from the analogical set ensures that the process of adding increasingly dissimilar exemplars is halted as soon as those differences may cause a shift in category. Exactly when this happens depends largely on the input pattern. To categorize the input pattern finally, either the predominant category in the analogical set or the category of a probabilistically chosen member of this set is chosen. In our experiments, we adopted the former approach.

1.4 Assignment of main stress to Dutch words

1.4.1 Data and experiments

The experimental set-up used in all experiments consisted of a 10-fold cross-validation experiment (Weiss & Kulikowski 1991). In this set-up, the database was partitioned ten times, each with a different 10% of the dataset as the test part, and the remaining 90% as training part. For each of the ten simulations in our experiment, the test part was used to test generalization performance. The success rate of an algorithm was obtained by calculating the average accuracy (number of test pattern categories correctly predicted) over the ten test sets in the 10-fold cross-validation experiment.

In order to insert additional noise to the data, the datasets were subjected to the following procedure: for a given noise rate, every feature value and category in the dataset was replaced by another possible feature or category value with a probability amounting to the noise rate. A replaced value could be the same as the original one (with a probability depending on the number of different values for that feature or category). After noise addition to the dataset, the training and test sets were created in the way described above.

1.4.2 Task description

The task consisted of predicting the stress pattern of individual (non-complex) Dutch words. For example, the main stress of the word *panama* is on the first syllable: ['pa:na:ma:]. The task of determining main stress in Dutch is notoriously difficult. According to recent linguistic analyses of the domain, not more than 80% of Dutch monomorphemes are regular in metrical terms (see Daelemans et al. (1994) for an overview). As such, the problem is typical of many natural language processing tasks: regularities, subregularities and exceptions account for data that are ambiguous and noisy (from the point of the modeller: human or learning algorithm).

The experiments were conceived as follows: in a training phase, words were presented together with their target stress patterns. Next, the algorithm was tested with new words (i.e. words not encountered during training) the stress pattern of which the algorithm had to predict. More specifically, the data were presented to the algorithms as strings of phonemes (representing their pronunciation). Table 1.2 shows a sample of the training input for the words *acroniem* ('acronym'), *actie* ('action'), *actief* ('active') and *acuut* ('acute'), respectively.

A full discussion of data selection and encoding is irrelevant for this study, and can be found elsewhere (Daelemans et al. 1994). In the results reported here, we were not interested in optimal generalization performance, but in a comparison of different classifier systems and input conditions. Optimal performance on this task is reported in Daelemans et al. (1994) as well.

1.4.3 Results

Comparison between AM and LL's basic scheme

The first question to be addressed relates to the overall accuracy of AM as compared to the basic scheme of LL (*k*-nearest-neighbour matching with different values of *k*

Table 1.2 A sample of the training input. In the "Category" column, A means stress on the last syllable, B on the penultimate syllable, etc. The remaining columns show, for each of the three last syllables of a word, its syllable structure (onset, nucleus, and coda, respectively). When part of the syllable structure is absent, the symbol "=" is used. "A" denotes a short vowel, "a" a long vowel.

Word	Category	Antepenultimate	Penultimate	Last
acroniem	A	= a =	kr o =	n i m
actie	B	= = =	= A k	s i =
actief	A	= = =	= A k	t i v
acuut	A	= = =	= a =	k y t

and an overlap metric for symbolic features). AM clearly outperforms LL: AM attains a global success score of 80.5% while LL (k = 1) reaches a success score of 75.4%, a difference that is highly significant as assessed by a *chi*-squared test ($\chi^2 = 7.5663$, $p < 0.006$**). When we extend LL to take into account more neighbours than just the closest matching one, the difference in performance between AM and LL still remains highly significant. In Table 1.3 the results are displayed comparing the success score of AM with an implementation of LL that compares a test item with its nearest neighbour (LL−1nn), its two nearest neighbours (LL−2nn), its five and ten nearest neighbours (LL−5nn and LL−10nn).

Table 1.3 Comparison of success scores of AM and LL *k*-nearest neighbours: assessment of difference from AM.

System	Success score	$\chi^2 =$	$p <$
AM	80.5		
LL−1nn	75.4	7.5663	0.006 **
LL−2nn	75.8	6.4682	0.0110 *
LL−5nn	76.1	5.6971	0.0171 *
LL−10nn	75.1	8.4416	0.0037 **

From Table 1.3 it appears that AM is significantly more successful than LL, irrespective of the number of nearest neighbours considered in the latter algorithm. All comparisons of the success score reveal a significantly better performance for AM. The superior performance of AM does not appear to be resistant to additional noise in the data. When more noise is added, AM still outperforms LL in the conditions considered, but the difference is no longer significant (Table 1.4). The significance of the differences in performance between AM and LL, as assessed by a *chi*-squared test, is indicated in Table 1.4.

Table 1.4 Performance of AM and LL relative to different noise levels.

System	Noise level (%)				
	0	20	40	60	80
AM	80.5	60.3	48.1	38.3	35.1
LL−1nn	75.4 **	56.2	44.8	34.9	33.2
LL−2nn	75.8 *	56.2	44.7	37.5	33.3
LL−5nn	76.1 *	59.3	49.9	38.6	32.3
LL−10nn	75.1 **	60.5	48.0	39.9	32.9

The results in Table 1.4 indicate that when additional noise is introduced into the training data, the performance of AM becomes similar to the performance of LL. Even if LL only takes into account the single nearest neighbour of the test item, it does not perform significantly worse than AM. This observation holds irrespective of the amount of noise added to the training data as well as the number of nearest neighbours taken into account.

Comparison between AM and LL's augmented implementations

In Section 1.2, a number of enhancements to the basic LL algorithm were discussed. Two extensions were described: the basic LL scheme can be enriched with (a) a differential weighting of features using "information gain", and (b) a value difference metric which takes into account the overall similarity of classification of all examples for each value of each feature (MVDM). In this section we compare the performance of AM with that of LL augmented with (a) information gain (LL-IG), (b) MVDM (LL-MVDM) and (c) a combination of the two (LL-IG-MVDM). In the data reported, LL was tested in the condition in which only the single nearest neighbour was considered.

In Table 1.5, the success score of AM is compared with the performance of LL's basic scheme (LL), and the three augmentations of LL mentioned above. The comparison shows that only in its basic scheme does LL attain a significantly lower success rate than AM. All extensions of LL (taking into account only the nearest neighbour) yield success rates that are very close to those of AM, or in some cases even higher.

The results displayed in Table 1.5 pertain to a training set in which no additional noise is added. When additional noise is present, the comparisons of AM and LL do not show many discrepancies: in all conditions, there are hardly any results that can be marked as significantly different. The noise tolerance of AM is no more robust than the noise tolerance of LL: out of 16 comparisons only 3 yield a statistically significant difference (Table 1.6). This means that, at least for this task, AM is no more noise-tolerant than LL. Extended with IG and MVDM, LL attains a very similar success rate to AM. It should be noted, however, that we have only studied

Table 1.5 Comparison of AM and augmented versions of LL: assessment of difference from AM.

System	Success score	$\chi^2 =$	$p <$
AM	80.5		
LL	75.4	7.5663	0.006 **
LL-IG	81.8	0.5224	0.4559 NS
LL-MVDM	79.4	0.3774	0.5372 NS
LL-IG-MVDM	81.4	0.2626	0.6065 NS

Table 1.6 Comparison of AM and augmented versions of LL: assessment of difference from AM when noise is included.

System	Noise level (%)				
	0	20	40	60	80
AM	80.5	60.3	48.1	38.3	35.1
LL	75.4 **	56.2	44.8	34.9	33.2
LL-IG	81.8	57.3	42.5 *	38.2	34.6
LL-MVDM	79.4	55.5 *	44.1	36.3	34.4
LL-IG-MVDM	81.4	54.4 **	46.3	36.5	34.6

and compared overall success score, and have not, for example, compared the errors made by the different variants (in terms of error types or relative markedness).

1.5 Conclusion

An important limitation of the AM algorithm is that it requires exponential time in the number of attributes. When overcoming this using massive parallelism, the algorithm would be extraordinarily memory-greedy. Using a very economic scheme, explained in Skousen (1989), the number of processors required for a 22-feature problem would be larger than the 2^{16} processors currently available on the Connection Machine. In LL, processing time is linear in the number of features.

A second restriction is that AM can only usefully be applied to unordered symbolic or Boolean features: with numeric features or ordered symbolic features, the ordering is not taken into account during classification. LL is more general in that all types of features can be handled by a uniform distance metric based on distance in a Euclidean space.

In the experimental tests reported in this paper, it was shown that AM outperforms the most basic implementation of a Lazy Learner in predicting the stress pattern of underived words. The addition of more nearest neighbours to the set of memorized items a test item is compared with does not yield significant improvements: AM still performs better. However, this advantage disappears when additional noise is entered in the training data. It was also shown that augmented versions of the Lazy Learner (that incorporate feature weighting and/or value difference matrices) perform equally as well as AM even when additional noise is added in the training material. We conclude that, at least for this type of classification task, there is no clear motivation to use the complex and costly AM algorithm instead of the more general and less complex class of LL algorithms.

References

Aha, D. 1990. *A study of instance-based algorithms for supervised learning tasks.* Technical Report 90-42, University of California at Irvine.

Aha, D., D. Kibler & M. Albert 1991. Instance-based learning algorithms. *Machine Learning* **6**, 37–66.

Cardie, C. 1993. A case-based approach to knowledge acquisition for domain-specific sentence analysis. In *Proceedings, 11th National Conference on Artificial Intelligence (AAAI)*, Washington, DC. 798–803.

Chandler, S. 1993. Are rules and modules really necessary for explaining language? *Journal of Psycholinguistic Research* **22**, 593–606.

Cost, S. & S. Salzberg 1993. A weighted nearest neighbor algorithm for learning with symbolic features. *Machine Learning*, **10**, 57–78.

Daelemans, W. 1995. Memory-based lexical acquisition and processing. In *Machine translation and the lexicon*, P. Steffens (ed.), 85–98. Berlin: Springer.

Daelemans, W. & A. van den Bosch 1992. Generalization performance of backpropagation learning on a syllabification task. In *Proceedings of the Third Twente Workshop on Language Technology*, Twente, The Netherlands, 27–38.

Daelemans, W., S. Gillis & G. Durieux 1994. The acquisition of stress, a data-oriented approach. *Computational Linguistics* **20**, 421–51.

Derwing, B. & R. Skousen 1989. Real time morphology: symbolic rules or analogical networks. *Berkeley Linguistic Society* **15**, 48–62.

Friedman, J., J. Bentley & R. Ari Finkel. 1977. An algorithm for finding best matches in logarithmic expected time. *ACM Transactions on Mathematical Software* **3**, 209–26.

Kira, K. & L. Rendell 1992. A practical approach to feature selection. In *International Conference on Machine Learning*, Aberdeen, 249–56.

Kitano, H. 1993. Challenges of massive parallelism. In *International Joint Conference on Artificial Intelligence*, Chambéry, 813–34.

Quinlan, J. 1986. Induction of decision trees. *Machine Learning* **1**, 81–106.

Quinlan, J. 1993. *C4.5: Programs for machine learning*. San Mateo, Calif.: Morgan Kaufmann.

Salzberg, S. 1991. A nearest hyperrectangle learning method. *Machine Learning* **6**, 251–76.

Skousen, R. 1989. *Analogical modeling of language*. Dordrecht: Kluwer.

Stanfill, C. & D. Waltz 1986. Toward memory-based reasoning. *Communications of the ACM* **29**, 1212–28.

Weiss, S. & C. Kulikowski 1991. *Computer systems that learn*. San Mateo, Calif.: Morgan Kaufmann.

2

Analogy, computation and linguistic theory

STEFANO FEDERICI AND VITO PIRRELLI[1]

2.1 Analogy, linguistic theory and generality

In computational linguistics, generalization by analogy can be defined as the inferential process by which an unfamiliar linguistic object *O* (called the "target object") is seen as an analogue of more familiar objects (the "base objects"), so that whatever piece of knowledge is acquired about the latter can be used to deal with the former too (Owen 1990). A fundamental property of generalization by analogy is its flexibility: that is, its capacity to deal successfully with a variety of different problems (in this context, a variety of linguistic phenomena), with not much built-in knowledge being required (e.g. concerning general structural properties of words, sentences, etc.). The problem is that, even in a relatively well-understood linguistic domain such as morphology, it is not as yet clear how powerful generalization by analogy should be for the huge variety of word formation processes attested across different languages to be conveniently and adequately captured.

1. This paper is the outcome of a joint effort. However, for the specific concerns of the Italian Academy, S. Federici is responsible for the first two subsections of section 2.2.3, for section 2.3.1 and the Appendix; V. Pirrelli is responsible for sections 2.1, 2.2.1, 2.2.2, the last three subsections of section 2.2.3, sections 2.3 and 2.4.

Our approach to the problem is somewhat pragmatic and computationally oriented: we start from the assumption that generalization by analogy is a relatively "weak" inferential procedure which does not have to rush to premature conclusions on the basis of few instances of attested evidence only (few base objects); as a result, its algorithms should not require much computational power. If this assumption is correct, generalization by analogy is a relatively slow, passive process of registering and accumulating (properties of) linguistic objects (e.g. words) by being exposed to a large number of them (a representative set of base objects). In our view, an analogy-driven algorithm should not be expected to outdo an expert linguist in extracting the right amount of linguistic knowledge from a couple of carefully chosen examples. Rather, it should wait for the right sort of evidence to appear, before a relevant analogy is acquired from a set of unselected examples. Incidentally, this mirrors the process of gradual acquisition of language by a child: its errors, its error-finding capabilities.

What we have implemented is a self-modelling system which learns, incrementally,[2] the analogies of the linguistic objects it is exposed to, in order to acquire generalizations about future unknown instances of similar objects. After the system has been trained, it can be tested either in analysis or in generation. While most of the analogy-based systems we know of (e.g. Dedina & Nusbaum 1991; Sullivan & Damper 1992) use analogy as a heuristic for identification of the best analogues of the target in the dataset of base objects (a process usually referred to in the literature as "mapping"), we have been working on the assumption that analogy plays a fundamental role in the learning phase as well, in particular in the way the system structures its own knowledge and extracts from this the relevant generalizations. Not surprisingly, this move has important consequences for the kind of generalization the system is able to draw from acquired evidence: in particular we contend that "linguistic analogy" is not just a matter of pairwise similarity between the target and its best analogue only, but rather involves the whole complex network of "analogical relations" holding among the base objects themselves. In this sense, analogy is indeed a "distributed" process.

In what follows, we will highlight some of the key issues that an analogy-based system for morphological processing has to tackle, ranging from the nature of the linguistic generalizations to be inferred, to the sort of performance that it would be reasonable to expect from such a system. Finally, we will give indications as to how our approach has been extended to deal with yet other linguistic problems.

2.2 Analogy and computability

2.2.1 The linguistic object

For the present purposes, a "linguistic unit" is assumed to be a symbolic object,

2. This is probably one of the most apparent differences from statistically based approaches to analogy such as Skousen's (1989).

that is a two-level representation consisting of a "linguistic form" (say a string of characters making up a word form, a string of words in a sentence, etc.) and a "linguistic content" (e.g. a set of morphological features conveyed by the word form, a set of syntactic features, etc.) (Fig. 2.1).

linguistic form		**linguistic content**
credevano		*credere*
(they) believed	$\Longleftrightarrow$	third person plural imperfect indicative

Figure 2.1 *Form and content.*

Analogy works on both levels. In theory, it has to be flexible enough to deal with any type of surface linguistic object and with any type of linguistic representation. For the sake of concreteness, in what follows our approach to analogy-based learning will be illustrated by taking words as our linguistic units.

2.2.2 Learning words

Within our framework, learning words consists in (a) memorizing them as "full linguistic units" (in the form of the two-level representation shown above), for (b) these objects to be compared with already memorized objects (full base objects) and some "matches" between them to be extracted. These matches (also called "cores") are themselves stored in turn: they will be utilized, together with full linguistic objects, either in analysis or in generation. Clearly, other ways to extract matches could be entertained. To give an example, linguistic objects can be compared with already extracted cores in their turn, for smaller and smaller cores to be acquired, in a sort of inferential cascade. Our experience indicates, however, that the computational cost of this cascade largely overwhelms its advantages: the system learns more quickly but its network grows far more quickly. In the long run, a slow learner performs as well as a quick one, since smaller cores are eventually extracted by comparing two linguistic objects that are different enough from each other (Pirrelli & Federici 1991).

2.2.3 Harnessing combinatorial explosion

When, where and how shall an analogy between two (or more) linguistic objects be looked for? The fact that two words share the same ending is not always indicative of a morphological relation holding between them. Unconstrained application of analogy across the lexicon of a language leads to combinatorial explosion of possible matches. This section is devoted to a consideration of sensible ways of constraining linguistic analogy.

Preconditions on the triggering of analogy

A linguistically plausible constraint is that the analogy between two word forms is relevant *iff* it is accompanied by an analogy at the level of their linguistic content. In other words, linguistic analogy involves symbolic objects as a whole, or, put in a nutshell, linguistic analogy is a symbolic relationship. This assumption has important consequences on the working of analogy as such. In our system (see Fig. 2.2), there is no possible way of matching, say, *red* and *spotted*, since there is no shared part of their linguistic representation that would license the extraction of a common ending core (*-ed* in this case).

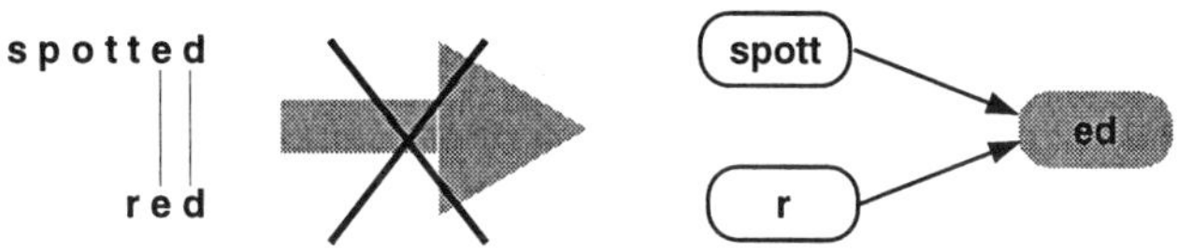

Figure 2.2 *Illegal analogical matching.*

Having defined the necessary condition for a linguistically relevant analogy to be looked for, in the next section we move on to a consideration of the possible ways in which the analogy in question can be extracted.

The matching algorithm

Any formalized notion of linguistic analogy must address the problem of *how to match* a new, unknown form of a base object (say a word form which had never before been encountered by the system) with already known forms of the same kind (e.g. word forms about which the system has already acquired some knowledge). For what concerns us here, this sort of matching applies to strings of characters, as opposed, say, to phonological segments. The "string-matching" algorithm we have been working on for modelling analogy can be worded as follows (a more formal description of the string-matching algorithm can be found in the Appendix).

> Start from the left end of both (the form of) a target and the base object and scan them rightwards; *extract*, along the way, all characters which appear in both, and *in the same order*.

To be more concrete, take the Italian infinitive word forms *invecchiare* ('to age'), an inchoative verb derivative of the adjective *vecchio* ('old'), and *ingiallire* ('to yellow'), again an inchoative verb which derives from the adjective *giallo* ('yellow'); or the Arabic pair *kulayb* ('little dog') and *kalb* ('dog') as in Figure 2.3.

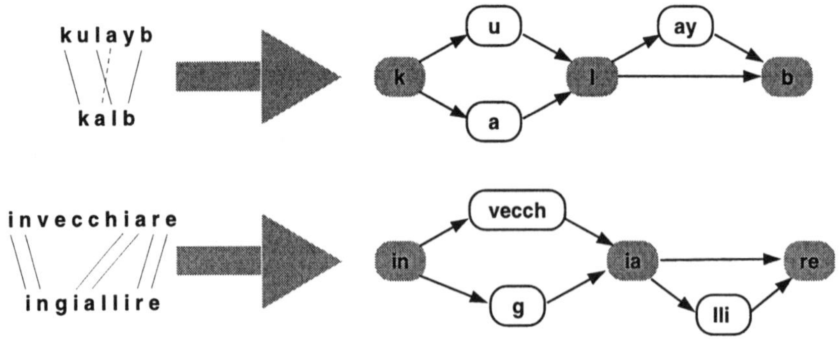

Figure 2.3 *More analogical matching.*

In the Arabic example, the shared portion of meaning ('dog') triggers the extraction of a tentative stem. The meaning 'dog' is thus associated with the match *k–lb*. The remaining portions of morpholexical features of the two word forms are associated with the substrings left out of the match (respectively, *u–ay* and *a*). Note that the two *a*s which are linked by a dotted line will *not* be extracted in the same pattern as *k–lb*, since they are ordered differently relative to the position of *l* (in the target, *a* follows *l*, but in the base *a* precedes it). In the Italian example, the shared morphological feature "infinitive" triggers the extraction of a (pseudo-)circumfix which, incidentally, contains some word-internal "noise", the string *ia*, on which more will be said later on (see Section 2.3.2 and Fig. 2.12).

An obvious advantage of constraining the matching routine is that we reduce considerably the number of possible cores to be extracted. On the more negative side, we are not able to track down analogies whose order in the base is interchanged relative to the order in the target, as indicated in the mapping between *un-redo* and *re-un-pack* to the left of the arrow in Figure 2.4a. This by no means implies that phenomena such as "inversion" or "metathesis", as in the Rotuman example in Figure 2.4b, are beyond the reach of our approach to analogy.

In Rotuman,[3] noun definiteness is expressed through inversion in the order of the last two segments (characters) of the word in its indefinite form. In fact, given our algorithmic definition of string matching, we are able to match only two linguistic objects which show the same order of interchangeable characters, as in the example in Figure 2.4c, where the common ending of two indefinite nouns is identified appropriately and extracted accordingly. The productive morphological relation between, say, *pa* and *ap* in the word for 'pigeon' in Rotuman is accounted for paradigmatically, and not derivationally as traditionally done in "item and process" frameworks (Hoeksema & Janda 1988), as explained later (see p. 22).

Finally, our matching algorithm excludes the possibility that a character is mapped onto a null character (to account for "deletion" phenomena). In a familiar context, deletive mapping would be helpful to derive an English singular noun from its plural

3. An Oceanic language spoken in Fiji.

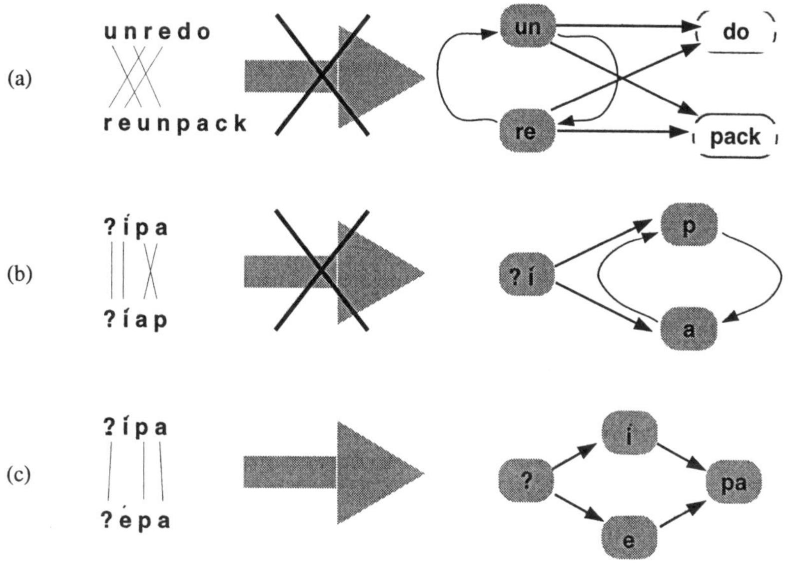

Figure 2.4 *Analogical treatment of inversion.*

form (*dogs* → *dog*). Later on we will show how it is possible to do this without deletion, and why the solution we propose is psycholinguistically more plausible besides being computationally more tractable.

The search for the best match

Assume that the target object can be matched against the set of base objects in more than one way: will every possible match be stored as a new piece of acquired information? It seems reasonable to give preference to those matches which are linguistically more significant. Irrelevant matches would then be discarded with marginal loss of information, if any. From an analogy-based perspective, however, there is no obvious way to tell linguistically significant matches from linguistically irrelevant ones simply by looking at a linguistic object considered in isolation. First, crude cut-off principles do not always work: for example, we know that not all languages present a "concatenative" morphology, the main consequence of this being that one cannot *a priori* prefer matches that consist of continuous substrings of characters over discontinuous ones (see our Arabic example above): for nonconcatenative languages, discontinuous matches are indeed descriptively more appropriate.

Second, we decided not to resort to any form of *a priori* knowledge made available to the analogy-based system by building it within the system's inferential algorithm: e.g. a "switch" (Cook 1988) that tells the matching routine that the morphology of the input language to be dealt with is either concatenative or nonconcatenative. In our view, the cognitive value of an analogy-based algorithm for incremental language learning is strengthened when and if the amount of language-specific information required for its convergence is reduced to a minimum.

We shall next consider two ways out of the problem of finding the best match: either temporarily storing all possible extracted cores in the learning phase, and then assessing their linguistic validity *a posteriori*; or choosing the best match immediately, in the light of the evidence available here and now. We call the first approach "*a posteriori* pruning", the second "dynamic pruning".

***A posteriori* pruning** Suppose that the system has already extracted all possible cores from the evidence available during learning. *A posteriori* pruning means pruning after learning takes place, and consists in looking at the times each extracted core is successfully used when the system is asked, after training, to analyse the same test corpus used for training (or, alternatively, to generate the set of word forms used in training on the basis of their abstract linguistic representations). Note that, in this checking phase, the system is not allowed to use full word forms, which are learned by rote anyway and would make this step trivial, but only extracted cores. Cores which are never used, or which never provide conclusive evidence in support of the correct linguistic representation in analysis (or the correct word form in generation), are eventually discarded. *A posteriori* pruning is thus a form of validation of the extracted matches or cores by testing their effectiveness in analysis or generation. An advantage of this approach is that it does not require any *ad hoc* limitation of the matching algorithm: nonetheless spurious cores will not remain in the dataset of acquired knowledge indefinitely, and will stop using up memory resources as soon as their contribution to the performances of the system is proved null. The obvious drawback of this strategy is that, when asked to match a new target object against its base objects, the system will keep on using the same "blind" matching routine. In other words, the system knows eventually which extracted cores are more relevant, but never learns how to avoid looking for irrelevant matches.

Dynamic pruning An attractive alternative to *a posteriori* pruning is to make the system able to learn not only what analogies to look for, but also *where they are most likely to be found* in the input string. Assume that the system is able to store already extracted cores in such a way that some important generalizations holding over them emerge incrementally as a by-product of this process. Assume further that the system can evaluate the linguistic relevance of new matches at run time, by testing how they fit the general patterns that have already emerged from stored items. The assumption can finally be made that the best possible match to be stored, out of a set of several suitable candidates, is just the one which best fits existing stored patterns of regularities.

In our system, linguistic objects are stored dynamically as "paradigmatic patterns" of analogies consisting of "nodes" and "links" between them, as illustrated in Figure 2.5.

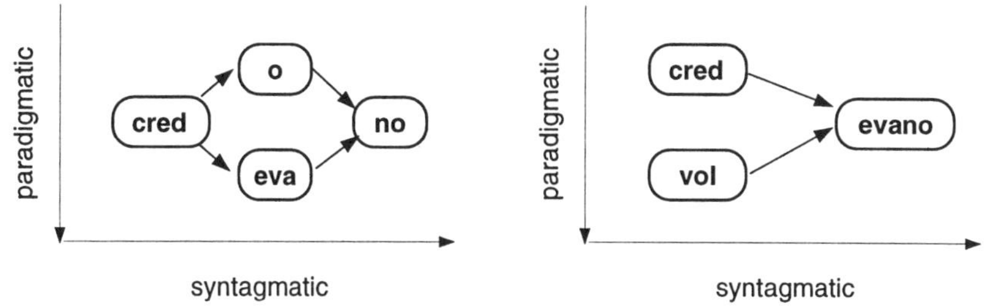

(a) Intralexemic (b) Interlexemic

Figure 2.5 *Intra- and interlexemic links.*

Figure 2.5a shows a paradigmatic pattern resulting from the comparison of the two linguistic units *credevano* ('they believed') and *credono* ('they believe'). The word-initial *cred*, common to both strings, is factored out and represented as a single node, which starts the paradigmatic pattern. The two strings then diverge, and the two different substrings in complementary distribution are represented as distinct nodes which are both accessible from *cred*. The pattern finishes with a common ending, which is again expressed as a single node. Links between nodes, depicted as arrows in the figure, indicate the syntagmatic relations between substrings, that is, the way they appear trailed one after the other in a word. In the case at hand, these links relate two word forms of the same lexeme (the Italian verb *credere*), and are accordingly referred to as "intralexemic" links. The vertical axis, on the other hand, expresses the paradigmatic dimension of available alternants, that is, the information concerning which (sub)strings are in complementary distribution with respect to the same syntagmatic context, i.e. with respect to the common (discontinuous) core *cred–no*. Accordingly, we say that the two alternants *o* and *eva* are "intralexemically related".

Figure 2.5b illustrates the paradigmatic pattern resulting from the overlapping of *credevano* and *volevano* ('they wanted'). This time, links relate word forms of two different lexemes (*credere* and *volere*), and are dubbed "interlexemic" nodes (Carstairs-McCarthy 1992). Now, the alternants *cred* and *vol* are said to be "interlexemically related".

Note that in both cases paradigmatic links are always left-to-right, that is, they neither loop back to previous nodes, nor go from one node to its paradigmatic alternant. This is due to the constraints imposed on string matching, and considerably reduces the expressive power of the resulting network, which will never look like the looping networks in Figures 2.4a and b.

In learning a new word, in order to build the relevant paradigmatic patterns, the system extracts all possible matches between the new item and already existing base objects; if more than one match shares the same set of morphological features, then the match selected for storage in the dataset of acquired knowledge is the one with more paradigmatic connections (links) with other items in the dataset, whether interlexemic or intralexemic. To be more concrete, suppose that the word form *cambiato* ('changed') has been stored together with its features (past participle of *cambiare*, masculine singular), and suppose further that the word form *odiato* ('hated') and its features (same as *cambiato*, except for the lexeme: past participle of *odiare*, masculine singular) are learned (Fig. 2.6).

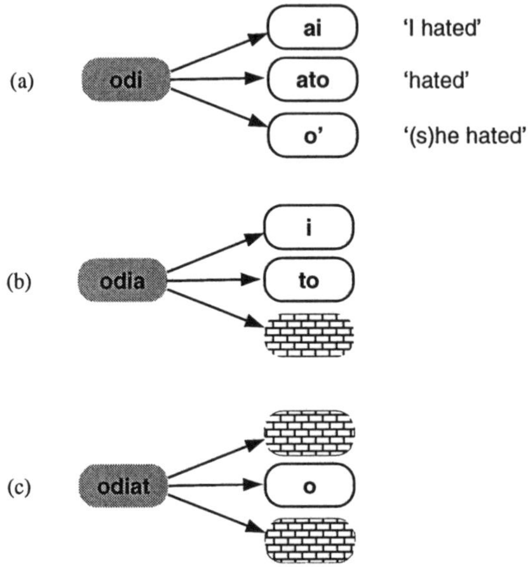

Figure 2.6 *Paradigmatic alternation.*

The system will then extract, among other things, the matches *iato*, *ato*, *to* and *o* as conveying the features "past participle, masculine singular". In this case, *ato* is likely to be preferred over the others as the best match, since it is intralexemically related to more other suffixes. This situation is graphically represented in Figure 2.6, where *ato* has more paradigmatic links than its interlexemic alternants *to* and *o*, and will eventually be preferred over them (a brick wall indicates non-existence of a suitable alternant).

In our vision of things, paradigms are flexible structures which can tentatively be extended on the basis of the available evidence. This is illustrated in Figure 2.7a, where the (learned) Italian word forms *compra* ('(s)he buys'), *ama* ('(s)he loves') and *amiamo* ('we love') are analogically structured in paradigmatic patterns: each node contains a string whose morpholexical content (*comprare*, third-person singular, etc.) is expressed by the attached label. Assume that *compra* is not yet part of the evidence available to the system, and is witnessed in input as a target word. Although *cant* and *a* have never been seen together, the system is able to find an available paradigmatic path between the two, zigzagging through the set of both inter- and intralexemic links available at the learning stage pictured in Figure 2.7a, as indicated by the arrow. More technically, if a certain stem shares an interlexemic link with another stem, then the former will inherit (dynamically, at run time) all the latter's intralexemic links, which are eventually exploited at run time to analyse a word form for which the system lacks direct evidence. We call this form of dynamic inheritance "paradigm extension".

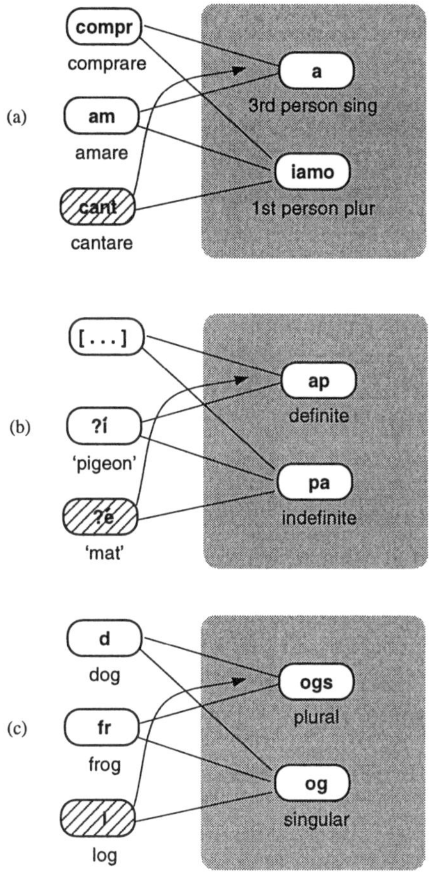

Figure 2.7 *Paradigm extension.*

Incidentally, the reader will note that paradigm extension can be resorted to in order to account for how metathesis can be used productively in Rotuman (see p. 19). In Figure 2.7b, the sequences *pa* and *ap* are intralexemically related in that they occur within the same word *?í* ('pigeon'). Given the interlexemic link between *?í* and *?é* ('mat') in Rotuman, both sharing word-final *pa* in their definite form, it is reasonable to extend this link intraleximically and account for the plausible paradigm-driven generalization that all *pa*-ending definite nouns in Rotuman end in *ap* in their indefinite form. Note that no algorithm for inversion is required to capture this generalization. The system will not try to account for inversion through the mapping between the two forms of 'pigeon' (both definite and indefinite), by deriving one from the other. On the contrary, it will wait until the ordered match *pa* emerges from two lexically unrelated forms such as *?épa* ('a mat') and *?ípa* ('a pigeon') which are both specified for indefinitiveness. Finally, Figure 2.7c illustrates our treatment of apparently deletive alternations: the unknown singular form of a word whose plural is known (*dogs*) can indeed be inferred by paradigmatic analogy with a rhyming word (*frogs*) whose singular form is known. This inference is weaker than the process of deriving *dog* from *dogs* through deletion of word-final *s*, but is in keeping with well-known findings of psycholinguistic research, according to which English-speaking children learn noun pluralization on the basis of rhyming words (Berko 1958).

To conclude this section, an altogether different strategy for pruning, and certainly a cruder one than the paradigm-driven approach illustrated here, should briefly be mentioned. It consists in choosing, always and only, the longest match out of all candidates. However linguistically blind it may be, this strategy yields good results. While a paradigm-driven heuristics is more economical in terms of stored matches, the use of the longest match makes the system more reliable for the analysis of those word forms whose stem is not known, but whose affixes are familiar, so that some predictions about the morphological features of the word forms in question can be made: we call this type of analysis a "partial morphological interpretation" of an unfamiliar word form (see below for more on this). Linguistically plausible matches work well when and if the word to be analysed can be covered in its entirety. However, they do not give reliable hints for good guesses.

The computational complexity of paradigm extension If string matching were unconstrained, and all resulting matches were extracted and stored, the number of potential interlexemic and intralexemic links (in the worst case), for N equal to the number of different learned word forms, and L equal to the number of characters in a word form, would be given by (1).

(1) $$\mathcal{O}\left(\sum_{i=1}^{N}(i-1)\times 2^L\right) = \mathcal{O}\left(N^4 \times 4^L\right)$$

This means that, when the system is learning the ith word form, it could potentially extract up to 2^L matches,[4] by comparing it with each of the $i-1$ word forms learned up to this stage (i.e. $(i-1)\times 2^L$ matches). In this way we can create up to $\left((i-1)\times 2^L\right)^2$ links. This number reduces to a maximum of $\mathcal{O}\left(N^2\right)$ when we use string matching as defined above (p. 19) and we store only the best match.

Actually, the computability of an analogy-based approach to language is given confirmation by the fact that, as we found in all our tests, the growth rate

4. This upper bound is comparatively low, given an average word length of about 6 characters per word in Italian: hence, it can be replaced by a constant k.

approximates a linear function of *N* (Fig. 2.8). In fact, we found that the morphology of language presents a relatively poor combinatorial complexity in terms of analogical relations: the same relations are repeatedly used and thus learned comparatively quickly, although their number is probably greater than the number of linguistic units commonly assumed by current grammatical theories (Pirrelli & Federici 1991).

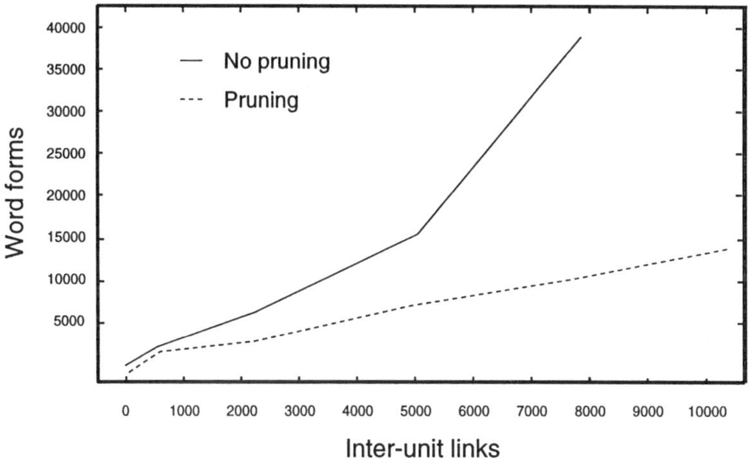

Figure 2.8 *Number of inter-unit links by learned word forms. Space complexity is* $\mathcal{O}(N^2)$.

The use of learned evidence in word analysis

How is a learned network used in word analysis? The system attempts to cover the word form in input either with a full learned word form if it exists (remember that both full word forms and extracted cores are stored and interconnected), or with a possible sequence of smaller matches. To give a simple example, the unknown string *logs* can be fully analysed by matching it onto the node containing word-initial *l* in the bottom left of the network in Figure 2.7c, and onto the *ogs* node, which can be accessed paradigmatically from *l* (as shown by the arrow).

The way matches are to be sequenced in a word is expressed, as we have seen, by paradigmatic links. If a complete coverage of the input word form is not possible, then the longest possible coverage is attempted by using those matches which are fully contained in the input word form. By doing this, a partial morphological interpretation is attempted. If more than one sequence of matches fits the input word form while converging on the same interpretation, that interpretation is yielded by the system. On the contrary, if they provide incompatible interpretations, then the longest match wins out over the other.

Linguistic theory and the analogy-based view

The reader will note that, in an analogy-based network, nodes are not always morphemes in the classical Bloomfeldian sense (Bloomfield 1933), in that they cannot be understood (and interpreted) in isolation, but only in the context of their paradigmatic links. Accordingly, *l* in Figure 2.7c is not the stem of *log* as such, but only the minimal string which distinguishes the word form *logs* from the rhyming *dogs*, or, in other words, which turns the meaningless *–ogs* into a unique meaningful symbolic unit of English (the plural form of the noun *log*). Generally speaking, more can be found through analogy-based matching than a simple indirect confirmation of rule-based accounts of morphological phenomena. To give another example, the regularity that many verbs which end in *ink* in English are strong verbs and present ablaut alternation, is something within the reach of an analogy-based account: *ink* is indeed extracted by our network, and represents an important node for interlexemic, paradigmatic extension as shown in Figure 2.9 (Pirrelli & Federici 1994b). Nonetheless, *ink* is certainly not a morpheme in any conceivable traditional use of the term.

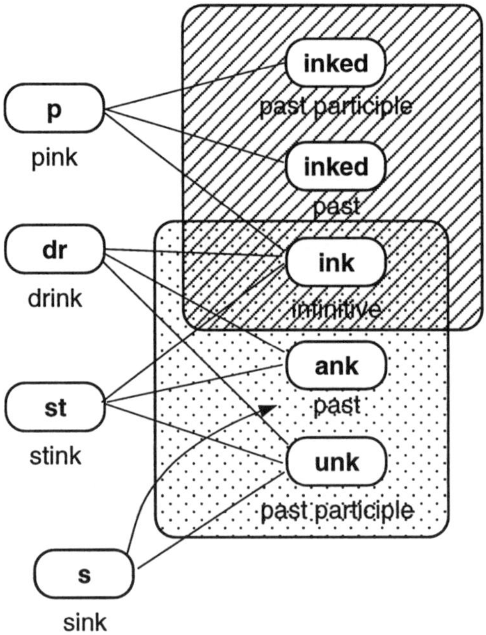

Figure 2.9 *Ablaut alternation: the analogy-based view.*

A final point is worth raising in this context. It is commonly assumed that there is only one way to assign a structural representation to a symbolic object (say, by splitting it into its components). Any violation of this principle is generally frowned upon in linguistic circles and pointed out as a bracketing paradox of some kind. In morphology, bracketing paradoxes are virtually ubiquitous, as witnessed by a word form such as *macro-economist*. Morphotactic and phonological reasons (Siegel

1979) support the structure (*macro*)(*economy*(*ist*)) as in Figure 2.10a, while lexico-semantic evidence is rather in favour of (*macro*(*economy*))(*ist*) as in Figure 2.10b, which captures the fact that a macro-economist is an expert in macro-economy.

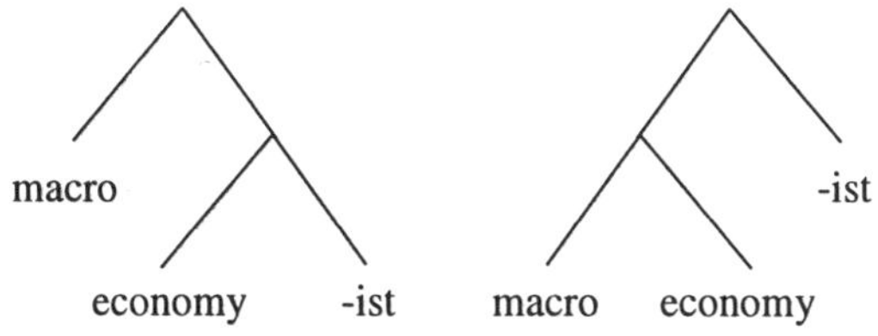

(a) (b)

Figure 2.10 *A bracketing paradox in morphology.*

The two structures are not compatible, but indeed both are morphologically justified, or justifiable. This is a problem in traditional accounts. However, if language is looked at as the network of analogical relations holding between linguistic objects, then it can be the case that the same object is analysed in more than one way, when more matches fit the target, depending on what sort of analogies the system can resort to. If *macro-economy* is already in the dataset of base objects, then *macro-economist* will be brought back to it and (*macro*(*economy*))(*ist*) will be yielded as the system's response; on the other hand, if *economist* is attested, and *macro-economy* is not, the latter is likely to be the best analogue of the target *macro-economist*, and the analysis (*macro*)(*economy*(*ist*)) is attempted. This does not have to worry us, as long as consistency is ensured at the level of morphological interpretation: structural information is no longer part of this interpretation, but rather reflects the analogical "history" of how the system relates a target word to its acquired knowledge.

To conclude, the analogy-based view of morphology apparently reverses the traditional morpheme-based assumption that a complex word is a function of the meanings conveyed by its constituents: on the contrary, word-internal units receive their interpretation from the (paradigmatic) context they are embedded in.

2.3 Performance

2.3.1 How well does analogy work?

MorphEUS is a self-learning, analogy-based architecture in which most of the ideas illustrated so far have been implemented. Accuracy rates of its performance in dealing with Italian morphology are shown in Figure 2.11. A non-pruning version of MorphEUS is compared with a pruning version: with pruning, MorphEUS is certainly slower in its parsing abilities, but its inferential weakness is rapidly made up for as learning progresses.

We tested the MorphEUS architecture in linguistic domains other than morphology (Table 2.1). As a stress assigner, our algorithm attains 93% accuracy after 40 000

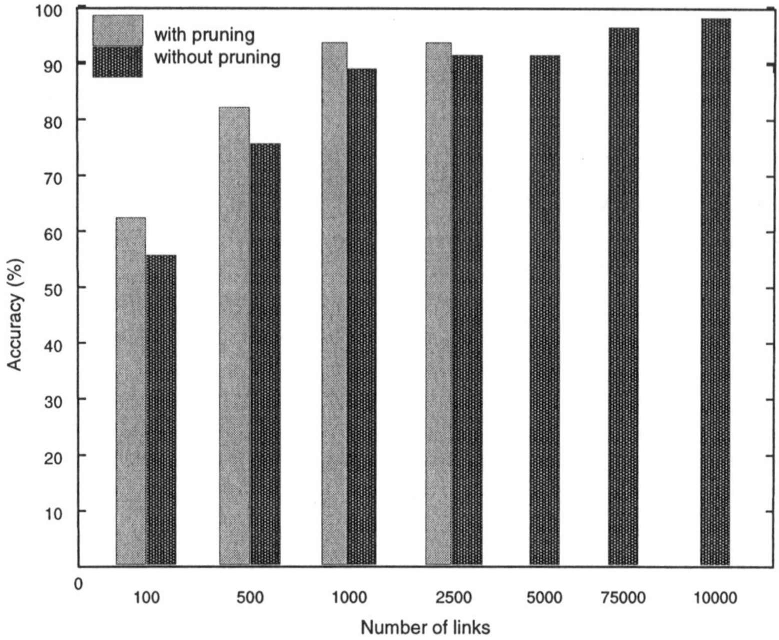

Figure 2.11 *MorphEUS success rate with and without pruning.*

training words (Federici & Pirrelli 1993). As a syntactic disambiguator (tagger), it manages to select the right part-of-speech tag out of the set of available candidates by looking at a three-word context (trigram) in the 95% of cases, after a training of 2000 trigrams (Pirrelli & Federici, 1994a). We also used the basic analogical principles of MorphEUS to deal with the interpretation of subject and object in Italian sentences, attaining 98% accuracy after a training sample of 360 selected sentences (Montemagni et al., Ch. 3). Finally, a multilingual analogy-based transcriber was developed whose accuracy on Italian names (99%) is far better than anything achieved by either statistics- or rule-based grapheme-to-phoneme software (Federici & Pirrelli 1995)

2.3.2 Self-amending capabilities

Analogy is prone to errors. For our purposes, two main categories of errors are:

- errors due to "background noise": the system extracts matches which are longer than they should be, due to the fortuitous overlapping of two word forms which are "too similar";
- errors by "overshooting": the system extracts a match which is shorter than it should be, due to the poor overlap between, say, a regular word form and an irregular one (e.g. between the English past tenses *changed* and *trod*).

Table 2.1 Performances of analogy-based systems for different tasks.

Task	System	Success rate
Morphological lemmatization	MorphEUS (Federici & Pirrelli 1993)	96%
TAG disambiguation	AnTaEUS (Pirrelli & Federici 1994a)	95%
Word generation	GenUS (Pirrelli & Federici 1994c)	75%
Stress assignment	Accent (Federici & Pirrelli 1994)	93%
Subject/object assignment	Roler (Montemagni et al., Ch. 3)	98%
Graph–phoneme transcription	PhoTEUS (Federici & Pirrelli 1995)	99%

The first thing to be observed here is that both of the above must be somewhat exceptional cases: were they systematic, they would amount to a linguistic regularity and should not worry us in the least. The second point is that having stored these sorts of errors in the network could lead to inaccurate system responses in analysis or generation. In fact, in the long run, the system is bound to get rid of these mistaken matches. Let us consider background noise first.

As pointed out above, longer matches are preferred in analysis since they take into account longer stretches of an input word form; however, if these matches contain noise, that is, if they are the result of fortuitous analogies, they will also contain, besides relevant substrings, noisy substrings, that is, substrings which should be associated with either another lexeme or other features (they should be included in other cores than the one in question). To be more concrete, let us turn back to the match between *invecchiare* and *ingiallire* discussed on p. 19 above.

Clearly, the match *in–ia–re* (Fig. 2.12a), associated with the feature "infinitive", although longer than *in– –re*, cannot be combined with the word-internal stem *giall*, since the latter already contains the characters *-ia-*; nor can it be combined with other stems, for that matter, since there are no Italian stems with an *-ia-* internal "gap". For this reason, we can say that *in–ia–re* lacks paradigmatic strength. Whichever type of pruning we resort to, we can be confident that the proper match *in– –re* (Fig. 2.12b) is bound to be preferred in Italian, as soon as enough morphological input evidence is provided during learning for the system to be able to cover a word form such as *ingiallire* in its entirety. Obviously, this will not be the case in Arabic.

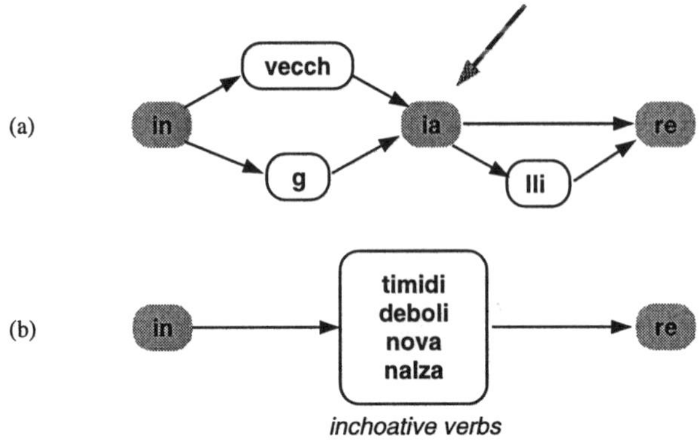

Figure 2.12 *Background noise.*

Errors by overshooting are even simpler to deal with (Fig. 2.13). "Overshot" matches are always shorter than correct matches. It follows that they will always be overridden by the latter in analysis, where the longer fully contained match is always given preference.

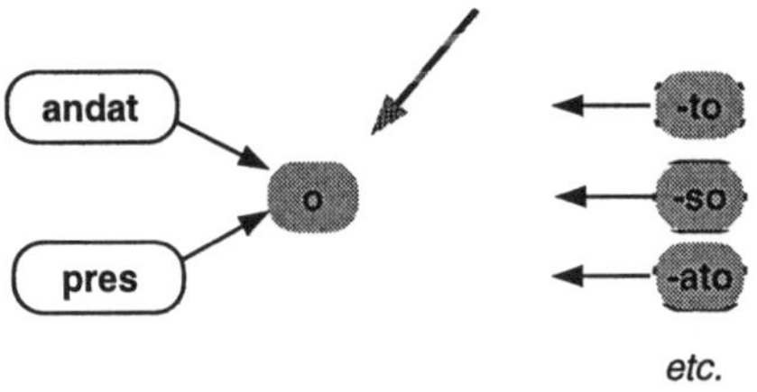

Figure 2.13 *Overshooting.*

2.4 Conclusions

In general, analogy seems to prefer redundancy to linguistic simplicity (or linguistic economy): more, partially overlapping, patterns, each grouping a few linguistic objects only are preferred to few, huge patterns, each of which accounts for all such objects at once (according to the most general rule). To give but one concrete example, analogy relates all *og*-ending singular nouns with their corresponding *ogs*-ending plural counterparts, and so on and so forth for a variety of endings, rather than relating all singular nouns to all plural nouns, no matter how they end. The last generalization is captured indirectly, by considering all small classes simultaneously. This is the "price" we paid to make analogy computable.

It is an interesting fact that psycholinguistic accounts of morphological processing have often emphasized the importance of hybrid linguistic representations in the mental lexicon, so that a certain complex word is purported to receive more than one morphological structure in the mind (Caramazza et al. 1988). Derwing (1990) goes so far as to claim that multiple morphological representations ensure efficacy of child language learning: what cannot be generalized over through one representation for lack of positive evidence to the child, can eventually be generalized by using a different strategy.[5]

On the computational front, as to the precise set of constraints to be enforced for harnessing the combinatorial explosion of all possible matches, our conclusion is that this choice may vary, depending on the types of application one has in mind and the nature and extension of the input one is dealing with: partial morphological analyses are more effectively tackled through a certain type of pruning ("choose the longest match") rather than another ("choose the paradigmatically strongest match"). Paradigmatic constraints make the learning process slower, but more reliable. Clearly, this point does not exclude a further theoretical possibility, certainly worth considering: namely, that the human ability to spot a relevant analogy in a given linguistic context may also be sharpened by cognitive factors other than purely linguistic ones.

Appendix

The list intersection operator ($\sqcap$) is recursively defined on the length of the match, s, between two strings a and b:

(a) length(s) = 1:
a_i, b_i, $s \in V^*$, let $a = a_1 s\ a_2$ and $b = b_1 s\ b_2$:
$a \sqcap b = s$

(b) length(s) = n+1:
a_1, b_1, $s \in V^+$, a_2 and $b_2 \in V^*$, if $\exists\ s_0 \in V^+$, $x\ V$ such that length(s_0) = n and $s = s_0 x$,
let $a = a_1 x a_2$, $b = b_1 x b_2$
$a_1 \sqcap b_1 = s_0$:
$a \sqcap b = s$

Example:
1437 $\sqcap$ 1307 = 137
but 1763 $\neg\sqcap$ 1307 $\neq$ 137

5. For example, Derwing contends that the child's choice of the appropriate allomorph for noun pluralization in English can be determined on the basis of either the final rhyme element of the stem or the final consonant of the root alone.

References

Berko, J. 1958. The child's learning of English morphology. *Word* **14**, 150–77.

Bloomfield, L. 1933. *Language*. New York: Holt.

Caramazza, A., A. Laudanna & C. Romani 1988. Lexical access and inflectional morphology. *Cognition* **28**, 297–332.

Carstairs-McCarthy, A. 1992. *Current morphology*. London: Routledge.

Cook, V. J. 1988. *Chomsky's universal grammar: an introduction*. Oxford: Blackwell.

Dedina, M. J. & H. C. Nusbaum 1991. Pronounce: a program for pronunciation by analogy. *Computer Speech and Language* **5**, 55–64.

Derwing, B. L. 1990. Morphology and the mental lexicon: psycholinguistic evidence. In *Contemporary morphology*, W. U. Dressler, H. C. Luschützky, O. E. Pfeiffer & J. R. Rennison (eds), 249–65, Berlin: Mouton de Gruyter.

Federici, S. & V. Pirrelli 1993. Stressing by analogy: the elicitation of accentual patterns through analogy-based networks. *Proceedings of the Onomastica Technical Workshop*, London, 33–8.

Federici, S. & V. Pirrelli 1994. The compilation of large pronunciation lexica: the elicitation of letter-to-sound patterns through analogy-based networks. *Papers in Computational Lexicography: Complex '94*, Budapest, 59–67.

Federici, S. & V. Pirrelli 1995. Analogia, apprendimento automatico ed elaborazione del linguaggio naturale. *AI*IA Notizie* **2** , 27–30.

Hoeksema, J. & R. D. Janda 1988. Implications of process-morphology for Categorial Grammar. In *Categorial grammars and natural language structures*, R. T. Oehrle, E. W. Bach & D. Wheeler (eds), 199–247, Dordrecht: Reidel.

Owen, S. 1990. *Analogy for automated reasoning*. New York: Academic Press.

Pirrelli, V. & S. Federici 1991. An analogical way to language modelling: MORPHEUS. *Acta Linguistica Hungarica* **41**, 235–63.

Pirrelli, V. & S. Federici 1994a. Context-sensitivity and linguistic structure in analogy-based parallel networks. In *Current issues in computational linguistics*, C. Martin-Vide (ed.), 353–62, Amsterdam: Elsevier.

Pirrelli, V. & S. Federici 1994b. Corpus-based acquisition of inflectional paradigms in Italian. In *CSNLP 1994: 3rd Conference on the Cognitive Science of Natural Language Processing*, Dublin.

Pirrelli, V. & S. Federici 1994c. "Derivational" paradigms in morphophonology. In *COLING 94: The 15th International Conference on Computational Linguistics*, Kyoto, Japan, 234–40.

Siegel, D. 1979. *Topics in English morphology*. Boston: Garland.

Skousen, R. 1989. *Analogical modeling of language*. Dordrecht: Kluwer.

Sullivan, K. P. H. & R. I. Damper 1992. Novel-word pronunciation within a text-to-speech system. In *Talking machines: theories, models and designs*, G. Bailly & C. Benoit (eds), 183–95, Amsterdam: North-Holland.

3
Constraints and preferences at work: an analogy-based approach to parsing grammatical relations

SIMONETTA MONTEMAGNI, STEFANO FEDERICI AND VITO PIRRELLI[1]

3.1 Introduction

Identifying the relations of subject and object in Italian is not a trivial task. The question (1) can be translated in English either as (2a), where Maria is the loved entity, or (2b), where Maria is the lover.

1. This paper is the outcome of a joint effort. However, for the specific concerns of the Italian Academy, S. Montemagni is responsible for sections 1, 2, 3.4 and 4, S. Federici is responsible for section 3.3, V. Pirrelli for sections 3, 3.1, 3.2 and 5.

(1) *Chi ama Maria?*

(2) a. Who loves Maria?
b. Whom does Maria love?

The answer to this question involves the simultaneous consideration of a number of different linguistic and extralinguistic factors. These factors can be distinguished on the basis of

- their predictive power ("constraints" vs "preferences"); and
- for what concerns linguistic factors only, the level of linguistic description they belong to (phonological, morphological, syntactic, semantic, pragmatic).

In most computational models, these factors are usually treated in different modules according to their nature, and used in different ways: i.e. the typical role of constraints is to build up linguistic representations, while preferences are commonly used to rank already built linguistic representations from the more likely to the less likely ones.

In this paper, we propose the architecture and working of a computational framework that provides a unified treatment of all of these factors where constraints and preferences are treated on the same footing and the distinction between different levels of linguistic description is blurred.

3.2 The problem

As already pointed out, in Italian the identification of subject and object relations is by no means a trivial task. Consider (3)–(7), and in particular the functional interpretation assigned to their nominal constituents.

(3) *I bambini leggono il libro.*
THE CHILDREN READ-plur THE BOOK
'The children read the book.'

(4) *Il libro, leggono i bambini.*
THE BOOK READ-plur THE CHILDREN
'The children read the book.'

(5) *Il bambino legge il libro.*
THE CHILD READ-sing THE BOOK
'The child reads the book.'

(6) *Carlo ha assunto la bambinaia.*
CARLO HAS APPOINTED THE BABYSITTER
'Carlo appointed the babysitter.'

(7) *I lavoratori hanno convinto i sindacati.*
THE WORKERS HAVE CONVINCED THE UNIONS
'Workers convinced the unions.'

In (3), subject–object identification (SOI) hinges on subject–verb agreement: the first nominal constituent *i bambini* ('the children'), which agrees in number and person with the third-person plural *leggono* of the verb *leggere* ('read'), is the subject, and the second nominal constituent *il libro* ('the book'), which does not concord with the verb, plays the role of the object.

Sentence (4) represents a different permutation (OVS) of the same constituents as (3). This example shows that in Italian a change in the ordering of the constituents does not affect the sentence interpretation which, in the case at hand, remains the same as in (3).[2]

Consider now sentence (5), where both nominal constituents concord with the verb, and the role of agreement as a distinctive factor for unique SOI is neutralized. When agreement is neutralized, other factors need to be resorted to. In the case at hand, it can be argued that, for lack of decisive syntactic evidence, it is the lexico-semantic knowledge about the verb *leggere* and the semantic restrictions imposed by the verb on its arguments which effectively guide SOI. *Leggere* selects a human subject and a readable object: in (5), *bambino* ('child') and *libro* ('book') respectively satisfy these restrictions.

In sentence (6), agreement fails again to mark unambiguously subject and object relations. A further difficulty here is that the lexico-semantic knowledge about the verb *assumere* ('appoint') and its arguments is rather unhelpful: with *assumere*, both subject and object should be human. SOI here is probably helped by the world-knowledge assumption that a babysitter is more likely to be appointed than to appoint someone else.

Sentence (7) is even more difficult, as both agreement and semantic restrictions are neutralized. *Lavoratori* ('workers') and *sindacati* ('unions') both agree with the verb, and are both human (or human-like in the case of *sindacati*). Moreover, world knowledge adds very little that might be useful to our task. Thus, in order to find the most likely interpretation for this sentence, we need to know the context in which it has been uttered, for example that the workers were trying to convince the unions about something. Finally, without knowledge of context, the interpretation of this sentence can rely on other cues, such as word order and prosodic contour combined together. Apparently, this is in contrast to what was said before, namely that word order does not provide conclusive evidence for SOI. Yet, this statement holds when word order is considered in isolation. However, when combined with prosodic information, word order can be used to identify the most likely interpretation. The sequence NP–verb–NP, combined with a prosodic contour where no particular emphasis is placed on either constituent, is commonly interpreted as SVO. On this basis, in (7) *i lavoratori* is the more likely subject and *i sindacati* the more likely object.

These examples are discussed in order to give the reader a flavour of the variety of factors which come into play for SOI in Italian; a thorough consideration of them all,

---

2. In passing, it should be noted that not all constituent orderings are equally frequent in Italian: their use varies according to the particular discourse situation. The evidence provided by the ordering of the nominal constituents with respect to the verb is not conclusive for SOI.

however, would go far beyond the scope of this paper. Put in a nutshell, these factors vary along different dimensions: i.e. their predictive power in the identification task; their linguistic or extralinguistic nature; for linguistic factors only, the level of linguistic description they relate to. Figure 3.1 projects this classification onto a two-dimensional space, where the horizontal axis represents the nature of these factors as a gradation from linguistic to extralinguistic ones, and the vertical axis shows their role in the SOI process, as constraints or preferences.

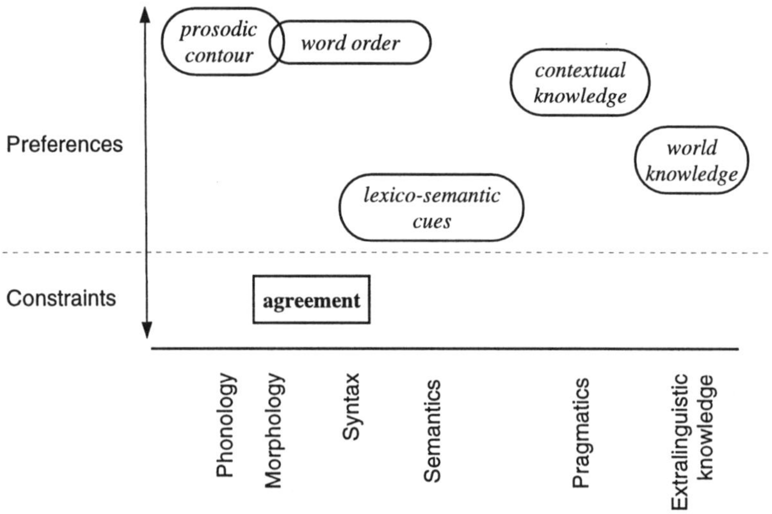

Figure 3.1 *Hybrid system architecture.*

In the diagram, it is shown that subject–verb agreement is a morphosyntactic constraint which represents a necessary, but not always sufficient, condition for identifying grammatical relations in Italian. When this constraint is neutralized "auxiliary" factors are generally relied on. In contrast to constraints which represent yes/no logical conditions, auxiliary factors or, in more appropriate terms, preferences, define tendencies, which, as such, can be violated. In the space of preferences, a factor in a lower position plays a stronger role for SOI, e.g. lexico-semantic preferences imposed by a verb on its arguments provide stronger evidence for SOI than constituent order or prosodic contour. The diagram, however, represents a static picture of the situation: i.e. only the typology of factors is accounted for, but their interaction remains neglected (see the stronger role played by prosodic contour and word order when combined together).

How is the distinction between constraints and preferences modelled in traditional natural language processing architectures? In the case of stratificational models, constraints and preferences, due to their different predictive power, are usually enforced in different modules, ordered in such a way that preferences come into play after constraints have failed to produce a unique analysis; thus, the role of preferences is that of selecting the most likely analysis among the possible ones (see Voutilainen et al. (1992) or Bennett & Paggio (1993) for an illustration of this kind of interaction between constraints and preferences). Both constraints and preferences are classified according to the level of linguistic description they pertain to: hence, depending on their nature they are treated at different levels. Like constraints, preferences can be syntactic (Kimball 1973; Frazier & Fodor 1978), lexico-syntactic (Ford et al. 1982), lexico-semantic (Fass & Wilks 1983), as well as pragmatic (Hirst 1987).

It should be observed that this architecture does not guarantee that an ambiguity which arises at a given level of analysis can be solved by preferences pertaining to the same level: for instance, the morphosyntactic ambiguity observed in (5) is solved through preferences based on lexico-semantic knowledge. In cases like this one, the ambiguity is carried over to further processing stages, and the resulting overgeneration is carried over through different modules until the module containing the relevant disambiguating cues is reached. Moreover, and more importantly in this context, if preferences are separated on the basis of their linguistic nature, the interaction between preferences specified in different modules is difficult to account for; this is to say that preferences cannot always be evaluated separately, level by level. All these facts led us to develop an alternative approach to constraints and preferences, where they are both treated on the same footing, regardless of the linguistic level they are associated with from a descriptive point of view.

3.3 The system

In this section we will illustrate the architecture and functioning of a computational environment where the task of SOI is modelled as a process of conflict resolution, triggered by the simultaneous activation of multiple constraints/preferences which may give contradictory indications about possible SOIs. The working environment (Federici 1991; Pirrelli & Federici 1991) is an extendible, parallel network that learns how to detect subject and object roles in a sentence on the basis of the knowledge acquired from a training corpus of sentences whose subject and object are explicitly indicated. The general principles underpinning the system are detailed in Federici & Pirrelli (Ch. 2).

The system is illustrated starting from a description of input and output representations (Section 3.3.1), to then considering its learning algorithm (Section 3.3.2), its inferential routine (Section 3.3.3) and its behaviour in the subject/object identification phase (Section 3.3.4).

3.3.1 Representation

The input to our system is not a raw sentence but a canonical representation of its constituent structure, which has been produced by a simple rule-based shallow parser (Montemagni 1995). In this canonical representation the sentence constituents are given in a conventional order: the verb first, then the two noun constituents in their relative order. As we will see below, information about the linear ordering of the constituents in the sentence is preserved through the use of indexes. During training, the input representation of a sentence is paired with its output representation, so that the system is taught how to associate them. In the response phase, the system is given the input representation alone, and is expected to yield the appropriate output.

Consider again sentence (3), repeated here for convenience: Figure 3.2 shows how its canonical representation looks in input.

(3) *I bambini leggono il libro.*

```
leggere/V leggere/V2 pers6/V2 . . . >>
   (V2/S leggere/S)(V2/O leggere/O)
bambino/N bambino/N1 pers6/N1 masc/N1 def/N1 . . . >>
   (N1/S bambino/S)(N1/O bambino/O)
libro/N libro/N2 pers3/N2 masc/N2 def/N2 . . . >>
   (N2/S libro/S)(N2/O libro/O)
```

Figure 3.2 *Canonical representation ("input pattern") of* I bambini leggono il libro.

In this representation, called an "input pattern", each sentence constituent is identified by a complex label expressing (a) its morphosyntatic category (e.g. `N` stands for "noun", `V` for "verb") and (b) its actual "position" within the sentence. Thus, `V2` means that *leggono* is the verbal constituent in second position within the sentence, `N1` that *i bambini* is the first nominal constituent within the sentence, and `N2` that *il libro* is the second nominal constituent. Note that while the verb index indicates the absolute position of the verb in the sentence, the noun indexes convey information about the linear precedence of noun constituents.

Each constituent is described by a set of features conveying linguistic information relevant to the task at hand; these features belong to different levels of linguistic description, ranging over morphosyntactic (e.g. agreement features such as person and number), lexico-semantic (e.g. the lexical head of the constituents in the sentence) and pragmatic (e.g. the topical position of the constituents) information. For each constituent, the set of features is distributed over two distinct groups: the left-hand side (LHS) features (those preceding ">>") and the right-hand side (RHS) features (those following ">>"). The former specify the lexical head of a constituent in its uninflected form, its morphosyntactic properties (person, number, gender, etc.), definiteness (in nominal constituents only) and, more generally, all other features which we might expect to be relevant for SOI. On the other hand, RHS features indicate the potential functional interpretation of each constituent when taken out of context: either as a subject or as an object. Note that, oddly enough, even a verb constituent can be interpreted as either subject or object. This has been done to deal with pro-drop languages like Italian, where the subject constituent can be omitted (e.g. (8)), as the subject's person and number can be recovered from the morphological ending of the verb (*leggono* is the third-person plural of *leggere*). Similarly, the feature O(bject) associated with the verb can be relevant when the object is realized as a clitic pronoun, which is treated, in our representation, as an affix lexically attached to the verb.

(8) *Leggono il libro.*
'They read a book.'

The reader will note that in the input pattern, the constituent structure of the sentence is uniquely defined, while the functional interpretation of its constituents is left open, as constituents are specified, by their RHS features, for both the subject and object roles (indicated by `/S` and `/O` endings). Hence, `N1/S` means that the first nominal constituent (`N1`) is a potential subject, `N1/O` that `N1` is a potential object, and so on. A further important detail of this representation is that `/S` and `/O` features are bracketed pairwise when they refer to the same constituent: the logical relation holding between them is an *and* relation, meaning that the entire condition between parentheses is false as soon as the information expressed by either parenthesized feature is false. In the system, this constraint is enforced through the notion of "ring" (see below).

Let us now consider the output representation of the same sentence (called the "output pattern") (Fig. 3.3).

```
leggere/V leggere/V2 pers6/V2 . . . >>
bambino/N bambino/N1 pers6/N1 masc/N1 def/N1 . . . >>
   (N1/S bambino/S)
libro/N libro/N2 pers3/N2 masc/N2 def/N2 . . . >>
   (N2/O libro/O)
```

Figure 3.3 *Output pattern of* I bambini leggono il libro.

The output pattern represents the solution to the problem left open by the input pattern: i.e. the output pattern makes a commitment as to what constituents are the sentence subject and object. In the RHS, inappropriate functional interpretations are simply cancelled out: e.g. in the example at hand, `V2/S`, `leggere/S`, `V2/O`, `leggere/O`, `N/O`, `bambino/O`, `N2/S` and `libro/S` all disappear. RHS features which are left are the functional interpretation of the sentence. In this way, the output pattern always represents a streamlined version of the input pattern. This implies that SOI, in our system, is basically modelled as a disambiguation procedure: to detect subject and object in a sentence means to eliminate false hypotheses concerning SOI. If the information conveyed by the feature `N1/O` is false, for example, then it should be eliminated; if it is true, it should remain in the RHS.

This way of modelling our task reflects the assumption that the network is a *tabula rasa*, i.e. that it does not know the first thing about subjects and objects, what they are, what constituents they should be assigned to, how many subjects there are in a sentence, how many objects, and things like that. This is something that the system has to find out by itself on the basis of the indications which are provided by pairs of input–output patterns during learning.

3.3.2 Learning sentences

Let us now consider how the input and output patterns of the sentence (3) are represented within the system's network. In the previous section, we saw that each feature in these patterns states a linguistic condition which is either true or false. Boolean features can be represented in a network as nodes (or units) which are either on (true) or off (false). Henceforth, we will refer to these feature units as "nodes".

From the point of view of our network, an input pattern is a set of activated nodes represented as grey discs in Figure 3.4 linked to one further node which belongs to the layer of so-called "hidden" nodes of the network.[3] In their turn, all grey input nodes activate their hidden node through excitatory signals (+ signals) which are propagated along forward links (straight lines in Fig. 3.4), called "input links".

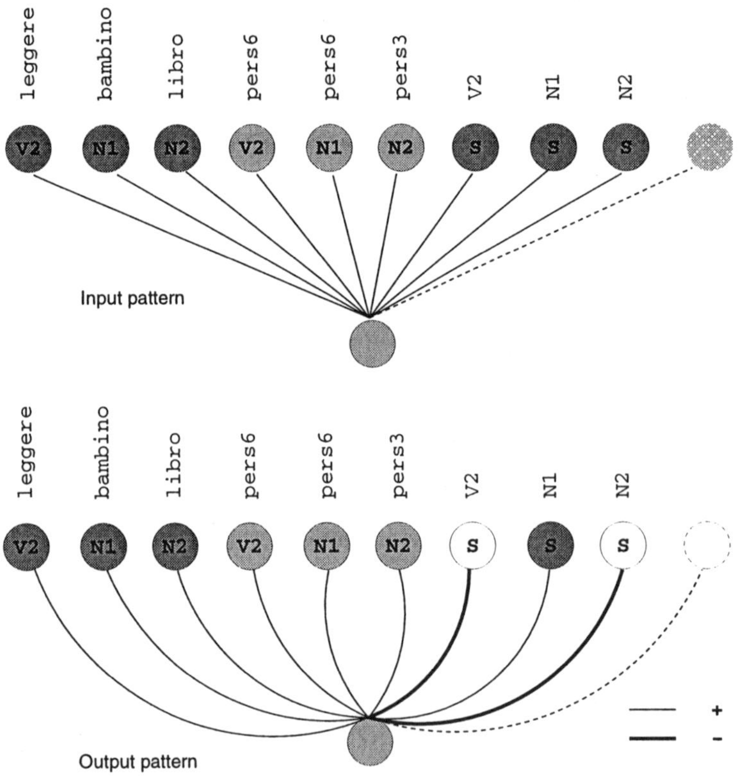

Figure 3.4 *Network structure for the input and output patterns of the sentence* I bambini leggono il libro.

The hidden node is linked back to its input nodes through backward links called "output links" (represented as arcs in Fig. 3.4): this network configuration is the

3. Note that, for the sake of readability, each pattern exhibits only some of its features; for example, in many patterns, only subject-related features are shown in the diagrams: the machinery described in these pages obviously extends to object-related nodes as well.

output pattern. Once created, an output link is given a polarity, that is, it will be either positive (if it conveys excitatory signals), or negative (if it conveys inhibitory signals): an output link never changes its polarity. In contrast to input links, which are always positive, output links can be either positive or negative. Negative output links (marked bold) are intended to turn off a node which thus becomes an off-unit[4] (represented as a white disc). Positive output links keep the node on (which thus remains an on-unit).

Finally, the *and* relation holding between parenthesized features in the RHS of the patterns, indicating feature codependency, is implemented in the network as a "ring"-like structure (Fig. 3.5) which is turned off as soon as one of its nodes is turned off.

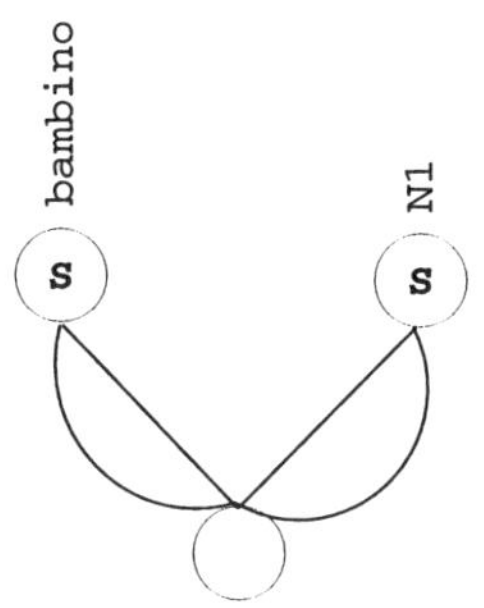

Figure 3.5 *"Ring" structure.*

As the system response is the set of input nodes which have been left on, we had no reason to create a separate layer of output nodes. This is to say that the input layer is also used to convey the system's output. The only difference between an input pattern and its corresponding output pattern rests then in the state of activation of the same nodes – activation which changes after the relevant hidden units have done their job.

The training of the network consists in showing pairs of input–output patterns. The learning of SOI by our network is modelled thus: each hidden node learns what type of signal should be returned to what feature nodes of its input pattern when the latter gets activated. This state of affairs is represented in Figure 3.6 by a so-called "learned pattern", which results from the combination of an input pattern with an output pattern.

4. Note, however, that the same node might be simultaneously supported by some other activated hidden node.

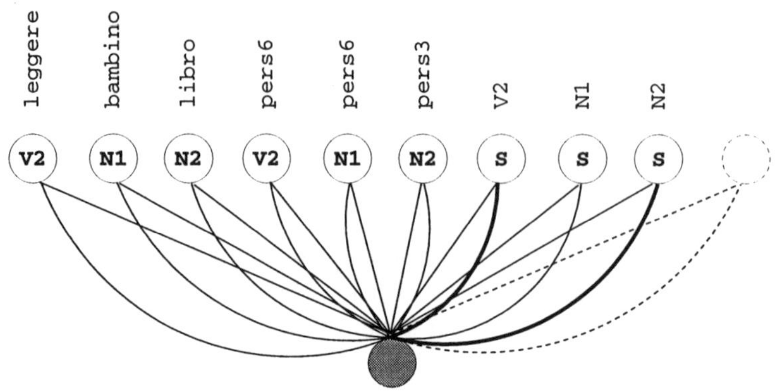

Figure 3.6 *Network structure for the learned pattern of the sentence* I bambini leggono il libro *(LP-1).*

3.3.3 Extracting core patterns

How are learned patterns used for SOI? If learned patterns like the one seen before were all the system knew about sentences, then only an already learned sentence could be correctly interpreted. This is due to the constraint, which has been enforced for reasons of computational efficiency, that a learned pattern is triggered in analysis when and only when it is *fully contained* within the pattern activated by the input sentence to interpret (see also Federici & Pirrelli, Ch. 2). But the system does more than this: it can carry out the SOI of new sentences by analogy to already known sentences. This section shows how this is done.

When two learned patterns have at least one positive output link and one negative output link in common,[5] then a third pattern is extracted from the two learned patterns and contains the common links and nodes shared by them. Thus, core patterns differ from learned patterns in that they have not explicitly been provided in input but they have been extracted by the system through its analogy-based inferential routine. The inferential routine can be illustrated through the following oversimplified steps, mimicking the gradual learning of constraints/preferences by the system.

Suppose, for example, that the new sentence (9) is learned by the system. The corresponding learned pattern (LP-2 in Fig. 3.7) and the learned pattern in Figure 3.6 (i.e. LP-1) will then give rise to the core pattern CP-A in Figure 3.8.

(9) *I topi mangiano il formaggio.*
'The mice eat the cheese.'

5. Two learned patterns are said to have one link in common if and when they share one particular link which, in both patterns (a) has the same polarity, and (b) is linked to the same input unit.

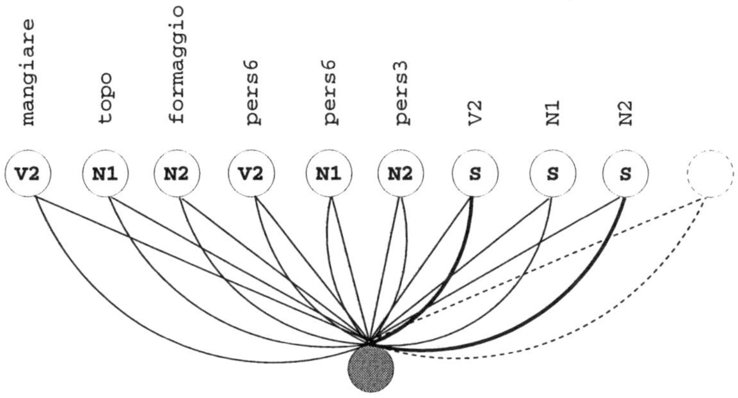

Figure 3.7 *Network structure for the learned pattern of the sentence* I topi mangiano il formaggio *(LP-2).*

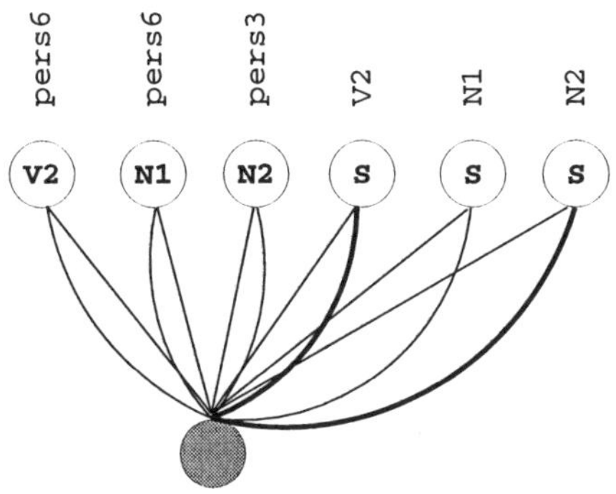

Figure 3.8 *The extracted core pattern CP-A.*

CP-A expresses the following generalization: in an NP–verb–NP structure where the first NP and the verb are marked as `pers6` and the second NP is marked as `pers3`, the first NP is the subject (see the positive output link supporting the activation of the `N1/S` node); note the inhibitory output links excluding the other possible interpretations (turning off, for instance, the `N2/S` and `V2/S` nodes). This pattern corresponds to a straightforward rule of agreement in Italian: every time a nominal constituent and a verb agree on the feature third-person plural (indicated as `pers6` in the figure), that nominal constituent is the subject of the sentence if the other nominal constituent is `pers3`, i.e. if it disagrees in person and number with the verb. If compared with the usual formulation of the agreement rule, this generalization is rather weak. First, it is position-dependent; and second, it is restricted to the combination of features `pers6`, `pers6`, `pers3`. We believe that the possibility of expressing weak linguistic constraints such as this one is not a drawback of the system, but rather gives it the leeway to capture and encode extremely subtle and articulated conditions.

The same CP-A will be used by the system for the interpretation of sentences like (10), where the NP1 *i lavoratori* and the V2 *hanno contestato* ('contested') are both marked as pers6 and the NP2 *il sindacato* ('the union') as pers3.

(10) *I lavoratori hanno contestato il sindacato.*
'The workers contested the union.'

From the examples in Section 3.2, we have seen that whenever agreement is neutralized, other factors are to be resorted to: so far the system has learned what before was classified as a constraint. Consider now (11).

(11) *Il libro legge il bambino.*
THE BOOK READ-sing THE CHILD

CP-A cannot apply in this case, since it is differently specified as to the agreement features: here, all constituents are marked as pers3. Assume now that the system learns the appropriate SOI for this sentence, shown in the learned pattern LP-3 (Fig. 3.9).

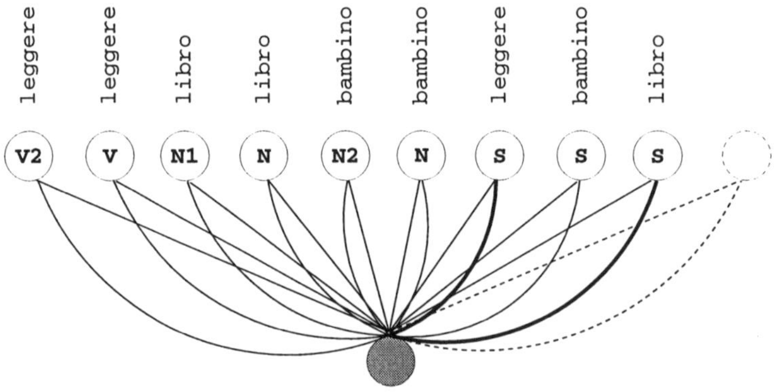

Figure 3.9 *Network structure for the learned pattern of the sentence* Il libro legge il bambino *(LP-3).*

At this point, by comparing this learned pattern with LP-1 (Fig. 3.6), the system is able to isolate, among others, another core pattern: CP-B (Fig. 3.10). Unlike the CP-A, which was based on morphosyntactic information only, CP-B contains purely semantic information, namely that the child *bambino* is a possible reader and the book *libro* is typically read (regardless of morphosyntactic features). In particular, CP-B corresponds to what we have previously classified as a preference, and in particular a semantic preference.

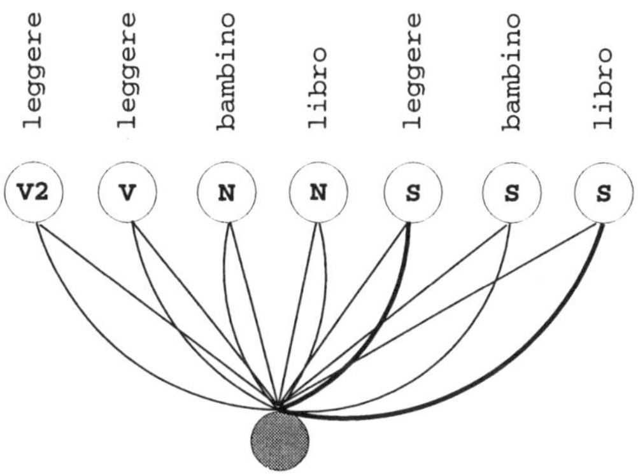

Figure 3.10 *The extracted core pattern CP-B.*

This CP-B will be used to decide on the appropriate SOI for a sentence such as (5) (repeated here for convenience). Like in the previous case, no morphosyntactic core pattern is available to assign the correct interpretation to (5), because of the mismatch between the agreement features of the input sentence and those contained by the core patterns available to the system at this stage.

(5) *Il bambino legge il libro.*

So far, we have seen a core pattern corresponding to a morphosyntactic constraint (CP-A), and another corresponding to what previously has been classified as a semantic preference (CP-B). However, it is very often the case that core patterns combine preferences and constraints, which are of a different nature. Let us now illustrate a more realistic pattern which has been extracted once the sentences (5) and (12) have been learned. The corresponding learned patterns are respectively the LP-4 and LP-5 in Figure 3.11.

(12) *Le ragazze leggono i libri.*
'The girls read the books.'

By matching LP-4 and LP-5, the core pattern CP-C is extracted (Fig. 3.12). This core pattern contains the information that books are typically read, if they are `NP2`: here, factors pertaining to different levels of linguistic description converge on the same SOI. From now onwards, any sentence containing the verb *leggere* in the second position, an `NP2` whose uninflected form is *libro*, and an `NP1` (unspecified as to its lexico-semantic content), will be interpreted by the system as having the `NP1` as the subject of the sentence, for lack of stronger evidence to the contrary. This is what we call "generalization by analogy".

Note that, in our system, we generalize over learned patterns only, i.e. core patterns are extracted by comparing learned patterns only. In principle, core patterns could be extracted by comparing learned patterns with already extracted cores, or core patterns with other core patterns. This would speed up the learning process, since smaller and more general cores would be extracted at an early stage. But, on the other hand, this would end up cluttering the network with a number of useless

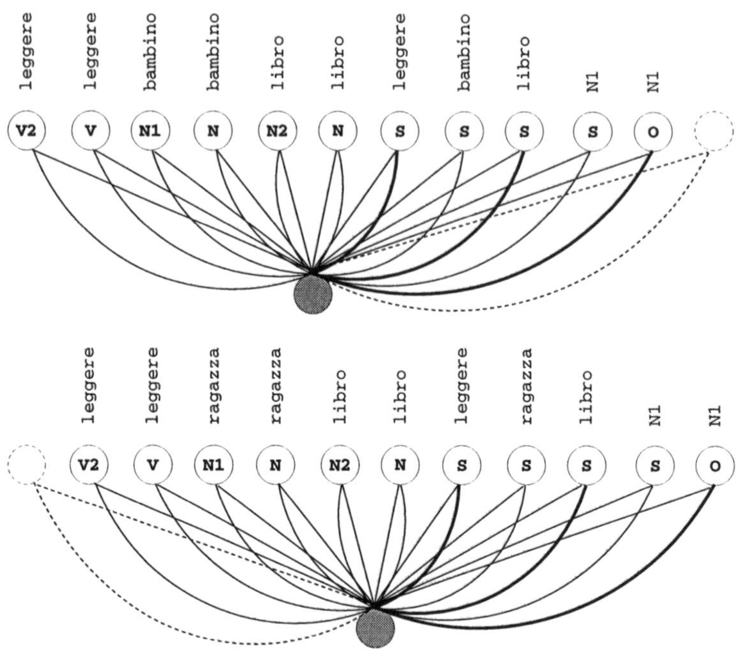

Figure 3.11 *Network structure for the learned patterns LP-4 (*Il libro legge il bambino*) and LP-5 (*Le ragazze leggono i libri*).*

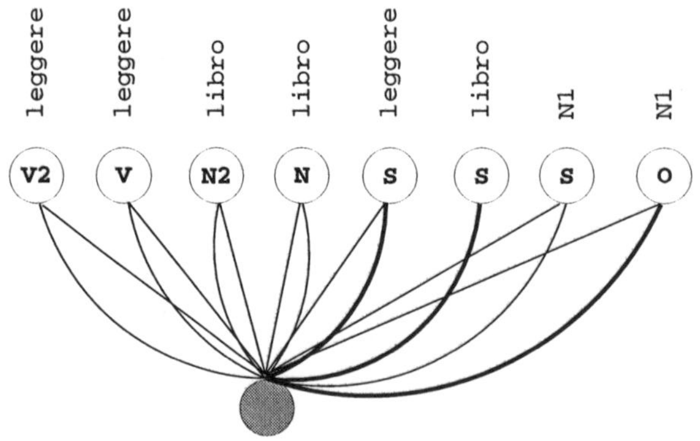

Figure 3.12 *The extracted core pattern CP-C.*

subcores. It is our opinion that, in the long run, relevant small core patterns are extracted nevertheless from learned patterns which differ significantly from each other (see Federici & Pirrelli, Ch. 2).

3.3.4 How are learned and core patterns used for SOI?

Core patterns, once extracted, are stored and used for SOI together with ordinary learned patterns. Like ordinary learned patterns, core patterns are triggered in analysis if and only if they are fully contained within the pattern activated by the input sentence to interpret. This constraint is illustrated in Figure 3.13, where common input nodes are shown twice (once for each pattern), and are given the same index. In this case the partially activated pattern is excluded (conflict is on nodes 5 and 6).

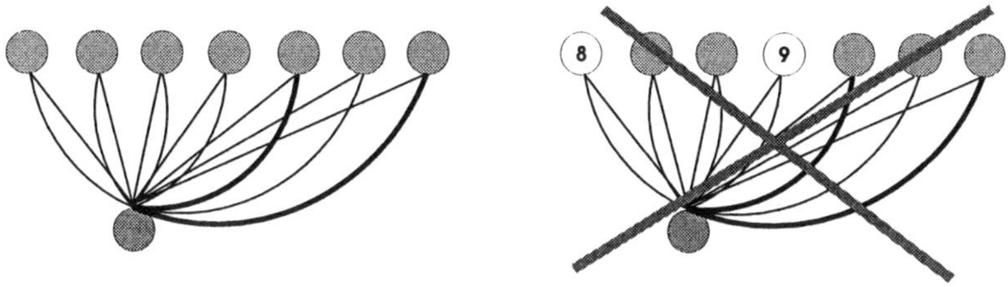

Figure 3.13 *Fully activated patterns always win out.*

Two fully activated patterns are in conflict with each other when their common links, if any, differ in polarity, that is, when they disagree on SOI. In case of conflict between two or more activated patterns, the longest activated pattern wins out, as illustrated in Figure 3.14 (conflict is on nodes 7 and 8).

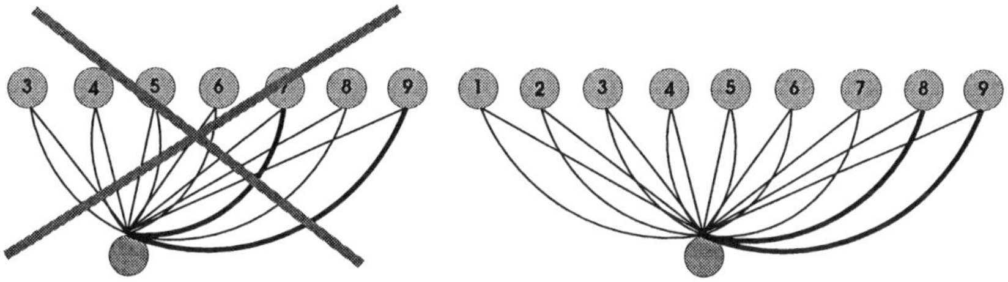

Figure 3.14 *Among fully activated patterns, the longest activated pattern always wins out.*

If there is more than one longest core pattern, then we are faced with a "stalemate". The stalemate situation can be pictured as follows. Let us assume that there are two mutually incompatible extracted cores of the same length: one which interprets, for instance, `NP1` as the subject, the other which interprets `NP1` as the object; these two cores inhibit each other. Other strategies, then, should be found for the system to yield its SOI: in cases like this, paradigmatic extension (as illustrated in Federici & Pirrelli, Ch. 2) is triggered, as shown in Figure 3.15 (conflict is on nodes 7 and 8 again).

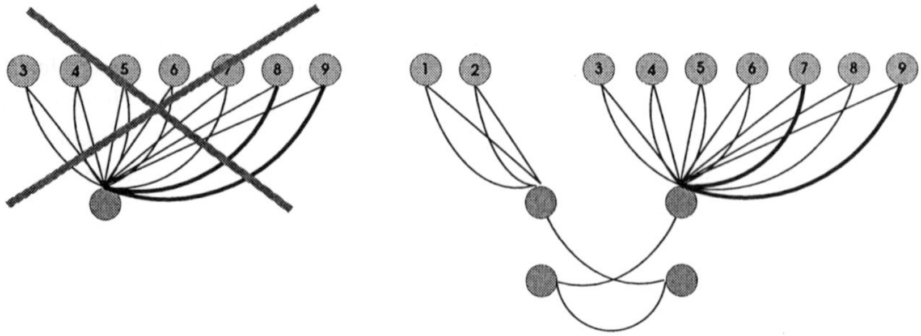

Figure 3.15 *Among longest activated patterns, the more paradigmatically activated one wins out.*

If the stalemate cannot be solved, all available interpretations are yielded by the system in its current version. In principle, statistically based heuristics could be used in this case to select the more likely interpretation.

3.4 Performance in SOI

The system has been trained on 360 sentences, grouped in 60 sets of six sentences each. Within every set, each sentence differs from the others in the ordering of the constituents only (not morphologically nor lexically), so that all the six possible permutations of these constituents are represented, as in (13), representing all possible translations of 'The children read the book'.[6]

(13) a. *I bambini leggono il libro.* SVO
b. *Il libro leggono i bambini.* OVS
c. *I bambini il libro leggono.* SOV
d. *Il libro i bambini leggono.* OSV
e. *Leggono i bambini il libro.* VSO
f. *Leggono il libro i bambini.* VOS

After training, the system was then tested on a corpus of 360 sentences. Some of them were just different combinations of the lexical choices already attested in the training sample. Some others contained unknown words. Note, however, that none of the sentences already encountered during training was used for the test. In fact, it was pointless to expose the system to already known sentences, because of the constraints mentioned in the previous section:

- the system's response is always based on *both* cores *and* learned patterns (that is, learned sentences);

6. It should be noted that in Italian different permutations of subject, verb and object are pronounced with different prosodic contours. Yet, this kind of information is unreliably encoded at the written level: punctuation, which is often used to render the prosodic contour, also serves other purposes (e.g. boundary marker, conjunction), and cannot be interpreted as an unambiguous prosodic marker.

- a winning pattern is always the longest fully activated one.

Obviously, no fully activated pattern can be longer than the learned pattern corresponding to the sentence itself. Then convergence is always guaranteed when a previously learned sentence is shown again.

In our test, the system identified the correct interpretation in 98% of the cases. Most of its failures were due to lack of knowledge about how words semantically or lexically co-select each other. Improvements of the results can in principle be achieved by enlarging the coverage of the training sample. This can be done in two different ways:

- by adding new sentences to the training sample;
- by adding specifications concerning the semantic properties of words.

We are currently working on the second extension, which we think would be crucial since we want our system to be able to generalize its knowledge on the basis of semantic information (which for the time being is only represented by the lemma), and thus to cope with words which it has never seen before. For this specific purpose, we are currently adding, for each sentence constituent, features corresponding to more general semantic labels expressed intensionally or extensionally, i.e. in the form of either semantic features or hyperonyms or synonyms.

3.5 Conclusions

In this paper, we have argued that in Italian it is difficult to draw a clear-cut distinction between constraints and preferences when it comes to subject–object identification. This difficulty is rather language-specific (for instance, in English SOI ambiguities never arise.[7]

Our account differs from more traditional approaches in that it treats constraints and preferences on the same footing, regardless of the linguistic level they are associated with from a descriptive point of view. In our system, both constraints and preferences are treated as clusters of nodes and features which are activated and operate according to the same principles. Thus, in our view, the difference between constraints and preferences is not one of kind but of gradation. What differs between the two is only their range of application:

- a core pattern that is never disconfirmed is a "constraint";
- a core pattern that can be disconfirmed in some cases is a "preference".

7. Whereas in English word order plays the role of a constraint for SOI, we saw that it does not function in this way in Italian where agreement is the only constraint to rely on for SOI. This could usefully be extended to deal with linguistic problems whose resolution involves the interplay of a wide range of factors, the predictive power of which cannot always be defined *a priori* (e.g. PP attachment).

Actual extracted core patterns often combine constraints and preferences which can both be of a different nature. Preferential cores that are never disconfirmed when simultaneously activated can be considered as forming a constraint in its own right.

As a last general remark, we would like to point out that this account calls into question the existence of a direct relationship between linguistic descriptions and their computational modelling. In linguistic theory, subject and object are traditionally classified as syntactic functions. However, from this it should in no way follow that the process of identifying subject and object relations is to be computed on the basis of syntactic information only. We saw that in Italian other factors, involving levels of linguistic description other than syntax, contribute decisively to this process. These factors are more effectively taken into account within a parallel computational architecture, where all of them are free to interact in a process of conflict resolution.

References

Bennett, P. & P. Paggio (eds) 1993. *Preference in Eurotra.* Luxembourg: Office for Official Publications of the European Communities.

Fass, D. & Y. Wilks, 1983. Preference semantics, ill-formedness and metaphor. *American Journal of Computational Linguistics* **9**, 178–87.

Federici, S. 1991. A self-expandable connectionist system for natural language processing. In *Proceedings of AAAI Spring Symposium*, San Diego.

Ford, M., J. Bresnan & R. M. Kaplan, 1982. A competence-based theory of syntactic closure. In *The mental representation of grammatical relations*, J. Bresnan (ed.), 727–96. Cambridge, Mass.: MIT Press.

Frazier, L. & J. D. Fodor, 1978. The sausage machine: a new two-stage parsing model. *Cognition* **6**, 291–325.

Hirst, G. 1987. *Semantic interpretation and the resolution of ambiguity.* Cambridge: Cambridge University Press.

Kimball, J. 1973. Seven principles of surface structure parsing in natural language. *Cognition* **2**, 15–47.

Montemagni, S. 1995. *Subject and object assignment in Italian.* PhD thesis, UMIST, Manchester.

Pirrelli, V. & S. Federici, 1991. An analogical way to language modelling: MORPHEUS. *Acta Linguistica Hungarica* **41**, 235–63.

Voutilainen, A., J. Heikkila & A. Anttila, 1992. *Constraint grammar of English. A performance oriented introduction.* Publication No. 21, Department of General Linguistics, University of Helsinki.

Part II
Connectionist methods

4
Towards a hybrid abstract generation system

MARIA ARETOULAKI

4.1 Setting the scene

In this paper, an alternative architecture is described for a subsymbolic hybrid NLP system that generates abstracts of texts. Traditional AI symbolic processors, namely morphological, syntactic, semantic and pragmatic analysis and synthesis modules (Section 4.4) are co-ordinated with a standard back-propagation Artificial Neural Network (ANN). The novelty of this network lies in its combination of *selected* information from all these standard modules and using it for pragmatic decisions. More specifically, it assigns degrees of importance to clauses in a text, as a first step towards automated abstract generation. Those with the higher scores are the ones that will be used in the summarization of the text. The high-scoring clauses are subsequently processed by symbolic generation modules which output the abstract, after having performed a number of lexical, syntactic and pragmatic operations on these clauses. The ANN and the related training and testing experiments are described later on in the paper (Section 4.5).

ANN models have enjoyed a resurgence of enthusiasm in the last decade, even for NLP tasks (see Section 4.3.1). It is not parallelism with the human brain, however, that gives ANNs their advantage, but rather their success at learning to solve realistic and complex problems. It seems that this alternative to traditional AI is proving very promising after a dead-end had been reached with pure symbolic computation (Section 4.2).

Purely connectionist systems have to date been used mainly for just one of phonological, morphological or syntactic analysis.[1] Some have dealt with semantics and a few with local disambiguation tasks (see Section 4.3.1). In contrast, the present network is used for the pragmatic treatment of whole texts. However, it is operating in a symbolic environment. As a consequence of the system flowchart, many different factors, both linguistic and extralinguistic, are *collectively* considered.

Abstracting is the process whereby a series of ordered, cohesive and coherent utterances is reduced to a relatively few propositions which convey the core messages of the corresponding text. Thus, in an abstract, peripheral details are ignored, while more general statements are used as its building blocks. The degree of generality often determines how important a sentence of the source text is in the composition of its summary. Nevertheless, numerous other criteria have to be taken into consideration as well, which render the overall task quite complex.

The great majority of abstracting systems operate on domain keywords and lexical pattern matching (cf. Mauldin 1991; MUC-5 1993). Nevertheless, such techniques can only have success with standardized technical or news documents of predetermined structure, vocabulary and semantics, e.g. telex messages (Young & Hayes 1985). In order for such systems to be robust in realistic situations involving unrestricted text of any domain, many other sets of knowledge have to be employed. This additional knowledge, in turn, can only be acquired by means of less superficial textual analysis.

4.2 Where has symbolism failed?

NLP systems typically have *modular* architectures, where symbolic processors for lexical, morphological, syntactic, semantic and some heuristic pragmatic analysis are called upon, usually in this exact order. This ensures "debuggability", flexibility, and updatability for the whole system. Nevertheless, the fact that there are separate stages of analysis without any interaction or co-ordination between them entails *overgeneration* of hypotheses and solutions of equal acceptability weights, not to mention the waste of computational effort. A wide-coverage prototype of this practice is the Core Language Engine (Alshawi 1992). In addition, such systems usually only tackle a limited number of pragmatic and semantic problems: this may be focus identification and tracking for anaphora resolution, discourse structure analysis and prediction, or user plan and goal determination and satisfaction. When a wider range of pragmatic aspects are being dealt with, the system is prohibitively slow. As a

1. Despite the special difficulties posed by the third type of processing.

consequence, an application of this type of system in the summarization of hundreds of texts cannot be of practical value.

For this reason there has been a shift towards domain keyword and lexical pattern recognition for summarization and other content retrieval and selection tasks. Vocabulary and phrase-structural analysis of domain corpora eliminates the need for large and complicated grammars, or even elaborate disambiguation techniques and pragmatics. Moreover, unknown words are just ignored or assumed to be proper names in the presence of the appropriate patterns. This is in contrast to traditional symbolic systems, which are prone to failure when faced with unknown, altered or incorrect input, due to the arbitrariness and rigidity of their knowledge. All these features inherent to the current statistics-based information-retrieval paradigm safeguard computational efficiency and usability in realistic situations (Scholtes 1993).

The Message Understanding Conferences (MUCs) have given ample examples to date of such fast and quite effective implementations, which certainly outperform "academic" text-understanding systems, despite high error rates. For instance, FASTUS (Appelt et al. 1993), in MUC-4, employs a set of nondeterministic finite-state automata for keyword and domain pattern recognition, as well as some "pseudosyntactic" analysis of noun and verb phrases. The output of the system is a number of "merged" templates for each text, describing the main incidents reported therein. Although the grammatical and semantic coverage is limited, it is just enough for the processing, in minutes, of 100 newspaper articles on Latin American terrorism, after a development cycle of just three and a half weeks. Indeed, it has been shown at these conferences that systems which insist on full parsing and more generic lexica and ontologies display the worst performance. This is why there has been a realization of late that text extraction is quite different from text understanding.

Another example of this sublanguage-based methodology is the DIDEROT information extraction system (Cowie et al. 1993), as presented at both MUC-4 and MUC-5. It was developed in a longer period, two years, but its coverage is also wider, since it can handle two domains (micro-electronics and joint ventures), and two languages (English and Japanese). Instead of finite-state automata, Prolog rules and facts are used, derived from statistical, corpus-based, lexicalized grammatical information. Other than that, the same processes are involved: name, date, keyword and noun phrase recognition; partial parsing based on domain-specific lexical patterns; semantic frame merging; and template generation with the relevant information.

In all such systems, co-reference resolution is usually dealt with by means of *ad hoc* manually encoded heuristics. Even when discourse analysis is introduced, however, the results are not impressive. In a different context (Lucas et al. 1993) an attempt was presented to develop a tool for the automatic summarization of full Japanese texts. Apart from keyword distribution across chapters, a detailed structural thematic analysis was performed over whole textbooks, in order to identify the important parts of a book and the dominant keyword patterns therein. This, however, was only done manually on three scientific books, and no algorithms have as yet been written to test the related interesting, but intuitive, formalizations. Moreover, the research was guided in part by the frequent presence of standardized opening and closing particles that Japanese appears to possess.

Consequently, it appears that both pure and incisive, and superficial statistics-based symbolic approaches have the following weaknesses:

- Pragmatics is not adequately accommodated, which means that the systems involved are incomplete and application-dependent.
- The rules and knowledge used, as well as the knowledge representation itself, are more often than not *ad hoc*, especially as regards the extralinguistic levels (Chalmers et al. 1992).
- They are generally unable to learn and reuse resources or successful solutions to past problems. Even IR systems such as the above cannot apply domain knowledge and heuristics to new domains successfully, but need to be tuned by retraining their statistical components accordingly (the "porting" problem).

The present *hybrid system* and the ANN therein (see Sections 4.4 and 4.5) have, at least partially, overcome most of these problems:

- Although the overall system is modular, its individual symbolic processors are guided by the trained ANN in performing a partial analysis of the input, and thus avoid overgeneration of solutions. The network has been trained separately with different sets of data that can be computed by the symbolic modules. Those datasets which induce the best performance in the network have been kept as the only ones to be relevant in the determination of importance, and, thus, as the only ones that need to be considered by the symbolic processors.
- The outputs of all the modules are used in parallel by the network, so that the multiplicity and interdependence of the linguistic and pragmatic aspects are respected and re-established.
- Only a single solution is given each time by the ANN, extremely efficiently, despite the diverse types of information involved.
- The system has general applicability; individual domains can be catered for after a limited amount of additional training of the network.
- No heuristic or other rules are fed to the ANN, only real data it generalizes upon.
- The network is very robust, as it never fails to find an approximate solution fast, however unfamiliar the input. This is why ANNs are so popular with the pattern recognition community (cf. Section 4.3.1). In contrast, symbolic methods are less flexible as regards the actual form of the data.
- The knowledge representation formalism is uniform and neutral in the network, namely 0s and 1s, irrespective of the formalisms used by the symbolic processors.

- The ANN is able, by its very architecture and function, to learn inductively and constantly, as is evident from the gradual improvement in its performance during training (cf. Carling 1992).

All these characteristics indicate that connectionism could very well be a viable approach to the processing of such a multidimensional object as the pragmatics of language in general, and the determination of sentence importance for summarization purposes in particular. They also point towards the indispensability of the PDP paradigm in the context of a generic, knowledgeable, but practical and efficient NLP/abstracting system.

4.3 The need for a hybrid system

ANNs are especially good at dealing with unfamiliar or noisy input, after having being trained with related data. The average success rate can reach 95%. Still, some researchers, connectionists themselves, acknowledge the fact that ANNs should better be used in conjunction with symbolic AI processors at this stage of their development (e.g. Fogelman-Soulié 1992; Shavlik 1992). There are three main reasons for this suggestion:

(a) *Precise computations*, such as lexical and morphological analyses, are not the strong point of ANNs. These are already successfully carried out by symbolic processors. Nevertheless, NLP in general involves dealing with the fuzzy, the imperfect and the incomplete rather than the precise, so connectionism is more suited to the analysis of higher levels of language.

(b) *Input size variation* decreases the robustness of ANNs. Sentence length, however, is constantly changing in a text. Thus, a preprocessor would be needed to "normalize" the data. Alternatively, features could be used that depart from the individual word level: attributes that relate to the thematic roles in a sentence (e.g. agent, patient, goal); features which specify the speech act performed by a clause (request for information or action, explanation, contradiction); features that refer to the main verb (tense, aspect, means, location); and so on.

(c) *New classes* of input data cannot be identified unless the ANN is retrained from scratch. A new semantic/pragmatic feature, for example, will be ignored by the network if it has not been incorporated in the training data.

These problem areas suggest that the embedding of ANNs in a symbolic environment would be really beneficial to both approaches. This is why the task of the present neural network is to co-ordinate different types of data computed by symbolic processors, discover and learn recurring patterns therein, and thereby acquire the ability to distinguish those patterns that contribute to the importance of a sentence in a text from those that do not. Hence, a considerable part of this research is the isolation of the most "relevant" linguistic and extralinguistic features, as regards text summarization.

4.3.1 Previous work on connectionist NLP

ANNs have been extensively used for the following NLP tasks: speech recognition and generation (e.g. Sejnowski & Rosenberg 1986), letter and word perception and generation (e.g. McClelland & Rumelhart 1981), sentential deep-case identification (e.g. McClelland & Kawamoto 1986), word disambiguation in context (e.g. Ide & Veronis 1990). Lately, there have also been considerable advances in the fields of syntax and semantics, with work on parsing, which has always posed special challenges to connectionism (e.g. Bennett 1988), compositional semantics (e.g. Touretzky 1989), or even inference (e.g. Diederich 1990).

Nevertheless, *"holistic" pragmatic* NLP tasks have rarely been considered as an ANN implementation. A reason for this may be the very fuzzy nature of pragmatic rules and cues themselves. No unified account of pragmatic phenomena has ever been agreed upon, despite the multiplicity of formulated theories. Still, throughout the work described here, a holistic approach towards utterance understanding and contextualization has been adopted. As a consequence, it is believed that all levels of information in a text, morphology, syntax, semantics, and the blanket term of "pragmatics", are equally and cumulatively important in language comprehension. What this means is that these levels cannot and should not be separated when analysing a text or even a sentence and a phrase.

A step towards higher-level connectionist NLP is Miikkulainen's (1992) script processing system. Hierarchical neural network modules perform specific tasks serially in an integrated environment. Stereotypical stories are parsed, classified according to the script scheme, and stored in an episodic memory. The system is able to infer events or role fillers that have been omitted in the input text. It can also paraphrase the whole story, including all the missing information as well. Moreover, it can answer questions about the story by accessing the episodic memory and retrieving the corresponding "trace". Nonetheless, the system has been trained with *ad hoc* three-sentence stories that conform to three script types, and nine tracks, themselves quite arbitrary. Although it is proven that there can be a full NLP system made up completely of co-operating ANNs, the system cannot deal as yet with real-world texts that, more often than not, do not conform to the specific script expectations or even to the lexical patterns learned. Consequently, such an approach would not be suited for the summarization of unrestricted text.

In contrast to pure connectionist systems, some *hybrid* architectures have been more practical and effective. For example, Wermter's (1992) SCANning understander scans unrestricted book titles, using a symbolic processor for surface syntactic analysis and keyword extraction, and classifies them according to ten semantic categories by means of a recurrent "plausibility" network. An extra layer keeps track of the preceding context of each word and, thus, contributes to its disambiguation in cases of generalized usage. The performance of this ANN is really impressive, reaching 96% success on average. However, it only operates on individual, or groups of, lexical items, having learned their frequency and semantic correlation in the different domain title corpora. Although very pragmatic and successful, this system could not be applied, as it stands, to higher-level, multidimensional, tasks that require domain-independent criteria.

4.4 The hybrid architecture of the abstract generation system

As shown in Figure 4.1, the summarization system proposed here consists of standard symbolic (morphological, syntactic, semantic and pragmatic) processors which look for specific features and information in the input text. These then assume a binary form by means of an encoder.

An ANN takes the selected encoded features as input and outputs two values which represent the relative degree of importance and unimportance, respectively, of the clause. The higher of the two values (with a range between a = 1 = positive and 0 = negative) is taken as the answer of the network. As already noted, importance has a relative meaning in this implementation. It is defined as indispensability in the composition of a succinct but comprehensive abstract.

Finally, symbolic generation modules collect the clauses that have been classified as important and perform a number of syntactic and semantic alterations on them. It is thus ensured that the resulting text is coherent and cohesive. Alterations include: the conjunction of main, as well as secondary, sentences; the substitution of anaphoric expressions for full noun phrases; the elimination of certain relative clauses and their replacement by prepositional or adjectival phrases (cf. Maybury 1990).

4.5 The feed-forward back-propagation ANN

A back-propagation network (Rumelhart et al. 1986a) has been employed, with an input, an output and a single hidden layer. Approximately 80 possible candidate input features have been identified, but to date only subsets of these have been considered. Since only two activation values are of interest, relating to whether a proposition is important or unimportant in the summarization process, there are just two output units. Both input and output values range from the minimum 0 to the maximum 1 (encoded as "a").

The 80 candidate inputs represent linguistic and extralinguistic features. Thus, morphological and syntactic, semantic and pragmatic information is represented. "Agent number" is an example of the morphological type with syntactic and semantic implications. Main verb "tense" and "aspect" are examples of syntactic attributes with morphological realizations and semantic/pragmatic consequences. "Agent quantification" and "cardinality" are semantic features with lexical and syntactic realization and pragmatic implications. "Elaboration", "Repetition" and "Contrast" are some of the pragmatic features encoding "speech-act"-like functions of

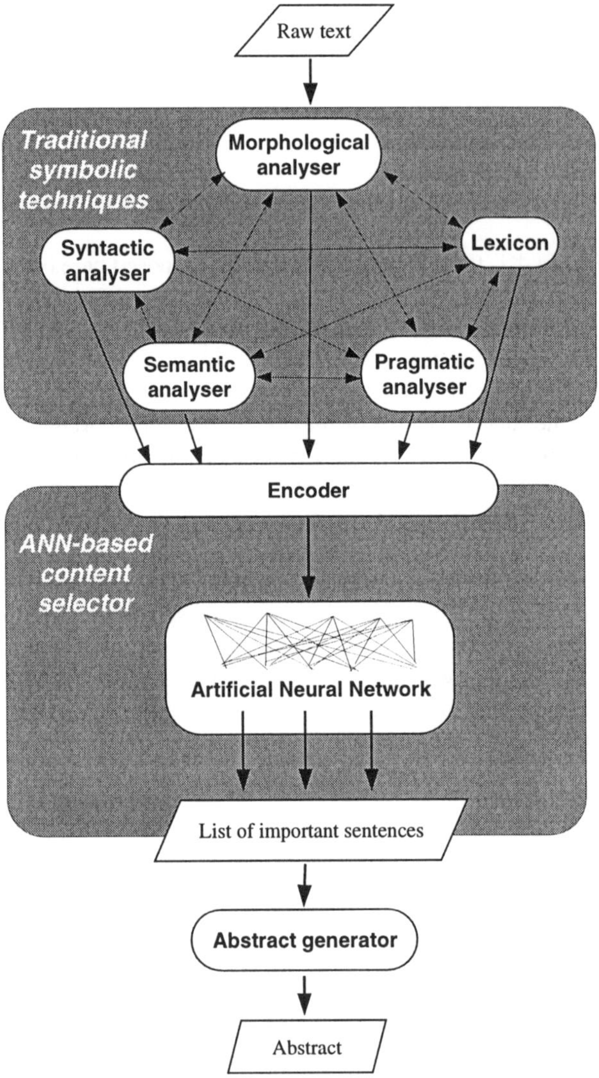

Figure 4.1 *Hybrid system architecture.*

the clause processed, which also have lexical, semantic, syntactic and morphological aspects. It becomes apparent that the majority of the 80 attributes cross boundaries in the traditional crude classification of language levels and belong to more than a single category. So, in computing the value for these features, both lexical and structural, and contextual information is used. The ANN does not accept specific values for the features; what is encoded is whether the feature is applicable or not, or whether it is specified in the clause or elsewhere in the text.

In the first ten series of experiments, the data employed consisted of whole sentences as they appear in real-world texts. However, in the future, individual clauses will be encoded separately. In this way, only the important ones, whether main or secondary, will be processed by the generation modules in the construction of the abstract. Accordingly, there are two features in the candidate set recording the presence of a secondary and a main clause, respectively, attached to the one currently being analysed. Thus, multiple embedding and conjunction of such clauses can be accommodated.

The input features have been selected in a non-systematic fashion. Most of them have been individually exalted by various pragmatic theories and system developers. Their relative importance, or at least influence, in language understanding is more or less evident. The number and the predication of a noun, for example, determines the way later pronouns are disambiguated depending on whether they are of the same number and compatible predication, or not. Similarly, the presence of a conditional means that whatever proposition is accompanied by it only holds if the conditional itself is true. And yet the exact role each feature plays is not at all clear. This is why attempts have been made here to run the ANN with various combinations of these 80 features so as to empirically evaluate the relative importance of each. Those features which cause a degradation in the network performance could be discarded or maybe modified, while the others will be corroborated. In a sense, a big set of "solutions" to pragmatic problems was compiled and the ANN has been delegated the task of deciding which are the "fittest" or more *relevant* ones for the summarization task.

4.5.1 The experiments

All experiments are being carried out on the PlaNet PDP platform (Miyata 1991). In the first instance, only 5 out of the set of 80 features were employed, namely:

(a) *Focus change* (a or 0); this records a shift from topic A in the previous sentence to topic B, or to a subtopic of A, in the current one (Grosz 1977).
(b) *Explanation* (a or 0) and
(c) *Contrast* (a or 0) are both rhetorical types of relation holding between two different sentences or two clauses in the same sentence (cf. Mann & Thompson 1987).
(d) *Generalization* (a or 0) is a reference to permanent states or habitual, recurring events, rather than individual, unique instances of them.
(e) Finally, *Title* (a or 0) specifies whether or not a clause is a title or subtitle in the input text.

These features were chosen out of the whole set as the most obviously influential, because they relate to the structure of the discourse and its emphasized topics. The associative nature of neural networks renders the specific order of the feature presentation in the input layer irrelevant, as long as it remains consistent across all input patterns (i.e. for all sentences).

Initially, the training and test data were based on 100 sentences taken from a variety of newspaper and scientific articles. These sentences had been encoded as strings of 0s and as depending on the corresponding values for the above five features. These strings constituted the input activation values for the network. The difference between the training and the test data is that the former also include a second column of digits for the two manually predetermined output activation values. These represent "importance" (0 or a) and "unimportance" (0 or a), and they have to be "guessed" by the network when not present. Example training sentences, with their input and output activation value vectors, are the following:

(1) Our object is to introduce contexts as abstract mathematical entities with properties useful in Artificial Intelligence.
a00a0 a0 [important]

(2) On the mountain highway that snakes northeast from Tirana toward the Serbian border, a white-knuckled drive of 120 miles takes more than eight hours over remnants of pavement originally laid by Communist Youth Brigades in 1947.
aa0a0 0a [unimportant]

The 10-fold cross-validation technique was adopted, whereby the overall dataset is divided into ten different subsets of test data (Weiss & Kulikowski 1991). Consequently, 10 different combinations of 90 training and 10 test sentences were employed in turn for each series of experiments. When the two sentences above were being used as test data, they were represented by just the vector on the left-hand side, with the input activation, i.e. a00a0 and aa0a0, respectively. The network had an overall 65% success rate with these five features.

In a second series of experiments, a sixth feature was added, "Goal specification", and the network performance improved, reaching a 69% success rate. Subsequently, four more were added, to make up a total of ten inputs: "Time specification", "Passiveness", "Quantification" and "Manner". Now the ANN attained an 86% success rate. This is significant, given that the great majority of the feature patterns were indecisive as regards importance. What this means is that most patterns were appearing just once in the training data and, consequently, the importance judgement was not representative of the overall behaviour of the specific pattern. This is where ANNs seem to outperform the corresponding decision-tree analyses.

Nevertheless, success could not be claimed until a larger test set had been used. So, this time 12 features were used for the encoding of 1100 sentences by three individuals. Moreover, apart from the aforementioned linguistic and extralinguistic features, a series of "meaningless" features were employed for the encoding of the same sentences. This was done for validation purposes. Examples of such features are: "The second letter of the third word is a vowel", "The fourth word has more than one *s*" and "The first word ends in a consonant". Instead of different sets of 10, between 900 and 1000 sentences were tested this time, after the network had been trained with the same initial 100 sentences, which are distinct from the test set. The corresponding success rates ranged from 55.9% to 59.0%. As regards the "meaningless" features, the success rate lay between 49.2% and 50.2%, which is no better than chance.

The next step taken was to establish the relationship between the training and the test data size and its effect on network performance. It was ensured that the training data set consisted of sentences encoded by all three individuals. As shown in Figure 4.2, the success rates are generally low for the relevant features, with the exception of the cases for 250 and 700 training data sizes, which gave two of the highest rates, 58.4% and 58.2%, respectively. This could mean that 250 sentences are sufficient for future training that gives results as good as if 700 sentences had been used. In addition, the graph suggests that the drop in performance with training sizes greater than 500 may be due to the *over-training* of the network. At any rate, despite the mediocrity of the results for the relevant features, the success rates for the trivial ones were even lower: around 50% and never exceeding 54%.

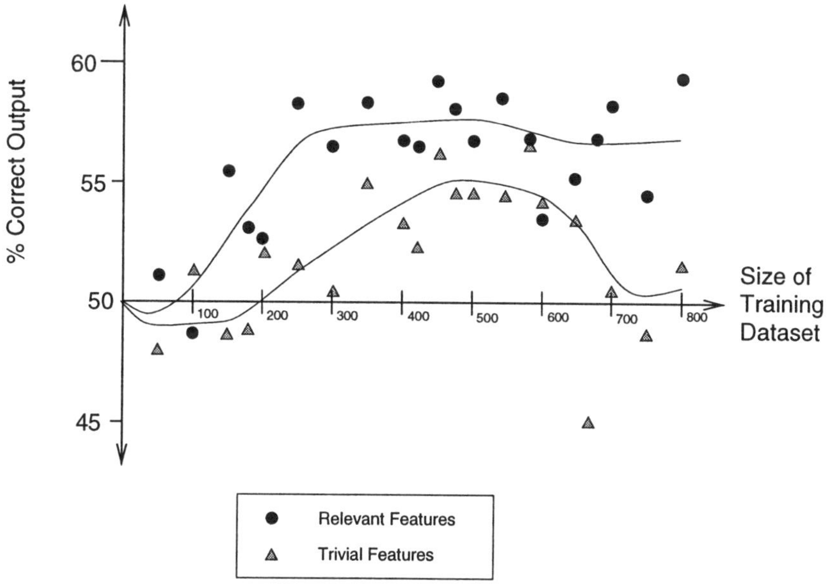

Figure 4.2 *The effect of the training data size on performance: training for 600 cycles and testing on untaught data.*

4.6 Conclusion and future work

In this paper, a hybrid architecture has been described for a system that generates abstracts of unrestricted texts. Symbolic morphological, syntactic, semantic and pragmatic processors have their selective results encoded in binary form in an interface to a high-level ANN. The ANN takes the encoded feature values for each sentence of the text and computes two output values determining the relative degree of importance and unimportance of the sentence currently analysed, in the summarization of the whole text it belongs to. Finally, symbolic generation modules collect the sentences that have been judged as more important than not and output the abstract of the initial text after applying a number of syntactic and semantic modifications on them.

A central claim of the paper is that ANNs are ideal for the simulation and exploitation of the strong interaction between the diverse linguistic and extralinguistic factors in language comprehension. They have the potential for faring better than traditional symbolic techniques in such complex tasks as pragmatic decision-making. As natural language is *de facto* creative, ambiguous and imperfect, unpredictability is the rule rather than the exception, which renders symbolic systems extremely vulnerable. In contrast, ANNs can handle novel or noisy input, because they are able to learn through experience and generalize over what has been learned. And yet to date ANNs have mainly been used for lower-level NLP tasks that symbolic systems already do quite well, and not for pragmatics or discourse analysis.

In the immediate future, further experiments have to be conducted with different combinations of 12 features from the 80-candidate set. Thus, the interdependence among the diverse features will be established more rigorously, and their relative influence in rendering a clause important will be clarified. Moreover, it may be the case that the number of features used so far is still quite small. Twelve features may not be enough to establish importance, hence an average success rate that is only 8.4% better than random. At least the features already used are not completely irrelevant, as was shown in the comparison of their success rates with those of the trivial features.

In addition, sentence encoding needs to be further *standardized*, so that discrepancies do not occur among the sentences encoded by one or another individual. This seems to have been the case up to now, rendering the data noisy. The noise is also increased by the fact that *diverse text types* make up the corpus: 52 news reports and scientific articles, of varying length and subject matter.

Finally, different topologies and network types have to be experimented with, e.g. the simple recurrent network. In this way, a comparison will be possible with the amount of generalization and the learning rate of the simple back-propagation network. To this end, conventional morphological, syntactic and semantic/pragmatic processors should be combined with the ANN, in order to produce a powerful hybrid system that outperforms either approach when adopted individually.

References

Alshawi, H. (ed.) 1992. *The core language engine.* Cambridge, Mass.: MIT Press.

Appelt, D. E., J. R. Hobbs, J. Bear, D. Israel, & M. Tyson, 1993. FASTUS: a finite-state processor for information extraction from real-world text. In *Proceedings of the 13th International Joint Conference on Artificial Intelligence (IJCAI-93)*, Chambéry, France, 1172–8.

Bennett, T. J. A. 1988. Self-organizing systems and transformational–generative (TG) grammar. *Cybernetics and Systems* **19**, 61–81.

Carling, A. 1992. *Introducing neural networks.* Wilmslow, England: Sigma Press.

Chalmers, D. J., R. M. French & D. R. Hofstadter, 1992. High-level perception, representation, and analogy: a critique of Artificial Intelligence methodology. *Journal of Experimental and Theoretical Artificial Intelligence* **4**, 185–211.

Cowie, J., L. Guthrie, W. Jin, R. Wang, T. Wakao, J. Pustejovsky & S. Waterman, 1993. CRL/BRANDEIS: description of the DIDEROT system as used for MUC-5. In *ARPA Proceedings of the 5th Message Understanding Conference (MUC-5)*, Baltimore, Md., 161–76.

Diederich, J. 1990. An explanation component for a connectionist inference system. In *Proceedings of the 9th European Conference on Artificial Intelligence (ECAI-90)*, Stockholm, 222–7.

Fogelman-Soulié, F. 1992. Neural networks and Artificial Intelligence: competition and cooperation. Invited Lecture at the 10th European Conference on Artificial Intelligence (ECAI-92), Vienna.

Grosz, B. J. 1977. *The representation and use of focus in dialogue understanding.* Technical Note 151, SRI International, Menlo Park, Calif.

Ide, N. M. & J. Veronis. 1990. Very large neural networks for word sense disambiguation. In *Proceedings of the 9th European Conference on Artificial Intelligence (ECAI-90)*, Stockholm, 366–9.

Lucas, N., K. Nishina, T. Akiba & K. G. Suresh. 1993. *Discourse analysis of scientific textbooks in Japanese: a tool for producing automatic summaries.* Technical Report 93TR-0004, Dept. of Computer Science, Tokyo Institute of Technology.

McClelland, J. L. & A. H. Kawamoto, 1986. Mechanisms of sentence processing: assigning roles to constituents of sentences. In McClelland et al. (1986), 272–325.

McClelland, J. L. & D. E. Rumelhart, 1981. An interactive activation model of context effects in letter perception: Part 1, an account of basic findings. *Psychological Review* **88**, 375–407.

McClelland, J. L., D. E. Rumelhart & the PDP Research Group (eds) 1986. *Parallel distributed processing: explorations in the microstructure of cognition. Vol. 2: Psychological and biological models*, Cambridge, Mass.: MIT Press.

Mann, W. C. & S. A. Thompson, 1987. *Rhetorical Structure Theory: a framework for the analysis of texts.* Technical Report RS-87-185, USC Information Sciences Institute, Marina del Rey, Calif.

Mauldin, M. L. 1991. *Conceptual information retrieval: a case study in adaptive partial parsing.* Dordrecht: Kluwer Academic Publishers.

Maybury, M. T. 1990. *Planning multisentential English text using communicative acts.* PhD thesis, Cambridge University.

Miikkulainen, R. 1992. DISCERN: a distributed neural network model of script processing and memory. In *Proceedings of the 3rd Twente Workshop on Language Technology (TWLT-3) on Connectionism and Natural Language Processing*, Twente, The Netherlands, 115–24.

Miyata, Y. 1991. *A user's guide to PlaNet Version 5.6. A tool for constructing, running, and looking into a PDP network.* Boulder, Colo.: Computer Science Dept., University of Colorado.

MUC-5, 1993. *Proceedings of the 5th Message Understanding Conference (MUC-5)*, San Mateo, Calif.

Rumelhart, D. E., G. E. Hinton & R. J. Williams, 1986a. Learning internal representations by error propagation. In Rumelhart et al. (1986b), 318–62.

Rumelhart, D. E., J. L. McClelland & the PDP Research Group (eds) 1986b. *Parallel distributed processing: explorations in the microstructure of cognition. Vol. 1: Foundations*, Cambridge, Mass.: MIT Press.

Scholtes, J. C. 1993. *Neural networks in natural language processing and information retrieval.* PhD thesis, University of Amsterdam.

Sejnowski, T. J. & C. R. Rosenberg, 1986. *NETtalk: a parallel network that learns to read aloud.* Technical report No. 86/01, Dept. of Electrical Engineering and Computer Science, Johns Hopkins University, Baltimore, Md.

Shavlik, J. W. 1992. *A framework for combining symbolic and neural learning.* Technical Report 1123, Computer Sciences Dept., University of Wisconsin, Madison, Wis.

Touretzky, D. S. 1989. *Connectionism and compositional semantics.* Technical report, Computer Science Department, Carnegie-Mellon University, Pittsburgh, Pa.

Weiss, S. M. & C. A. Kulikowski, 1991. *Computer systems that learn: classification and prediction methods from statistics, neural nets, machine learning, and expert systems.* San Francisco, Calif.: Morgan Kaufmann.

Wermter, S. 1992. A hybrid and connectionist architecture for a SCANning understander. In *Proceedings of the 10th European Conference on Artificial Intelligence (ECAI-92)*, Vienna, 188–92.

Young, S. R. & P. J. Hayes, 1985. Automatic classification and summarization of banking telexes. In *Proceedings of the 2nd IEEE Conference on Artificial Intelligence Applications (CAIA-85): The Engineering of Knowledge-based Systems*, Miami Beach, Fla., 402–8.

5
Recurrent neural networks and natural language processing

HERMANN MOISL

5.1 Introduction

One of the many application areas of Artificial Neural Networks (ANNs) has been natural language processing (NLP), and various ANN approaches to language processing have been proposed (see Sharkey & Reilly (1992) for an overview and recent work). This paper concentrates on one which has been prominent in recent research: induction of language processing devices in synchronous recurrent distributed ANNs by exposure to symbol string environments (Castano et al. 1993; Elman 1990, 1991; Giles et al. 1990, 1991, 1992; Giles & Omlin 1993; Pollack 1991; Sanfeliu & Alquezar 1992; Servan-Schreiber et al. 1989, 1991; Sharkey & Sharkey 1993; Watrous & Kuhn 1992). Such nets have yielded promising results in language processing and in NLP more particularly, but there appears to be a problem in principle which renders them inadequate for general NLP. In terms of their architecture and string-processing dynamics these nets look very like strict finite-state automata (FSAs), where "strict" refers to FSAs in which there is no distinction between processor and memory (on which see, further, Schwarz 1992).

But one of the earliest and most enduring results in generative linguistics is that finite-state devices are inadequate for generating natural languages, with the consequence that the nets in question appear to be inadequate on theoretical grounds for NLP. The general argument of this paper is that the theoretical problem is only apparent, and that the adequacy of recurrent distributed nets for NLP is a purely empirical issue. The discussion is in two main parts. The first considers and rejects standard arguments against finite-state NLP, and the second sketches a general approach to finite-state NLP using one particular kind of recurrent ANN: the simple recurrent network (SRN).

5.2 Finite-state processing in NLP

NLP research has been and continues to be naturally associated with other disciplines that concern themselves with the study of human language: theoretical linguistics most obviously, but also the range of disciplines that come under the umbrella of cognitive science, for which theoretical characterization of natural language is widely seen as paradigmatic for understanding of cognition more generally. The argument of this section is based on the assumption that the aims of NLP and of these associated disciplines are fundamentally different. Mainstream linguistics and cognitive science regard natural language as an abstract object, and aim to explain it by developing maximally expressive and economical theories about it. NLP, on the other hand, is concerned with the design and construction of physical devices to process physical strings for some purpose. On the basis of this assumption, the current section argues that the objections in principle to finite-state NLP stem from a failure to keep these aims separate.

The more or less standard approach in non-ANN NLP, exemplified in Gazdar & Mellish (1989), is to implement a physical device on the basis of some preferred linguistic theory. That is, the grammatical categories, syntactic structures, and any structure-manipulating devices such as movement rules of the linguistic theory are incorporated into a language-processing algorithm, and that algorithm can then either be directly physically realized or simulated on a general-purpose computer. The result is a physical device whose behaviour is both completely specified by the linguistic theory and as fully understood as the theory itself. Moreover, as a purely practical matter, when simulation rather than direct realization is chosen – and it invariably is – the construction of the NLP device becomes no more difficult than design and coding of the algorithm: a compiler takes care of the rest. These are considerable advantages, but the fact remains that direct instantiation of linguistic theories is not a necessary approach to construction of NLP devices.

Given a physical system with an observable behaviour, what internal mechanisms produce that behaviour? This is the identification problem, and the answer, in Arbib's words, is this:

Even if we know completely the function, or behavior, of a device, we cannot deduce from this a unique structural description. . . . The process of going from the behavior of a system to its structural description is then not to be thought of as actually identifying the particular state variable form of *the* system under study. It is, rather, that of identifying a state variable description of *a* system that will yield the observed behavior, even though the mechanism for generating that behavior may be different from that of the observed system. (Arbib 1987: 38–9, emphasis original).

True, theoretical linguistics is concerned with natural language in the abstract, not with the language behaviour of individual systems/humans, but the identification problem nevertheless applies in that a class of systems is at issue: linguistic theory is a structural description of the class of natural language speakers.

This applies straightforwardly to the present discussion. Assume some function, say, a mapping from sentences to meanings. An NLP device realizes the function by pairing physical sentence representations with physical meaning representations. Such a device would be describable in terms of a processor which uses linguistic-theoretic ontology even though it did not physically instantiate that ontology but rather used some other mechanism. In other words, linguistic theory has no necessary implications for the design of NLP processors. In principle, then, the way is open for candidate NLP technologies, including devices with finite-state architecture such as recurrent ANNs. There are, however, some standard objections to finite-state architectures for NLP, and these will now be dealt with in turn.

5.2.1 Unbounded-length centre-embedding strings

One of the aims of syntactic theory is to characterize the range of natural language sentence structures as economically as possible without any necessary regard as to how those characterizations might relate to production and understanding of utterances by speakers in the real world. Some of these structures are characterized as recursive; because it imposes no physical realization constraints, syntactic theory permits an arbitrary depth of recursive embedding and consequently sentences of unbounded length, which renders the language in question an infinite string set. Now, Chomsky (1956) long ago demonstrated that finite-state devices are incapable of generating or processing the language a^nb^n, that is, a set of strings in which some unbounded number of a given symbol a is followed by exactly the same number of some other symbol b, where n is any positive integer. Since this string pattern is attested in natural languages in what are analysed as recursive centre-embedding structures, and since generative grammars do not specify limits on recursive structures, any NLP device has to be able to deal with unbounded centre-embedded strings. But this is impossible if the device is finite-state, and so finite-state devices are inadequate for NLP.

If, however, one is concerned not with abstract characterization of natural language but with constructing a physical NLP device, it is only necessary to consider the string set which the device can be expected to encounter in practice rather than the set it might encounter in principle. On that view, arguments against the finite-stateness of natural languages simply do not apply. In the real world there is no such thing as an arbitrarily deeply nested recursive structure, and no such thing as a string of unbounded length. These things have finite limits, and, seen in terms of what infinity is conventionally taken to mean, even the longest natural language strings are really very short. The difference between the theoretical linguist's and the NLP researcher's views of natural language comes down to this. A grammar with recursion generates an infinite string set as long as there is no bound on the application of that recursion. As soon as a bound is imposed the language which the grammar generates becomes a finite subset of the one generated by the unbounded version, which can be processed by a finite-state device (Hopcroft & Ullman 1979). There is consequently no reason why a finite-state device should not process any member of the class of natural languages.

None of this is new. Miller & Chomsky (1965: 464–83) recognized that the human language processor had to be finite-state, and the inevitable finite-stateness of physical NLP devices has since been generally accepted though rarely mentioned and sometimes, it seems, forgotten. Despite this, strict finite-state architecture has never, to my knowledge, been seriously entertained for NLP. The reasons for this have to do with the second and third objections, to which we now turn.

5.2.2 Capturing generalizations

Strict finite-state architecture differs from that of higher-order automata in automata theory in that the the higher-order ones have a processor–memory distinction (Schwarz 1992). If a bound is placed on the memory of such a higher-order device, it becomes functionally finite-state, that is, it can be simulated in terms of input–output behaviour by a strict finite-state machine. The only difference is that the two sorts of device use different algorithms to compute any given function on account of their different architectures. Advocates of finite-state NLP have preferred higher-order, bounded-memory architectures to the strict finite-state one explicitly on account of the former's explanatory advantage in relation to generative linguistic theory (Chomsky 1956; Miller & Chomsky 1965; Church 1980; Pulman 1986). If one's aim is explanation, then clearly a higher-order automaton with bounded memory is to be preferred. But the primary aim of NLP is construction of physical devices, not explanation, so the choice between higher-order, bounded-memory and strict finite-state architecture is in principle neutral.

5.2.3 Compositionality

Semantic theory in theoretical linguistics aims to associate linguistic expressions with meanings, given some definition of "meaning". This involves at least:

- assignation of meaning to the primitive expressions – the morphemes – of a given language;

- specification of how the primitive expressions relate to composite expressions – phrases and sentences – in that language;
- specification of how linguistic meaning relates to the world.

There are various approaches to these tasks; the one used for exemplification here, formal or Montague semantics (Cann 1993), has been and continues to be influential. Formal semantics defines the meaning of a sentence as its truth conditions: a sentence means what the world would have to be like for the sentence to be true. Truth conditions are defined relative to a "universe of discourse" which the semantic theory models. Such a model has two main parts:

(a) The entities of the universe of discourse are identified, and the relationships between these entities and the primitive expressions of the language, that is, the denotations of the primitive expressions, are defined; and

(b) How the denotations of composite expressions are constructed from those of primitive expressions is specified.

Part (b) is based on Frege's principle of compositionality, which says that the meaning of a composite expression is a function of the meanings of its component primitives and their manner of combination, and is defined using a grammar which both generates the sentences of the language in question, and associates a constituent structure with each sentence. The connection between syntactic structure and meaning is made by the rule-to-rule hypothesis, in which each syntactic rule is associated with a corresponding semantic rule which specifies the meaning of a composite expression in terms of its immediate syntactic constituents. In this way, syntax can be said to drive semantics in the sense that, given the meanings of the morphemes of a language, syntactic structure determines what sentences mean.

Compositionality has also been at the centre of a long-running debate in the cognitive science community, where the rival claims of an established "classical" approach to the study of cognition and those of the "connectionist" challenger are at stake (for recent discussion and extensive references see Dinsmore (1992) and Volume 4 of *Connection Science*). The classical position, forcefully put by Fodor & Pylyshyn (1988), is that, in order adequately to explain certain fundamental aspects of cognition, one requires the notion of the structured representation, that is, of a mental object consisting of primitive symbols arranged in a constituent structure with compositional semantics, and the notion of mental processes which interpret representations in a way that is sensitive to their structure; because they are by nature finite-state devices, ANNs cannot articulate or process representations with a constituent structure adequate for capturing the requisite generalizations about cognition. In response, connectionist cognitive scientists have worked to vindicate ANNs as a suitable alternative paradigm for cognitive theorizing by developing specifically connectionist accounts of compositionality, chief among them Smolensky's (1990) tensor product representation and van Gelder's (1990) functional compositionality, which is based on temporal rather than spatial structuring of constituents. Functional compositionality is exemplified in Pollack's (1990) RAAM architecture, and applied to NLP by Chalmers (1990) and Blank et al. (1992).

Central to both theoretical linguistics and cognitive science, then, is the idea of semantic interpretation of an expression on the basis of its syntactic structure. Now, it is universally agreed that natural language sentences have complex and varied structures. How, therefore, can a finite-state architecture which imposes a single, strictly sequential syntax on sentences be adequate for natural language semantics? The classicists in the cognitive science debate think that it cannot, and the connectionsts agree in that they found it necessary to develop compositional representational methods for ANNs. Nevertheless, I claim that compositionality has no necessary implications for NLP. The basis for this claim is, again, that explanation is one thing, and construction of physical devices another. Compositional semantics in natural language sentences depends crucially on the attribution of more or less complex syntactic structure to sentences. But sentences are abstract objects, and so are the structures attributed to them: both are artefacts of linguistic theory. Physical strings, whether spoken or written, have no structure apart from strict temporal or spatial sequence. One approach to implementing a sentence-to-meaning function is to map strings onto abstract sentences with abstract structures and to process these sentences in accordance with those structures, which yields a processor that is perspicuously related to linguistic theory as well as to structured meaning representations, but the identification problem says that this is not necessary. Since, for NLP, it suffices that the sentence-to-meaning function be realized by a device which pairs strings with physical meaning representations, another legitimate approach is to attempt to process strings in accordance with the structure we know for certain they have – strict sequence – using a processor with strict finite-state architecture.

5.3 Recurrent ANNs and NLP

Assuming the validity of the arguments in the preceding part of the discussion, the way is clear for development of an approach to NLP based on strict finite-state architecture. But, as the Celtic chieftain Calgacus is reputed to have said of the Roman invasion of Britain: "They made a desert and called it peace" (Tacitus, *Agricola*). Notions of complex phrase structure and associated compositional semantics provide intuitively accessible and theoretically well-developed ways of thinking about language and offer a basis for the design of NLP devices via the relationship between linguistics and computation which formal language and automata theory define. If one dispenses with these notions in NLP design, what will replace them? This section sketches a proposal for an alternative.

It is best to be clear at the outset that generative linguistic theory is not being challenged: for present purposes it is accepted as a characterization of what has traditionally been called "human linguistic competence". The issue is the relationship between linguistic theory and the physical processing mechanisms required for

NLP, and the argument is, in essence, that physical instantiation of computational architectures with the processor–memory distinction (Schwarz 1992) is unnecessary.

Generative linguistic theory defines a function from linguistic expressions – words, phrases, sentences – to meanings, given some definition of "meaning". An NLP device implements this function if, given a physical representation of an expression, it returns a physical representation of the associated meaning. Since natural languages are finite sets for NLP purposes, it becomes possible to define the function as a list of <expression, meaning> pairs, and for an NLP device to do nothing more than table lookup on a physical representation of the list. The proposal is to train a recurrent ANN with strict finite-state architecture to implement such a table lookup device. The discussion is in three parts: Section 5.3.1 designs a computer simulation of an ANN to associate strings with meaning representations; Section 5.3.2 presents test results and analysis of that ANN; and 5.3.3 briefly addresses some issues which arise from Sections 5.3.1 and 5.3.2.

5.3.1 Network design and implementation

The aim is to implement a mapping from linguistic expressions to meanings, given a finite set of expressions. This requires pairing of each expression of length 1 with a meaning, each expression of length 2 with a meaning, and so on up to some maximum length, as in Figure 5.1. Here, meanings are labelled "1", "2", "3", . . . ; the expression *the* means "1", *the man* means "2", *the man in* means "3", and so on.

	Meanings					
	1	2	3	4	5	6
Strings	the					
	the	man				
	the	man	in			
	the	man	in	the		
	the	man	in	the	tent	
	the	man	in	the	tent	slept

Figure 5.1 *String-to-meaning mapping.*

In view of the number of words in English and of the possible combinations of words up to some reasonable maximum sentence length, this approach may appear to require a very large number of meanings, but in fact there are exactly as many as that which generative linguistic theory would posit for the same expression set. Linguistic theory would generate the meanings more elegantly than an explicit listing by building them out of the meaning primitives assigned to morphemes, but elegance is not an issue here.

Like much of the grammatical induction work mentioned in Section 5.1, the net used to implement this mapping is a simple recurrent network (SRN), a discrete-time dynamical system whose architecture and processing dynamics make it straightforwardly interpretable as a finite-state automaton (for example, Arbib 1987: 24–6), as in Figure 5.2.

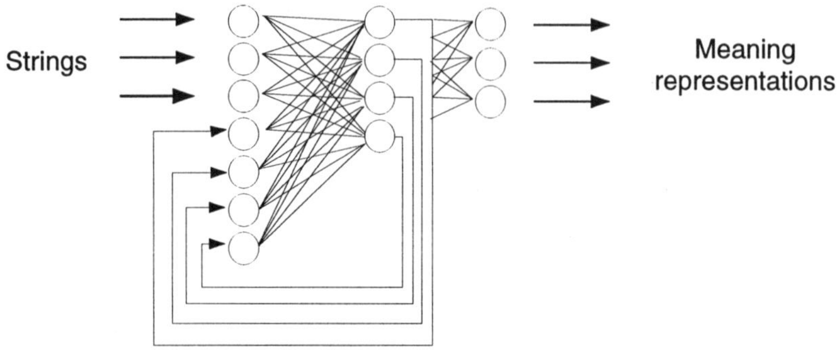

Figure 5.2 *SRN implementation of string-to-meaning mapping.*

The set of hidden-layer configurations is the state set. The connections between the input and hidden layers are the next-state function in that, for every combination of current input and current state, they generate a characteristic associated next state in the hidden layer. The connections between hidden and output layers are the output function in that, for every state of the hidden layer, they generate a characteristic output in the output layer.

The SRN is in principle a physical device with physical input and output signals, but as with virtually all ANN research practice, it is simulated on a conventional computer. The linguistic expressions and meanings, which are in principle to be represented physically, in fact need to be given a representation appropriate to the simulation. This means numerical vectors whose components represent features of the physical input and output signals. The frequently used "one-hot" encoding is adopted here, where each distinct input and output from the net is assigned a unique binary-valued vector in which one component is "1" and all the rest are "0". This is unrealistic for actual NLP work, where one would want to represent features of acoustic or visual input in some detail, but it suffices for present purposes. The result is a list of <binary-valued vector sequence, binary-valued vector> pairs which represent the linguistic <expression, meaning> pairs of the mapping.

The SRN is trained by repeated random selection of a pair from the list, and presentation of that pair to the net so that it can learn to associate the components using back-propagation; this continues until the learning error curve stops decreasing significantly. For example, training the net on the list in Figure 5.1 would proceed as follows:

1. Choose a pair, say <*the*, 1>: the vector representation of *the* is presented to the designated units in the first layer of the net, the vector representation of "1" becomes the target output, and back-propagation is applied.
2. Choose another, say <*the man*, 2>: the vector representation of *the* becomes the input and the vector representation of "1" the target output, then the vector representation of *man* becomes the input and the vector representation of "2" the target output, applying back-propagation in each case.
3. Similarly, for <*the man in*, 3>, *the* is associated with "1", *man* is associated with "2", and *in* with "3".

In this way, the net learns a mapping from strings to meanings: in all the Figure 5.1 strings *the* means "1", in strings 2–6 *the man* means "2", in strings 3–6 *the man in* means "3", and so on up to *the man in the tent slept*, which means "6".

5.3.2 Results and analysis

Results

The simulation was trained and tested on sets of up to 24 strings of maximum length 12, all of them of the declarative variety, such as (1), and learned the string–meaning function perfectly.

(1) The cat with the long tail sat on the mat.

Special attention was paid to the net's ability to handle long-distance dependencies, since this is always an issue in NLP research and has often – though erroneously – been regarded as a problem for finite-state processors. The net had no difficulty with maintaining dependencies across the distances so far required of it, (2)–(3), or the centre-embedding (4).

(2) The man in the boat by the shore sees.

(3) The men in the boat by the shore see.

(4) The car the man the woman loves drove stopped.

Analysis

For an SRN with n units in its hidden layer, the values which those units assume at any processing step constitute an n-component vector. Each such vector defines a point in n-space. For a test string of length a there are a hidden-layer configurations, and for b test strings there are c configurations as given in (5).

(5) $$c = \sum_{1 \ldots b} \sum_{1 \ldots a}$$

In the grammatical inference research mentioned in Section 5.1, it is usual to carry out a cluster analysis of these c vectors in order to gain some insight into network operation. These analyses have shown that the points are not in general haphazardly distributed in *n*-space, but cluster in regions of that space such that all the hidden-layer vectors which generate a given output are adjacent. Such clusters are usually interpreted as states of a finite-state machine which the net has inferred from string input, but this is an unnecessary abstraction. The component vectors of a cluster typically differ from one another to greater or lesser degrees, and an alternative interpretation, adopted here, is to assign a separate state to each distinct hidden-layer configuration. This results in a much larger finite-state machine for a given function, but corresponds more directly to physical reality.

The hidden-layer configurations which the trained net assumed in the course of string processing in the results reported above were subjected to cluster analysis, and the results were unsurprising: the hidden-layer vectors clustered in accordance with the target output, as above. Assuming, however, a separate state for every distinct vector, the analysis shows that there is a unique state for every <expression, meaning> pair. Thus, for the three strings (6)–(8), the state sequences for initial *the* and for *man* are identical in all three cases; thereafter (6) and (7)–(8) bifurcate, and (7)–(8) continue with identical state sequences for *in the restaurant ate*, at which point they too bifurcate; *ate his lunch* in (6) and (7), though lexically identical, have different state sequences; there are three distinct states for *lunch*.

(6) The man ate his lunch.

(7) The man in the restaurant ate his lunch.

(8) The man in the restaurant ate a sparing lunch.

By following the trajectory which each string generates in the state space, one can see that the net learns a distinct state sequence for every distinct string.

5.3.3 Discussion

Whether or not the approach proposed in Section 5.3.1 will be practicable, and what sorts of development are required, are empirical matters. At least two issues arise at this stage, however, both of them having to do with the assumed prior existence of an <expression, meaning> list and of a corresponding physical representation of it:

(a) Though theoretically possible on the grounds of finiteness, construction of an <expression, meaning> list for some natural language would be a huge and almost certainly infeasible task.

(b) Linguistic expressions and meanings are abstractions, and compilation of a list implies some physical representation scheme. Representation of linguistic expressions is well understood, but it is not at all clear what a physical representation of a meaning might look like; in the foregoing discussion "meaning representations" were simply variables instantiated by arbitrary vectors for the sake of argument.

Despite its theoretical validity, the architecture proposed in Section 5.3.1 emerges as impractical in the light of (a) and (b). The following development of that architecture is intended to address this. An increasingly favoured idea in connectionist research is that ANN-based systems be "hooked up" to the world with a range of sensors which transduce physical signals into a format amenable to ANN processing, thus providing input representations which relate to environmental regularities in a systematic way and thereby, it is hoped, allowing nets to behave in ways interpretable as semantically coherent (e.g. Peschl 1992; Pfeifer & Verschure 1992; Plunkett et al. 1992). The development of the NLP approach being proposed here is based on this idea (Fig. 5.3).

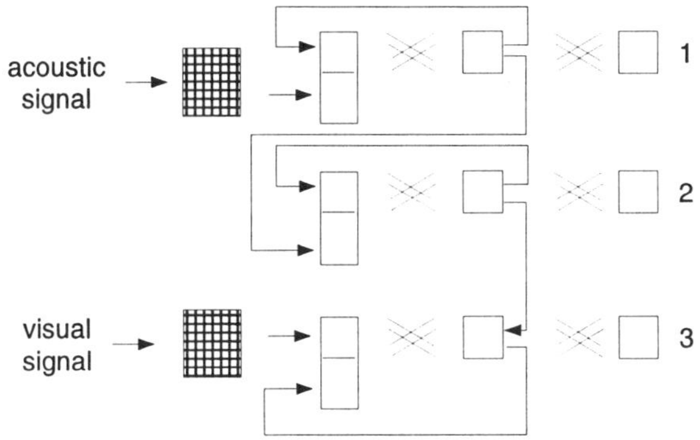

Figure 5.3 *Interconnected finite-state automata.*

The acoustic and visual components are the input sensors. Input to both is via Kohonen nets (represented by grids) which function as transducers from physical signals to 2-D topographic maps. In the acoustic component the map is input to an SRN which processes sequences of maps corresponding to time-sliced acoustic inputs. In the visual component the map of some visually perceived state of the world is input to a feed-forward ANN; this model takes no account of real-world dynamics at present, and an SRN is consequently not required. Between these two components is a feed-forward net ("link net") whose input layer is the hidden layer of the acoustic sequence processor, whose target output is the hidden layer of the visual processor, and whose hidden layer represents the association of the two. Training assumes sources of acoustic and visual input such that the two sorts of input would be perceived by a human observer as naturally related: (9) would be correlated with a state of the world in which a cat is sitting on a mat, and not with a crane lifting bricks.

(9) The cat sat on the mat.

This addresses (a) and (b) above as follows:

(a) Given an appropriate physical environment, the net learns to implement the expression-to-meaning function on-line and incrementally. There is no need to predefine an <expression, meaning> list.

(b) The net generates its own representations: expression representations are abstracted from acoustic input in the hidden layer of the acoustic SRN, and meaning representations develop in the link-ANN hidden layer in the course of training; the intention is that, at any stage of acoustic input, the link-net hidden layer should represent the meaning of the string up to that point, where "meaning" is understood in an impoverished sense appropriate to the restricted range of inputs.

5.4 Conclusion

This paper has argued that pessimistic assessments of the adequacy of recurrent ANNs for NLP on the grounds that they have a finite-state architecture are unjustified, and that their adequacy in this regard is an empirical issue. Whether or not the model can be developed for general NLP remains to be seen, but even as it stands it exemplifies the kind of radical departure from linguistics-based NLP that is possible once the supposed theoretical obstacles to finite-state NLP are removed. In particular, it departs from linguistics-based NLP in making no use of any syntactic or compositional structure beyond the purely sequential, and amounts to table-lookup mapping from strings to meaning representations.

References

Arbib, M. 1987. *Brains, machines, and mathematics*, 2nd edn. New York: Springer.

Blank, D., L. Meeden & J. Marshall 1992. Exploring the symbolic/subsymbolic continuum: a case study of RAAM. In *The symbolic and connectionist paradigms: closing the gap*, J. Dinsmore (ed.), 113–48. Hillsdale, NJ: Lawrence Erlbaum.

Cann, R. 1993. *Formal semantics: an introduction.* Cambridge: Cambridge University Press.

Castano, M., E. Vidal & F. Casacumberta 1993. Inference of stochastic regular languages through simple recurrent networks. In Lucas (1993), 16/1–6.

Chalmers, D. 1990. Syntactic transformations on distributed representations. *Connection Science* **2**, 53–62.

Chomsky, N. 1956. Three models for the description of language. *IRE Transactions on Information Theory* **IT-2**, 109.

Church, K. 1980. *On memory limitations in natural language processing*. Technical Report LCS/TR-45, Department of Electrical Engineering and Computer Science, MIT.

Dinsmore, J. 1992. *The symbolic and connectionist paradigms: closing the gap.* Hillsdale, NJ: Lawrence Erlbaum.

Elman, J. 1990. Finding structure in time. *Cognitive Science* **14**, 179–211.

Elman, J. 1991. Distributed representation, simple recurrent networks, and grammatical structure. *Machine Learning* **7**, 195–225.

Fodor, J. & Z. Pylyshyn 1988. Connectionism and cognitive science: a critical analysis. *Cognition* **28**, 3–71.

Gazdar, G. & C. Mellish 1989. *Natural language processing in LISP*. Wokingham, England: Addison-Wesley.

Giles, C. & C. Omlin 1993. Extraction, insertion, and refinement of symbolic rules in dynamically driven recurrent neural networks. *Connection Science* **5**, 307–38.

Giles, C., G. Sun, Y. Lee & D. Chen 1990. Higher order recurrent networks and grammatical inference. In *Advances in neural infromation systems 2*, D. Touretzky (ed.), 380–7. San Mateo, Calif.: Morgan Kaufmann.

Giles, C., D. Chen, C. Miller, H. Chen, G. Sun & Y. Lee 1991. Grammatical inference using second-order recurrent neural networks. In *Proceedings of the International Joint Conference on Neural Networks, IEEE 91*, Seattle, Wash., Vol. II, 273–81.

Giles, C., C. Miller, D. Chen, G. Sun, H. Chen & Y. Lee 1992. Extracting and learning an unknown grammar with recurrent neural networks. In *Advances in neural information processing systems*, J. Moody, S. Hanson & R. Lippmann (eds), 363–71. San Mateo, Calif.: Morgan Kaufmann.

Hopcroft, J., & J. Ullman 1979. *Introduction to automata theory, languages, and computation*. Reading, Mass.: Addison-Wesley.

Lucas, S. (ed.) 1993. *Grammatical inference: theory, applications, and alternatives*. London: IEE.

Miller, G. & N. Chomsky 1965. Finitary models of language users. In *Readings in mathematical psychology II*, R. Bush, E. Galanter & D. Luce (eds), 156–71. New York: John Wiley.

Peschl, M. 1992. Construction, representation, and the embodiment of knowledge, meaning, and symbols in neural structures. *Connection Science* **4**, 327–38.

Pfeifer, R. & P. Verschure 1992. Beyond rationalism: symbols, patterns, and behaviour. *Connection Science* **4**, 313–25.

Plunkett, K., C. Sinha, M. Moeller & O. Strandsby 1992. Symbol grounding or the emergence of symbols? *Connection Science* **4**, 293–312.

Pollack, J. 1990. Recursive distributed representations. *Artificial Intelligence* **46**, 77–105.

Pollack, J. 1991. The induction of dynamical recognizers. *Machine Learning* **7**, 123–48.

Pulman, S. 1986. Grammars, parsers, and memory limitations. *Language and Cognitive Processes* **1**, 197–225.

Sanfeliu, A. & R. Alquezar 1992. Understanding neural networks for grammatical inference and recognition. In *Advances in structural and syntactic pattern recognition*, H. Bunke (ed.), 75–98. Singapore: World Scientific.

Schwarz, G. 1992. Connectionism, processing, memory. *Connection Science* **4**, 207–26.

Servan-Schreiber, D., A. Cleeremans & J. McClelland 1989. Learning sequential structure in simple recurrent networks. In *Advances in neural information processing systems 1*, D. Touretzky (ed.), 643–52. San Mateo, Calif.: Morgan Kaufmann.

Servan-Schreiber, D., A. Cleeremans & J. McClelland 1991. Graded state machines: the representation of temporal contingencies in simple recurrent networks. *Machine Learning* **7**, 161–93.

Sharkey, A. & N. Sharkey 1993. Connectionism and natural language. In Lucas (1993), 20/1–10.

Sharkey, N., & R. Reilly 1992. *Connectionist approaches to natural language processing*. Hillsdale, NJ: Lawrence Erlbaum.

Smolensky, P. 1990. Tensor product variable binding and the representation of symbolic structures in connectionist systems. *Artificial Intelligence* **46**, 159–216.

van Gelder, T. 1990. Compositionality: a connectionist variation on a classical theme. *Cognitive Science* **14**, 355–84.

Watrous, R. & G. Kuhn 1992. Induction of finite state languages using second-order recurrent networks. *Neural Computation* **4**, 406–14.

6
Learning the semantics of aspect

GABRIELE SCHELER

6.1 Introduction

A common goal of theoretical linguistic work as well as Machine Translation (MT) research is the construction of semantic representations, which can be used as interlingual representations in the context of MT.

Constructing semantic representations is often controversial and results are difficult to evaluate, because little is known about what constitutes a semantic representation and what information it must contain. However, semantic representations are a useful concept when we have a specific language processing task. In different tasks, we may use the same or similar semantic representations to interface with different modules for further processing. In this work, we concentrate on the task of translation, and accordingly interface the semantic representation with a language generation module for another language. This task-oriented approach has the important advantage that the specific contribution of a semantic representation can be assessed and valued.

The main point of this paper is to show how we can extract semantic features, describing aspectual meanings, from a specialized syntactic representation.

The overall goal is to translate English to Russian aspectual categories, which cannot be handled well by rule-based MT. The reason is mainly that the constellations of contextual information that determine semantic content and accordingly morphological categories in another language are too numerous and too diverse to be used as triggers for rules.

In Figure 6.1, a model of the complete translation process is shown. It consists of:

- an input tagger which provides syntactic tags to the continuous input text and thus transforms it to the specialized syntactic representation;
- the transformation of the syntactic representation into the semantic representation, which is a *feature extraction* task;
- a universal (interlingual) set of semantic features describing aspectual meanings;
- the categorization of the individual aspectual meanings to the language-specific grammatical categories, which is a *pattern classification* task.

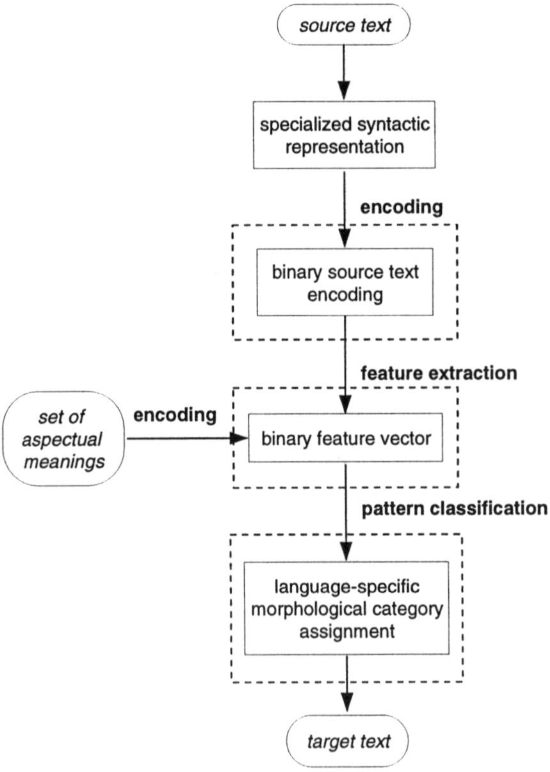

Figure 6.1 *Model of the translation process.*

A significant trait of the model is that the semantic-feature extraction process is realized by a specialized language processing module for dealing with aspectual information. This *vertical modularity* has been inspired by neurolinguistic research (Marshall 1988; McCarthy & Warrington 1988). Instead of the more usual horizontal modules for morphology, syntax, and lexical and sentential semantics, we use vertical modules that can be defined as areas of processing that combine, for example, temporal morphology, temporal adverbials, temporal semantics and temporal cognition. Thus we have a number of specialized modules dealing with time, aspect, space, etc. This means that we do not use a full syntactic representation, with all information that can be extracted by a parsing mechanism, but a specialized syntactic representation, containing in this case quantification of noun phrases (subject and direct object), lexical category of the verb with respect to aspectual properties, and temporal and modal sentential adverbs.

There has been earlier work which is related to the present one. Feature-based syntactic representations for pattern association with semantic representations have been used by McClelland & Kawamoto (1986) and St. John & McClelland (1990). Their models are used to deal with the association between syntactic cases and semantic roles. The semantic representations achieved were not interfaced with any other module. A combined interpretation and generation approach has been used by Miikkulainen (1990) for the analysis of relative clauses. There, the internal representation also consisted of situations and roles. Another vertical module was modelled by Munro & Tabasko (1991). Here locative prepositions were interpreted as spatial relations. However, the model lacked generalization in the creation of semantic representations.

The paper is structured as follows: the next section gives the motivation for the use of a feature-based semantic representation. Then the notion of specialized syntactic representation is further explained, and the grammar that has been used in setting up the representation is presented. The following sections contain results of experiments in interpretation, in generation, and in translation. In the conclusion, results are assessed and further questions are raised.

6.2 Interlingual (universal) semantic representation

In this section, we consider a representation for grammatical meanings which are relevant to the morphological forms progressive/simple in English and imperfective/perfective in Russian. It is thus primarily an *interlingual* representation, i.e. a representation that is not constrained by a single language, but captures semantic properties of more than one language. In principle, such a representation can be constructed to have *universal* properties, i.e. to capture the semantic distinctions that are used in any language, as this is a set that becomes exhaustive with the consideration of sufficiently diverse languages (cf. Comrie (1984) for a discussion of semantic universals). However, the set of features that we use here is shown to be sufficient for only two languages.

Namely, we can show that from such a feature the correct aspectual form of an English or Russian sentence can be predicted by presenting a classifier which computes the corresponding transformation function.

The representation has the form of a number of distinct representation dimensions and individual features, which are encoded in binary form. Descriptive work, exploring aspectual distinctions in many different contexts and collecting different uses and conveyed meanings has sometimes led to a formulation of aspectual meanings in terms of binary feature sets (Bondarko 1983; Breu 1980; Scheler 1984). Being the outcome rather than the starting point of research, these feature sets, however, were not validated for their capability of producing and predicting the correct morphology for a given sentence.

In model-theoretic approaches to aspectual semantics (Dowty 1979; Hinrichs 1988; Verkuyl 1993) the main effort consists in constructing logical representations for aspectual meanings. These representations are usually constructed for individual sentences, without paying attention to the functional dependency between overt morphological form and semantic representation and its computability.

We use simple feature–value representations instead of model-theoretic constructs for two reasons:

- The morphological form should be effectively computable from the semantic representation.
- Model-theoretic constructs, which capture inferences, are hardly necessary to perform an effective and correct translation. They seem to belong to another level of organization, a "deeper" semantic structure. However, feature-based representations can be constructed so as to have a natural logical interpretation, including inferential connections (cf. Scheler & Schumann 1995).

The set of grammatical meanings that have been used in these experiments consist of 15 dimensions like **habituality**, **event-extension**, **event-type**, **degree-of-completion**, **duration** and between two and five values for each of these features, such as for **event-type**: STATE, ATELIC-EVENT, TELIC-EVENT, CAUSE-STATE.[1]

Note that the set must contain the features for all semantic distinctions that occur in the training and test sets in order to produce good learning and generalization results. The feature set which has been obtained heuristically (cf. Scheler 1984) can thus be empirically validated.

It is also possible to use feature selection techniques for elimination of superfluous features or values (cf. Duda & Hart 1973). Elimination of features may be important for generalization to new patterns, to exclude generalizing on irrelevant information. However, such a pruning of the feature set has not been performed here.

This approach uses certain assumptions about the nature of linguistic categories. It is presumed that in the language production process a certain morphological category is selected by virtue of a certain active feature set of meanings pertaining to this category (features on a "semantic map"). This feature set comes into existence from

1. The complete list of features is given in Scheler (1994).

the cognitive and intentional states that accompany language production. Similarly, in interpretation, a certain morphological category creates a representation on the feature map.

6.3 Syntactic features for aspectual meanings

The idea of using a distinct syntactic representation is that for analysis linguistic input is fed into several specialized modules, which take the necessary information for their task and retransform it into a suitable form, probably in several steps.

As a starting point in this work we use a hypothetical intermediate representation, which can be gained from free text by a fairly simple tagger or parser. Relevant syntactic information has been selected in accordance with the detailed presentation in Scheler (1984), cf. Partee (1973), Vendler (1967). The categorizations presented here are all fixed lexical decisions and not contingent on the use of these words in a given sentence. This is in accordance with the principle of a unidirectional parser, and could be changed by the integration of the semantic-feature extraction module into an integrated (top-down/bottom-up) module for syntactic analysis. The syntactic representation contains six *slots*, i.e. place-holders for functionally different terms, and a number of *values* for each slot. The following description is the "grammar" of the specialized syntactic representation for aspectual meanings:

quantification of subject: SINGULAR-DEFINITE, PLURAL-DEFINITE, SINGULAR-INDEFINITE and PLURAL-INDEFINITE, as they are indicated by morphological marking on English noun phrases.

temporal adverbials: These are distinguished into classes according to the preposition (AT, FOR, ON) or conjunction (WHEN) used, and the type of noun that forms the head, such as *8 o'clock* or *three hours*. Words such as *now*, *today*, *yesterday* form a category of their own.

morphological verb markers: PAST/PRESENT, PERFECT/NON-PERFECT, PROGRESSIVE/SIMPLE.

sentential adverbs: These comprise:

- adverbs ALWAYS, SOMETIMES, X-TIMES (e.g. *five times*), USUALLY;
- adverbs such as SUDDENLY, JUST, as independent categories;
- adverbials of manner (*slowly*, *with great care*, *well*), which have been categorized into those indicating processual nature PROC-ADV, and those that do not and are neutral in this regard (ADV) and
- sentential negation (NEGATION).

quantification of direct object: SINGULAR-DEFINITE, PLURAL-DEFINITE, SINGULAR-INDEFINITE and PLURAL-INDEFINITE.

lexical verb classes: A list of verb classes sufficient for the chosen examples has been derived from Scheler (1984): TELIC-ACTION, ACHIEVEMENT,

ACTIVE-PERCEPTION, ATELIC-ACTION, PASSIVE-PERCEPTION, GRADUAL STATE-CHANGE, STAGES-OF-ACTIONS (*try*, *begin*, *finish*), STATE, MOTION.

This syntactic representation is transformed into a semantic feature representation with pattern association techniques. The semantic representation is the basis for the selection of an aspectual category in another language.

Initially, 49 patterns were created. From a standard English grammar (Thompson & Martinet 1969) a number of sentences were selected, exemplifying the different uses of English tenses and aspects. The results, especially for generalization, could be much enhanced, when several syntactic variants for the most salient examples were created. That is, examples were created to allow the classifier to determine the influence of minor syntactic changes on the semantic representations. Five variations on a simple sentence are shown in (1)-(5), together with their syntactic and proposed semantic representation.

(1) He has not done his homework.
NEGATION * SING-DEF TELIC-ACTION SIMPLE PERFECT PRESENT SING-DEF
past * * relational-to-present holistic * * * action existential telic negated * single non-habitual

(2) He was doing homework from 5 to 7.
* FROM-POINT-TO-POINT SING-DEF TELIC-ACTION PROG NON-PERFECT PAST PLU-INDEF
past * * non-relational processual * occurs-at-period-in * action referential atelic * * single non-habitual

(3) Sometimes he is doing his homework with much care.
PROC-ADV,SOMETIMES * SING-DEF TELIC-ACTION PROG NON-PERFECT PRESENT SING-DEF
* * * non-relational processual * * * action existential atelic * long-duration single habitual

(4) Right now all students are doing their homework.
* NOW PLU-DEF TELIC-ACTION PROG NON-PERFECT PRESENT SING-DEF
present * * non-relational processual extends-around * * action referential atelic halfway-through * single non-habitual

(5) Yesterday, Tom did his homework twice.
X-TIMES YESTERDAY SING-DEF TELIC-ACTION SIMPLE NON-PERFECT PAST SING-DEF
past hesternal * non-relational holistic * occurs-at-period-in * action referential telic completed * repeated non-habitual

This is a method which is well known in theoretical linguistic work (cf. for example Verkuyl (1993) on aspectology), and which is also much used in second-language learning, i.e. the attempt to implement a specific linguistic system onto an existing one. Possibly it is being used in first-language acquisition as well.

6.4 Results of experiments

6.4.1 Categorization of grammatical meanings (generation)

The first experiment concerns classification of grammatical meanings, i.e. learning and generalization of grammatical category assignment. A total of 63 semantic representations were used. Of these, 20 were created from English aspectual forms, 20 were created from Russian aspectual forms, and 23 were additional test cases.

The following encoding technique for the symbolic features was used: for each dimension, it was determined how many bits are necessary to code all possible values for this dimension. A neutral value ("*") has been added for each dimension. This results in 34 bits for the semantic representation.

The results are presented in Table 6.1. "Learning" concerns the correct assignment of categories by a neural net, which has been trained with complete input–output pairs. "Generalization" concerns the correct assignment of a category to an unlabelled input by the trained neural net. Generalization to test cases and training sentences from the other language have been indicated separately.

Table 6.1 Learning grammatical aspect.

Language	Learning correctness (abs = 20)	Test sentences (abs = 23)	Translation (abs = 20)	Generalization total (abs = 43)
English	20 (100%)	21 (91%)	17 (85%)	38 (88%)
Russian	20 (100%)	22 (96%)	19 (95%)	41 (95%)

The method used was "standard back-propagation" from SNNS (cf. Zell et al. 1993), presentation of patterns in topological order, five hidden units, two or three output units, input units as indicated, learning rate $\rho = 0.2$.

The results can be summarized as follows:

- Learning of the training set was easy, fully possible and quick for both English and Russian representations.
- Generalization to new examples was present and can be considered successful.
- There is not much difference between generalizations for additional test sentences and translations. This shows that category formation proceeds from arbitrary input patterns, as long as these are cognitively adequate and describe a possible state of affairs. The feature set is interlingual: no special language-specific feature sets are required.

6.4.2 Semantic-feature extraction (interpretation)

The syntactic representations, consisting of 6 slots with between 2 and 13 different values, have been translated into binary feature vectors, using the same technique as for semantic representations. The resulting coding has a length of 25 bits.

The architecture was again that of a feed-forward neural network, trained with standard back-propagation. A separate encoding level for the syntactic representation was included, i.e. a chance to recode the slot–value representation in an opaque way, which proved an asset in generalization (cf. Hinton (1986) for a discussion of recoding). The numbers of units in the different layers were 25–15–12–34.

The training technique used was cross-validation by leaving-one-out (cf. Weiss & Kulikowski 1991: 26–39) which is a preferential method for small samples of less than 100 patterns. Because semantic representations for the training set have to be created by hand, it is difficult to obtain large samples. However, as we shall see, the network learns well with small samples and can then generate additional semantic representations, which can be checked for their suitability by interfacing them with another task.

The network was trained with 48 patterns (2500 cycles) and then the remaining pattern was tested for generalization. A typical result for learning is shown in Table 6.2. This process was repeated 49 times, until all patterns had been tested. The results of generalization are also shown in Table 6.2. The third row (marked by †) indicates the results when we exclude "outliers", i.e. patterns with more than 10 errors.

Table 6.2 Learning and generalizing syntactic-to-semantic pattern association.

Phase	Total number of patterns	Correct (%)	Patterns with $n \leq 5$ errors (%)	Patterns with $n > 5$ errors (%)	Average errors per pattern
Learning	48	42 (87.5)	48 (100)	0	0.18
Generalization	49	5 (10.2)	35 (71.4)	14 (28.6)	3.81
Generalization†	46	5 (10.8)	35 (76.1)	11 (23.9)	3.23

The results show that learning, i.e. implementing the functional relationship, is no problem, as expected with a small training set. The figures on generalization show that some implicit rules on how to set semantic values given syntactic input have been abstracted. The task was not an easy one, and an average of three to four errors per pattern remained.

The results can be discussed as follows. Most information that is needed in order to determine semantic features for aspectual meanings is indeed local syntactic information and has been captured by the specialized syntactic representation. However, for most patterns certain features could not be uniquely determined. There are several strategies possible for a remedy.

One possibility would be to include more syntactic information. However, a careful analysis has shown that further information is usually drawn from the same set of aspectually relevant syntactic features (Scheler 1984). To give an example, the present-perfect of recency (PPR) (**proximity**:RECENT) is usually indicated by the adverb *just*. When *just* is missing, it is possible that a pattern is nonetheless somehow "similar" to other typical PPRs. However, one would expect this similarity to be expressed by the same lexical category of the verb (ACHIEVEMENT or TELIC-ACTION) and/or by the absence of a direct object, typical PPRs being of the type illustrated in (6). Therefore one would not expect to gain much by including more local syntactic information.

(6) a. He has (just) gone.
b. I have (just) eaten.

Another question is whether features of lexical content and situational context would improve performance. It is difficult to obtain reliable features describing situational context (but cf. Gallant (1991) for an attempt). Lexical content features would have to be imported from other analysing modules, a problem that has not been satisfactorily solved (cf. McClelland et al. (1989), Scheler (1989) for a proposal on lexical–syntactic interaction during processing). An analysis of the example sentences that were not well generalized would lead one to expect some improvement from the inclusion of a wider semantic context.

The third idea is to have the system modify the semantic representation from knowledge of the likelihood of semantic representations. Such knowledge could be incorporated into weights in lateral connections between the semantic feature values. To make a distinction between such knowledge from experience and the learning related to the present task requires a different learning method. In this way, performance would probably be significantly improved.

6.4.3 Translation of aspectual categories

The final experiment concerns the translation of aspectual categories, i.e. generation from the semantic representations that the system has found using unseen sentences.

The training set was first manually translated from English to Russian[2] to provide a measure of success for the automatic translation.

The generalized representations of the syntax–semantics mapping experiment (Table 6.2) were given to the Russian aspect classifier that had already been trained on semantic representations. The results are given in Table 6.3.

Table 6.3 Translation of aspectual categories using system-created semantic representations.

Phase	Total number of patterns	Correct (%)
Learning	48	47 (97.9)
Generalization	49	45 (91.8)

This shows that the errors were negligible in determining Russian aspect. The explanation for this successful performance is straightforward: the average error for

2. I wish to thank Dr Roman Terterjan for carefully checking all translations.

generalization was less than 4 bits out of 34. In addition, when neighbouring binary features are wrong, this is often only one error on the symbolic level. Accordingly, of the 15 features needed to determine a binary classification, only one or two were set differently than in the learning task. This is a level of error that the classifier can tolerate. Two of the misgenerated patterns were also "outliers" in the interpretation task.

This approach, which uses knowledge of meaning components and syntactic indicators is also contrasted with a "pure" neuronal or statistical approach, where English input is matched directly with Russian morphological categories, and a functional dependence is sought without further explicit representations.

In this experiment, syntactic representations for 49 English sentences were created, encoded in binary form, and labelled according to Russian morphology. The network consisted of 25–15–12–2 units and the training regime was the same as in the second experiment (Table 6.2). The results of learning and generalization are shown in Table 6.4.

Table 6.4 Translation of aspectual categories without explicit semantic representation.

Phase	Total number of patterns	Correct (%)
Learning	48	48 (100)
Generalization	49	38 (77.5)

Accuracy of assigning Russian aspect in generalization was better than chance (50%), but not good enough to be practically useful for translation or checking of grammatical correctness. It was significantly lower than the results using an explicit semantic representation, where 91.8% of generalized semantic representations, containing errors, were nonetheless correctly assigned to the Russian aspectual category.

We have seen that the semantic representations are redundant with respect to category assignment, in the sense that there are 15 features involved for a binary choice, and several features usually concur. The fault tolerance of the classifier allows the handling of slightly "corrupt" representations and still assigns the correct category.

Using explicit semantic representations as target structures for syntactic representations thus proves an asset in complex tasks like translation.

6.5 Conclusion

It has been shown that extracting semantic features for a specific area of meaning and generation of morphological categories is a task that is well suited to neural network models. Standard back-propagation is a useful method to determine whether the *problem specification* is correct, i.e. whether there are generalizable patterns involved and whether the problem has been put in such a way as to make a functional implementation feasible. For a closer look, we may want to consider techniques of coding and corresponding learning mechanisms more fully (cf. Scheler 1995). In this paper, however, we have been concerned with opening up an area of investigation, namely learning the assignment of overt morphological categories to their semantic specification. It could be shown that the proposed function is learnable and generalizable by a standard mechanism.

This approach is a considerable improvement over rule-based methods. The influence of diverse syntactic information on the semantic representation need not be manually analysed in detail in order to set up a great number of individual rules with different trigger patterns. Instead, the various aspects of the information in the syntactic representation are extracted and a semantic representaion is set up automatically. Generation is modelled as a pattern classification process, where a morphological selection is made on the basis of a semantic feature representation. This task could be shown to be easily solvable by a standard neural network. Accuracy in translation was tested with an intermediate, explicitly constructed, semantic representation. It was notably better than a purely statistical approach, where English and Russian output were coupled directly. The advantage of a fault-tolerant mechanism was evidenced by the fact that translation results are highly successful even from semantic representations containing errors.

We have considered a feature representation for aspectual grammatical meanings, a learned classifier for English and Russian morphological aspect and a transformer from a syntactic to a semantic representation. The trained system can be incorporated into an existing MT system as a specialized module which improves rule-coded translation of grammatical aspect and considerably reduces coding effort for new languages (only tagging input and back-propagation learning are required).

An important goal for further research is the translation of aspectual forms from continuous texts. For this goal, a syntactic tagger has to be added to the system. A similar system can then be used as a grammar checker for the correctness of aspectual forms.

References

Bondarko, A. V. 1983. *Principy funkcional'noj grammatiki i voprosy aspektologii.* Moscow: Nauka.

Breu, W. 1980. *Semantische Untersuchungen zum Verbalaspekt im Russischen.* Munich: Otto Sagner.

Comrie, B. 1984. Universals: form and function. In *Explanations for language universals*, B. Butterworth, B. Comrie & Ö. Dahl (eds), 87–103. The Hague: Mouton.

Dowty, D. 1979. *Word meaning and Montague grammar.* Dordrecht: Reidel.

Duda, R. O. & P. E. Hart 1973. *Pattern classification and scene analysis.* New York: John Wiley.

Gallant, S. I. 1991. A practical approach for representing context and for performing word sense disambiguation using neural networks. *Neural Computation* **3**, 293–309.

Hinrichs, E. W. 1988. Tense, quantifiers, and contexts. *Computational Linguistics* **14**, 3–14.

Hinton, G. E. 1986. Learning distributed representations of concepts. In *Proceedings of the Eighth Annual Conference of the Cognitive Science Society*, 1–12. Hillsdale, NJ: Lawrence Erlbaum.

McCarthy, R. & E. Warrington 1988. Evidence for modality-specific meaning systems in the brain. *Nature* **334**, 428–30.

McClelland, J. L. & A. Kawamoto 1986. Mechanisms of sentence processing: assigning roles to constituents. In *Parallel Distributed Processing: explorations in the microstructure of cognition*, D. E. Rumelhart, J. L. McClelland & the PDP Group (eds), 77–109. Cambridge, Mass.: MIT Press.

McClelland, J. L., M. St. John & R. Taraban 1989. Sentence comprehension: a Parallel Distributed Processing approach. *Language and Cognitive Processes* **4**, 287–335.

Marshall, J. C. 1988. Sensation and semantics. *Nature* **334**, 338.

Miikkulainen, R. 1990. A PDP architecture for processing sentences with relative clauses. In *COLING-90: Papers presented to the 13th International Conference on Computational Linguistics*, Helsinki, Vol. 3, 201–6.

Munro, P. & M. Tabasko 1991. Translating locative prepositions. In *Advances in neural information processing systems 3*, R. Lippman, J. Moody & D. Touretzky (eds), 598–604. San Mateo, Calif.: Morgan Kaufmann.

Partee, B. 1973. Some analogies between pronouns and temporal expressions in English. *Journal of Philosophy* **70**, 601–9.

Scheler, G. 1984. *Zur Semantik von Tempus und Aspekt, insbesondere des Russischen.* Magisterarbeit, Universität München.

Scheler, G. 1989. *Remarks concerning the interaction of grammar and semantics.* Technical Report, Computerlinguistik, Universität Heidelberg.

Scheler, G. 1994. *Extracting semantic features for aspectual meanings from a syntactic representation using neural networks.* Technical Report FKI-91-94, Institut für Informatik, Technische Universität München.

Scheler, G. 1995. *Neuronale Lernverfahren zur Modellierung der Semantik spatialer Ausdrücke.* Technical Report FKI-204-95, Institut für Informatik, Technische Universität München.

Scheler, G. & J. Schumann 1995. A hybrid model of semantic inference. In *Proceedings of the 4th International Conference on Cognitive Science in Natural Language Processing (CSNLP 95)*, Dublin.

St. John, M. & J. L. McClelland 1990. Learning and applying contextual constraints in sentence comprehension. *Artificial Intelligence* **46**, 217–57.

Thompson, A. J. & A. V. Martinet 1969. *A practical English grammar*. Oxford: Oxford University Press.

Vendler, Z. 1967. *Linguistics in philosophy*. Ithaca, NY: Cornell University Press.

Verkuyl, H. J. 1993. *A theory of aspectuality: the interaction between temporal and atemporal structure*. Cambridge: Cambridge University Press.

Weiss, S. M. & C. A. Kulikowski 1991. *Computer systems that learn*. San Mateo, Calif.: Morgan Kaufmann.

Zell, A., N. Mache, R. Hübner, G. Marnier, M. Vogt, K.-U. Herrmann, M. Schmalzl, T. Sommer, A. Hatcigeorgiou, S. Döring & D. Posselt 1993. *SNNS User Manual v. 3.1*. Institute for Parallel and Distributed High-Performance Systems, Universität Stuttgart.

7
Experiments in robust parsing with a Guided Propagation Network

PER WESTERLUND, DOMINIQUE BÉROULE AND MARTINE ROQUES

7.1 Introduction

Natural language parsers are usually adapted to textual input data, which strictly follows a set of grammatical rules (Sabah 1988). We are here interested in dealing with casual speech, which requires a high degree of robustness. The computational model used for this purpose is a parallel architecture developed in the framework of human–machine interaction, and which is based on a real-time working principle, coincidence detection. Applications of this processing principle to parsing have already been investigated, using different formalisms and focusing either on robustness (Jacquemin 1992) or on learning mechanisms (Roques 1994). The present paper concentrates on a formalism based on Guided Propagation Networks (GPNs) (Béroule 1990), proposing a parser which deals with different kinds of noise after having learnt syntactic structures from examples of correct sentences.

7.2 Guided propagation

7.2.1 Principles

The study presented here is based on the assumption that any event may be represented by a relative position in both space and time, within a topological memory. The recognition of a given event is then characterized by the activation of its associated memory location. This activation occurs during a certain time interval relatively to the activation of other memory locations, which leads to a "space–time representation". In GPNs, a set of characteristic space–time locations can be reached by an internal flow of signals. This flow starts from a "root cell" and can follow several divergent directions given by memory pathways which end in "event detectors" (EDs) (see Fig. 7.1). A given input pattern, made up of a series of stimuli, may guide the internal flow towards its associated pattern detector. Pattern matching is thus carried out through the measurement of possible spatial and temporal "coincidences" between internal and incoming signals.

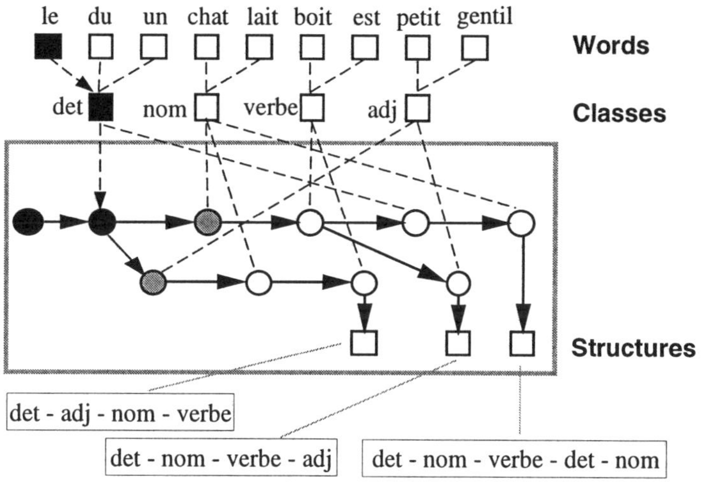

Figure 7.1 *Example of architecture of a Guided Propagation Network.* Event detectors (EDs) are represented by square cells. They form the system input (row of word detectors) at the top of the figure, which feeds the class detectors, and the system output (structure detectors) at the bottom of the figure. The structure detectors stand at the end of memory pathways composed of context-dependent (CD) cells. In the module, a tree of pathways starts from a root cell (to the left-hand side) which initiates the internal contextual signal. The first CD cell to the right-hand side of the root (displayed in black) is now fully activated by the "det" detector; two CD cells (displayed in grey) are "pre-activated", that is, stimulated below their threshold by contextual signals. This indicates the expectation of two possible next classes: "nom" or "adj". The next processing step will decide which pathway is chosen by the internal flow, depending on which word actually occurs.

7.2.2 The model

Cells

Coincidence detection between incoming signals (stimuli) and internal (context) signals is implemented by "context-dependent (CD) cells". Every CD cell i is thus possibly fed by two types of input: stimuli (S_i) and context (C_{i-1}). Event detectors (EDs) can be found at the network input (rows of "word detectors", "class detectors"), and at the output of each network module ("syntactic-structure detectors").

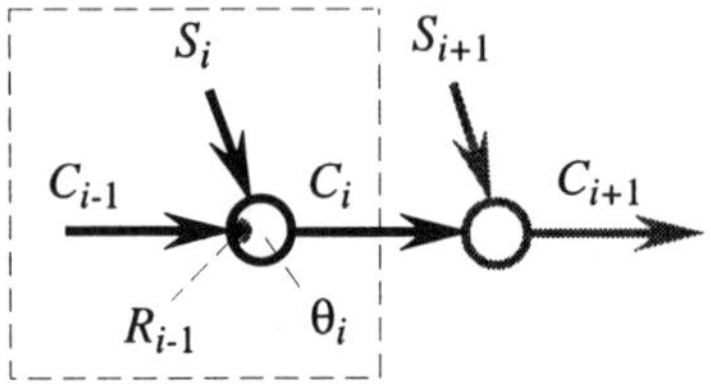

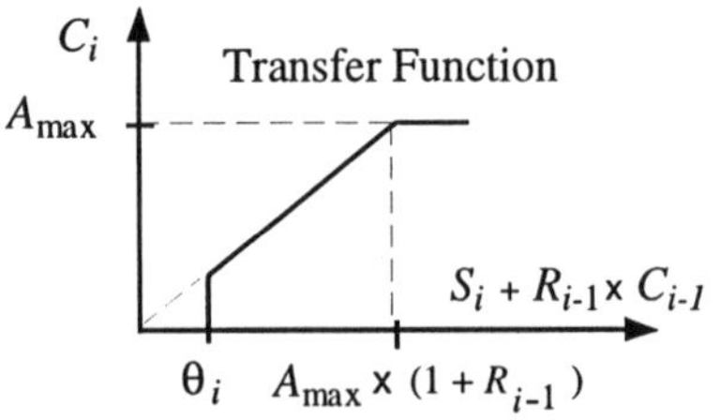

Figure 7.2 *Parameters of a cell involved in its transfer function which relates the amplitude of its output signal to its input.*

The basic parameters of a CD cell i (see Fig. 7.2) are:

- The ratio (R_i) between the contributions of the context and the stimuli. R_i corresponds to the contextual weight if the stimulation weight is equal to 1.
- The excitability (E_i), with which the threshold of the cell is defined as a ratio of the total possible input (the maximal stimulus and weighted context), as in (1):

$$(1)\ \theta_i = \frac{(S_i + R_{i-1} \times C_{i-1})_{\max}}{E_i} = \frac{A_{\max} \times (1 + R_{i-1})}{E_i}$$

  where A_{max} is the maximum value of the signal delivered by a cell.
- The time-delays which synchronize the input signals to the cell.
- The shape of the input signals is covered by three parameters: onset, duration (of the constant part) and offset (decreasing part of the signal), whose purpose is to provide tolerance of temporal distortions. When two signals

(i.e. stimulus and context) are fully synchronized at the level of a CD cell, their coincidence, which is evaluated through their summation, reaches a maximum value. Then, due to the decreasing value of the offset part, the bigger the temporal distortion between two signals, the smaller their sum. The possible coincidence between stimulation and context signals can thus be more precisely evaluated (Westerlund 1995).

There are three modes in which each cell can work:

- Restricted propagation: in this case, both context and stimuli are needed to activate the cell.
- Extended propagation: in this mode the propagation is "knowledge-driven", since the internal signals are sufficient to activate the cell.
- Forced propagation: in this mode, propagation is mainly driven by the data. The stimuli are strong enough for the cell to overcome its threshold.

The relation between the propagation modes and the parameters (R and E) is shown in Figure 7.3.

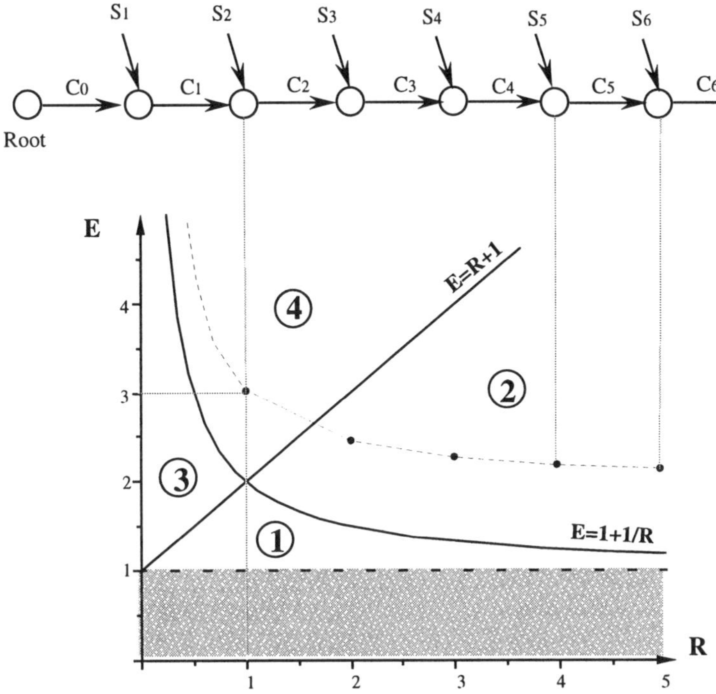

Figure 7.3 *The different propagation modes of cells which participate in a pathway, as function of their parameters E and R.* Area 1 refers to the "restricted propagation" mode, in which every cell is set during learning. Area 2 corresponds to the "extended propagation" mode. Area 3 is "forced propagation". Area 4 is "forced-extended propagation" mode. The parameters assigned to each cell here depend on its location along its pathway (at the top of the figure).

Pathways

The architecture of a network module is made up of pathways, which grow from the root. Two basic sprouting mechanisms are involved in the growth of pathways (Béroule 1988), as follows.

Learning may be triggered in the course of processing when EDs are activated without actually feeding the internal flow. If the time at which an ED gets activated coincides with the response of a CD cell, there will be a "generalization" (Fig. 7.4): a new link connects the ED to the CD. If this coincidence criterion is not satisfied, a new branch leading to a new CD cell is created from the last fully activated CD ("differentiation") (Fig. 7.5).

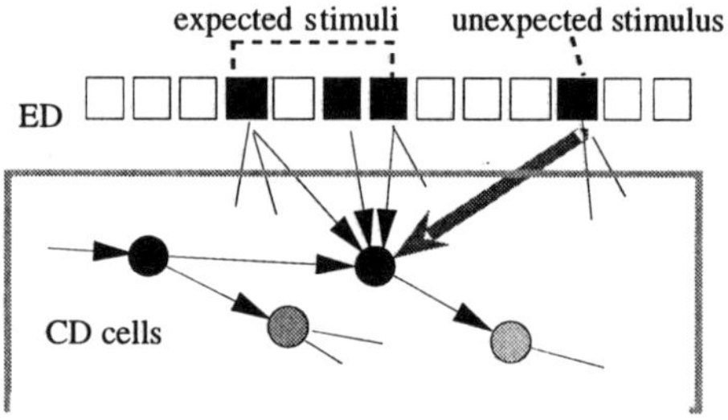

Figure 7.4 *The bold grey link has been created by generalization.*

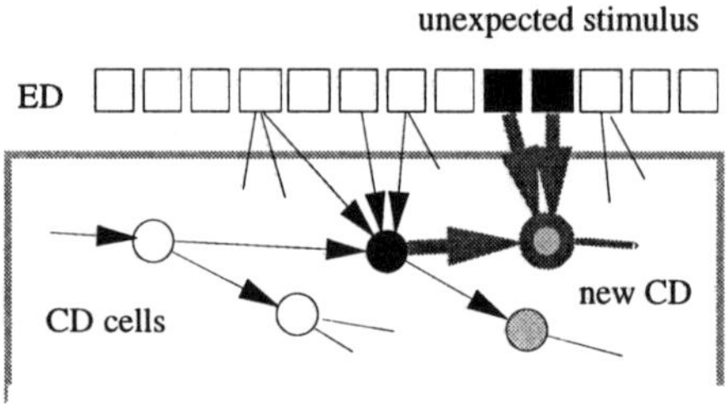

Figure 7.5 *The cell and the links shown in bold have been created by differentiation.*

Learning can then be continued through the selective "reinforcement" of useful pathways, in order for the network to code for the frequency of represented events. Alongside this long-term process, propagation can be temporarily facilitated within the network, in order for it to deal with noisy data. This is obtained through the modulation of parameters E and R at the level of every CD, moving them from the "restricted" to the "extended" propagation mode (see Fig. 7.3).

7.2.3 Robust parsing

For parsing natural language, the network includes two "peripheral" modules made up only of EDs. The first one responds to words, whereas the second one groups them into classes. The next modules represent syntactic structures that can be hierarchized: substructure detectors at the output of a first module can feed the pathways of a deeper module, inside which combinations of substructures are represented. There are basically two ways for the system to build such structured representations in relationship with the teaching strategy (Roques & Béroule 1991):

- by providing the network with complex structures, from which it may then extract substructures, using several possible criteria;
- by selecting a set of elementary sentences in order to build a first module. In a second phase, sentences that combine substructures of the previous set allow the system to create deeper memory pathways fed by the output of the first module. This process can be repeated again using sentences of increasing complexity.

Figure 7.1 shows an example of the architecture used for syntactical parsing.

In the experiments carried out for testing the network robustness, we did not use a hierarchy of modules. All the structures were represented in the same tree of pathways (Fig. 7.1). Once created through learning, these pathways could be fed by input sentences. If the network was given a sentence with a known structure, one of its pathways became fully activated. Every CD cell receives at the right time both context and stimulus signals, which leads to a maximum response of the ED located at the end of the pathway. But this scheme (Fig. 7.6) may be modified in several ways, depending on the distortion undergone by the input pattern.

Each of Figures 7.6 to 7.13 show the activity in time (represented on the *x*-axis) of the CD cells which constitute a memory pathway ($CD_1 \rightarrow CD_2 \rightarrow \ldots \rightarrow CD_5 \rightarrow ED$). From the top to the bottom of the *y*-axis may be found the activity of the five CDs and the final ED. The horizontal dashed lines indicate the cell threshold; the small marks on the baseline give the time at which the CD cell i delivers a contextual signal received by CD_{i+1} after a certain time-delay. The five stimuli S_1, $S_2, \ldots, S_5$ represent the five words of the input sentence.

7.3 Dealing with noise and distortions

The ultimate objective of this work is to deal with the output of a speech recognition module involving the irregularities of natural spoken language. The experiments currently being carried out are only concerned with an approximation of distortion, using a textual input.

Four types of noise were considered as irregularities in natural speech:

- unrecognized word (which can also be due to the deficiencies of the word recognition),
- inversion of two words,
- repetition of a word, and
- omission of a word.

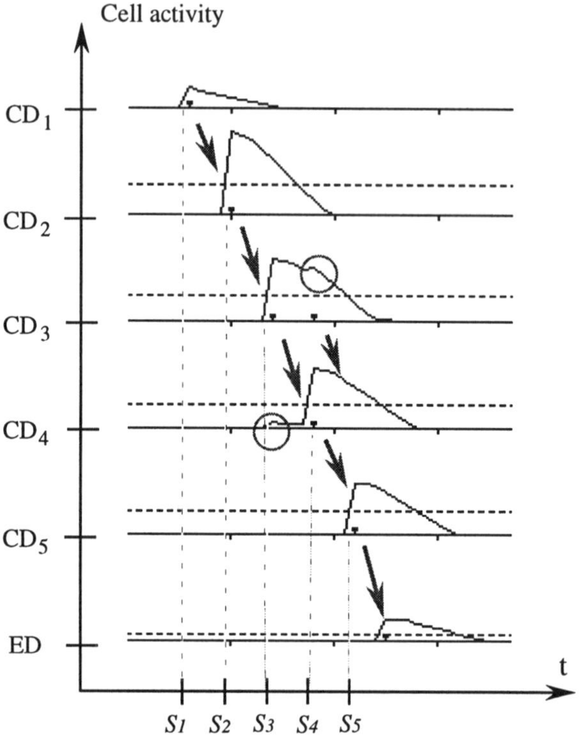

Figure 7.6 *Correct sentence.* The output value of the ED is here 100% of $A_{\max}$. It may be noticed (circles) that S_3 and S_4 activate both CD_3 and CD_4, via the "nom" class to which they both belong.

The basic corpus with which the network was taught was composed of 23 sentences with different syntactic structures, taken from a corpus used for the study of French intonation (Beaugendre et al. 1992). A program was designed to modify automatically a corpus according to the above distortions (Westerlund 1995). Each output file consisted of sentences that have been subjected to one type of distortion at a certain location. For instance, one of these files contained sentences in which the second word was replaced by a "#" character in order to simulate noise.

7.3.1 Formal aspects

Above a certain threshold θ_i, the transfer function of a cell i responds in a linear way to the positive transitions of the summed input signals. Accordingly, the cell output remains null while its input stays below its threshold, and is equal to the maximum $A_{\max}$ for the maximum input $A_{\max} \times (1 + R_{i-1})$.

In the simplified linear case, $\theta_i = 0$, the slope of the function is equal to $1/(1 + R_{i-1})$, and the output of the cell is given by (2).

$$(2)\ C_i = \frac{S_i + R_{i-1} \times C_{i-1}}{1 + R_{i-1}}$$

Replacing C_{i-1} by its value in the above recursive formula, we obtain the expression (3), in terms of a sum of weighted stimuli.

$$\begin{aligned}(3)\ C_n = & \frac{1}{1 + R_{n-1}} \times S_n \\ & + \frac{R_{n-1}}{(1 + R_{n-1})(1 + R_{n-2})} \times S_{n-1} \\ & + \frac{R_{n-1} \times R_{n-2}}{(1 + R_{n-1})(1 + R_{n-2})(1 + R_{n-3})} \times S_{n-2} \\ & \ldots \\ & + \frac{R_{n-1} \times R_{n-2} \times \ldots \times R_1}{(1 + R_{n-1})(1 + R_{n-2}) \ldots (1 + R_0)} \times S_1\end{aligned}$$

If C_n is the output of a pathway comprising n cells and which is therefore fed by n stimuli, the conditions (4) should follow.

$$(4)\ \forall i \in [1, n], S_i = A_{\max} \Rightarrow C_n = A_{\max}$$

In other words, if the pathway is fed by all its stimuli with a maximum value, its output should be maximum. This can be verified by replacing every S_i in (3) by $A_{\max}$, provided that $R_0 = 0$.

Further, $C_n = A_{\max}/p$ if $1/p$ of the stimuli are actually participating in the pathway activation. This should be true for the limiting case when only one stimulus activates the pathway, whatever its location in time and along the path.

$$\begin{aligned}(5) \quad C_n &= \frac{A_{\max}}{n} \\ (a) \quad &= \frac{1}{1 + R_{n-1}} \times A_{\max} \\ (b) \quad &= \frac{R_{n-1}}{(1 + R_{n-1})(1 + R_{n-2})} \times A_{\max} \\ &= \frac{R_{n-1} \times R_{n-2}}{(1 + R_{n-1})(1 + R_{n-2})(1 + R_{n-3})} \times A_{\max} \\ & \ldots \\ &= \frac{R_{n-1} \times R_{n-2} \times \ldots \times R_1}{(1 + R_{n-1})(1 + R_{n-2}) \ldots (1 + R_0)} \times A_{\max}\end{aligned}$$

The equality (5a) gives $R_{n-1} = n-1$, from which (5b) gives $R_{n-2} = n-2$, and so on until $R_0 = 0$.

According to this calculation, the distribution of contextual weights R_i follows an arithmetical progression along a pathway. This means that if every cell of a pathway has the same threshold, the more distant a cell from the beginning of the path, the more it will be driven by its contextual input. In order better to balance the respective contributions of S and C, the threshold can also be modified, following the curve that separates the context-driven mode from the other modes (see Fig. 7.3). Parameters E and R can thus be distributed along the curve (6),

$$(6)\ E_i = \frac{1}{1+R_i} + (E_{\text{param}} - 2)$$

where E_{param} is the excitability of the second cell of the path. The excitability of the first cell is infinity ($\theta_1 = 0$).

7.4 Experimental results

7.4.1 Growth rate

If the network is set in the "restricted propagation" mode, it can be enlarged whenever an input sentence does not match one of its internal representations, which may involve additional cells. The purpose of this test was to check whether the number of cells converged towards a certain limit, despite syntactic ambiguities of the input. The growth rate of a hierarchized network was thus measured in terms of number of words in the sentences, when it was given the same corpus several times. The result was that for n words there were about $0.7n$ cells, as shown in the left-hand part of Figure 7.7.

The growth of the network as a function of the number of classes is presented in Figure 7.8. The maximum number of classes used was 12. This number includes a division of the nouns into proper and common ones, of the verbs according to their form, and of the pronouns into relative and personal pronouns.

7.4.2 Tolerance to distortions

In order to carry out an experiment on network robustness, every CD cell was set in a robust mode, according to Figure 7.3. The network was then fed with distorted sentences. The result was the rate of sentences that were correctly parsed. The listing in Figure 7.9 was displayed while the software was running, trying to handle two unrecognized words at the beginnings of the sentences. In agreement with the theory, the activation value of the correct pathway corresponded to the ratio of unchanged items in the syntactic structure.

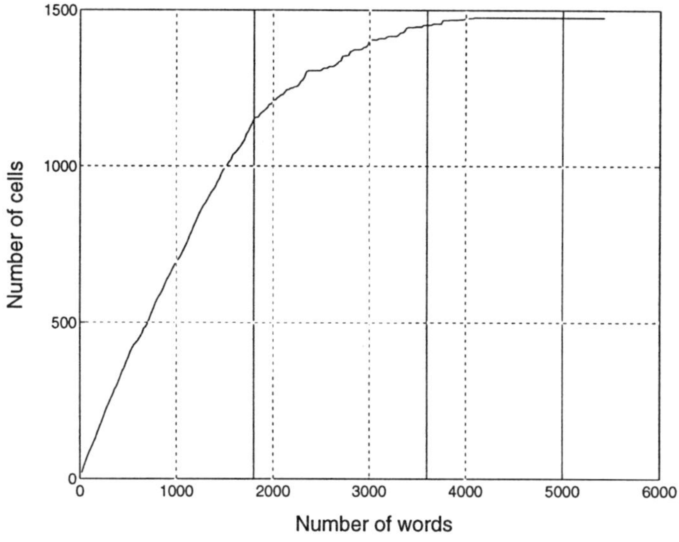

Figure 7.7 *The same corpus presented three times, as indicated by the solid vertical lines.*

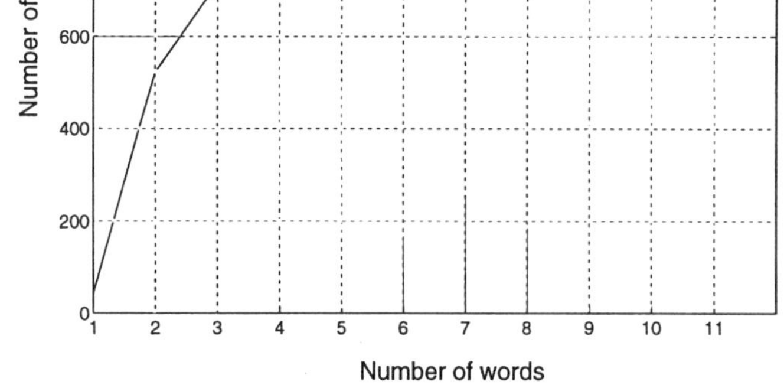

Figure 7.8 *The number of cells for different numbers of classes.*

```
Current word :   #
Current word :   #
Current word :   amère
.
PATHWAY 1 :   33.3 OK
nomp → vco → adj

Current word :   #
Current word :   #
Current word :   monde
Current word :   va
Current word :   bien
.
PATHWAY 1 :   33.3
nomp → vco → adj

PATHWAY 4 :   60.0 OK
adv → ppe → nom → vco → con

PATHWAY 5 :   36.0
ppe → vco → vpa → prp → nomp

Current word :   #
Current word :   #
Current word :   partis
Current word :   pour
Current word :   Paris
.

PATHWAY 5 :   68.0 OK
ppe → vco → vpa → prp → nomp
PATHWAY 1 :   33.3
nomp → vco → adj
```

Figure 7.9 *Listing displayed while software is running.*

The sequence of figures (from Fig. 7.10 to Fig. 7.13) illustrates how the normal activity of a pathway stimulated by its reference pattern (Fig. 7.6) was disturbed by several types of distortions. The input sentence was (7), in which *partis* may be a noun or a verb.

(7) *Ils sont partis pour Paris.*
'They have left for Paris.'

The corresponding structure is (8), where "ppe" is pronoun, "vco" conjugated verb, "vpa" verb participle, "prp" preposition and "nom" proper name.

(8) `ppe → vco → vpa → prp → nomp`

The legend for each figure is as described above (p. 101).

The shape of the stimulus signal was chosen slightly different from the contextual one, which had an onset of 0, a duration of 3 and an offset of 7, in order better to understand the graphical displays in the figures. The signal offset immediately follows the instantaneous onset, with a value of 8.

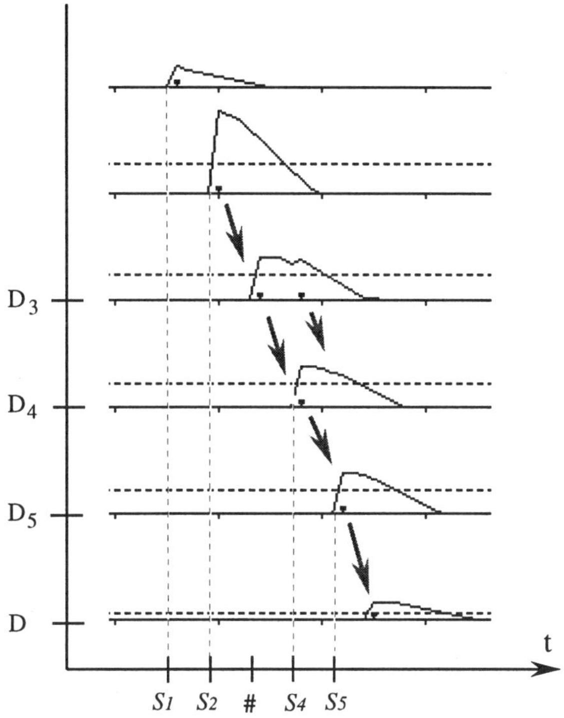

Figure 7.10 *Unrecognized word.* The third word is not found in the lexicon (*Ils sont # pour Paris*). The context signal generated by CD_2 activates CD_3 which is not stimulated at the same time by S_3 as it should be. But the context signal is weighted enough to cross CD_3 and propagate towards CD_4, which is stimulated at the expected time by S_4. The ED activity is 80% (4/5) of A_{max}, which is compatible with the fact that 4/5 of the complete sentence remains unchanged.

Software was designed to compare the output of the system with the correct analysis, according to the following algorithm: if the right structure belongs to the set of those which are the most strongly activated, the size *N* of this set is kept. The result for one sentence is either the inverse value of *N*, or 0 if the correct structure does not belong to the winners' set.

These numbers were then averaged over all the sentences in one corpus and the results presented in tables where the rows represent different kinds of distortion

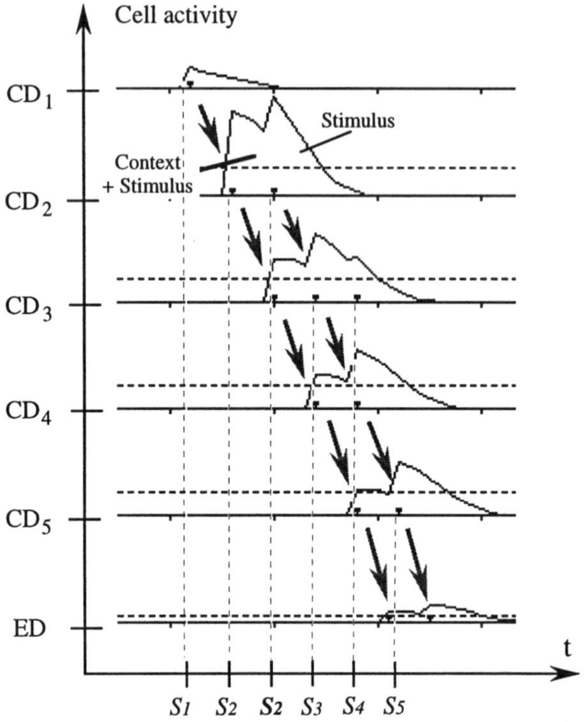

Figure 7.11 *Repeated word.* The second word occurs twice (*Ils sont sont partis pour Paris*). In this case, the initial flow of activity issued from CD_1 separates into two flows generated by the repeated stimulus, until the end of the pathway. The strongest flow activity that reaches the ED is 90% of A_{max}.

and the columns represent different positions of the distortion. The first column corresponds to the reference corpus, without distortions. It is given for the same sentences as those that are affected by the distortion. Inversion does not affect sentences composed of only one word.

The results shown in Table 7.1 were obtained with the following parameters:

Excitability: 3. This allows more than two-thirds of the structures to be distorted.

Contextual signal: its total duration must take into account a possible delay due to inverted words (see Fig. 7.13). Since the number of processing steps between the occurrence of two words is equal to 4, we let the offset start after 3 steps, with a long duration (8).

Stimulus: in the same way, the duration of a stimulus must be long enough to wait for a delayed context signal (see Fig. 7.12). The stimulus is given the same shape as the context signal.

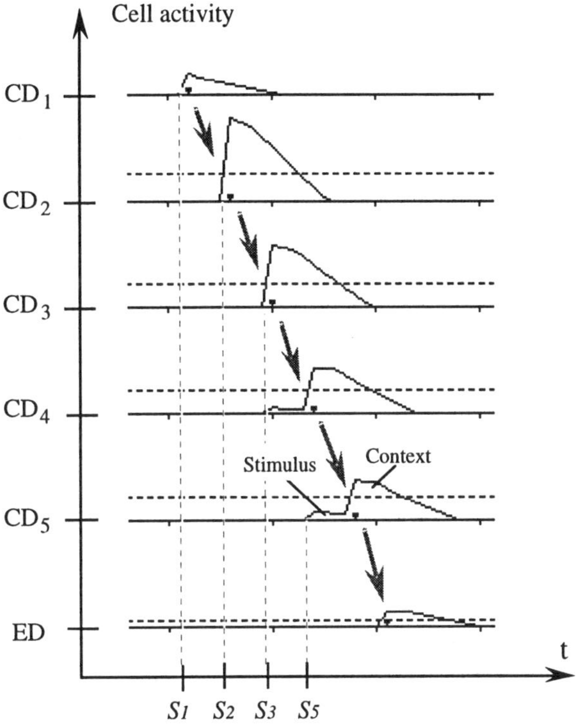

Figure 7.12 *Omitted word.* The fourth word of the sentence S_4 has not occurred (*Ils sont partis Paris*). But CD_4 gets activated under the only influence of the context signal generated by CD_3. The fifth word S_5 stimulates CD_5 earlier than expected, but its output signal roughly coincides with the context signal generated later by CD_4. It may be noticed that at the level of the fifth cell of the pathway, the context signal is 4 times stronger than the stimulus, due to the arithmetical progression of the context weight. ED's activity is 76% of A_{max}.

Table 7.1 Example of results.

Position	1	2	3	4	5	6	7	8
Reference	91	91	91	90	90	97	95	100
Noise	91	91	96	93	85	93	95	100
Inversion	89	93	83	74	69	97	82	100
Repetition	98	78	69	79	72	73	95	100
Omission	72	59	74	74	85	87	95	100

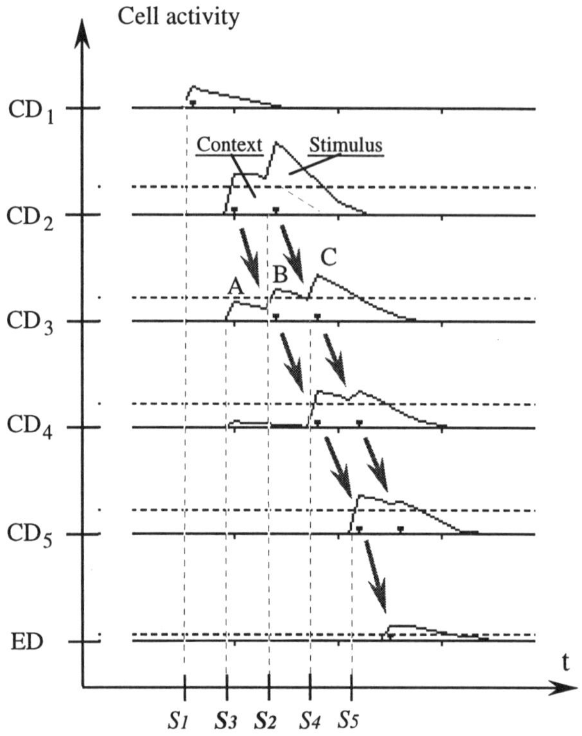

Figure 7.13 *Inverted words.* The input sentence is *Ils partis sont pour Paris.* There are two problems in this case, which are both settled thanks to the duration of the signals integrated by every cell. (i) S_3 occurs earlier than expected and thus cannot coincide with the context signal sent by CD_2. (ii) S_2 (Stimulus) occurs later than expected at the time when the value of the context signal (Context) sent by CD_1 starts to decrease (offset). CD_3 is stimulated too early by S_3 (A), then by the context delivered by CD_2 (B), and in the end by the combination "Context + Stimulus" of CD_2 (C). The ED is activated at 72% of A_{max}.

These results are displayed in Figure 7.14. It may be noticed that the earlier an omission or a repetition occurs in a sentence, the lower is the recognition rate. This can be related to the arithmetical progression of the contextual weights, which amplify a lack of activity due to a resulting time distortion – i.e. all the words after the distortion come later or earlier than expected – at the beginning of a pathway, as it is propagated towards the structure detector. On the other hand, a distortion at the end of a sentence is negligible compared with the weight of the contextual signal.

7.5 Conclusion

The experiments carried out in this study involved a corpus of textual sentences, from which several distorted versions were derived. Although not natural, the distorted

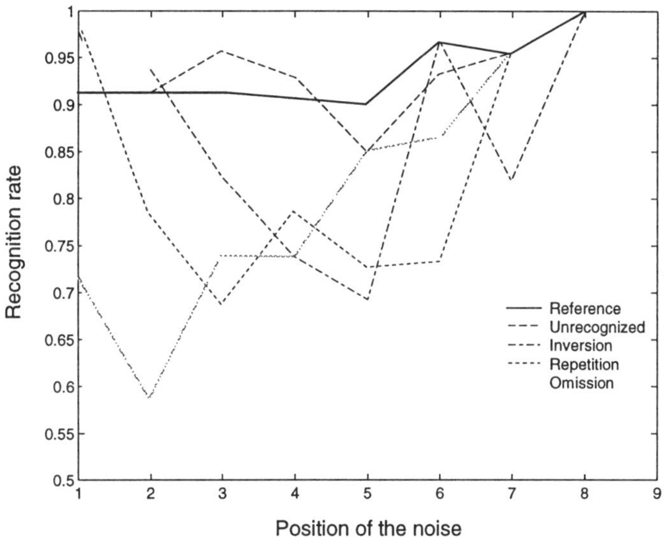

Figure 7.14 *The recognition rate as a function of the position of the noise.*

sentences allowed systematic tests to be performed, in order to evaluate the system robustness when submitted to a controlled input. A formalism was developed for the "matching score" given by the system output to account for the degree of distortion undergone by the reference syntactic structures.

A possible next step of this work could combine two aspects that have been separately addressed until now: the automatic hierarchization of the network, and robust recognition by a one-module network.

Together with decreasing the total number of cells, this would make progress towards the automatic parsing of casual speech, in which the same distortions as those undergone by words may also affect groups of words. In a hierarchized network, the output of the "substructure" module would be treated by a "structure" module in the same way as words are by the current one-module network. Inverted, missing, repeated or noisy substructures should then not prohibit the recognition of the structure to which they belong.

There remains to be included in the model an automatic local adjustment of the parameters during processing. In the current software simulation, the strength of the connections of a pathway are set once and integrate similar internal signals, although in natural language, the words in a sentence are not linked in the same way. For instance, the selective reinforcement of the connections that are used could account for the frequency with which two words occur together. In the same way, the tolerance of distortions provided by the shapes of the signals should vary in degree, taking into account examples of "allowed" and "forbidden" distortions. A forbidden distortion would then result in the decreased duration of a certain internal signal.

From a more general point of view, the expected ability of GPNs to deal with spoken natural language may result from both their adaptability and their robustness to distortions. But, as can be noticed in the experiments reported here, these two features involve different regulations of the cell parameters. In the "restricted propagation" mode, the internal contextual flow is focused enough for possible unexpected words to be "stored" at the right space–time location in the network, without supervision. After a preliminary learning phase involving well-formed sentences, the cells of the network are set in the robust mode, in which unexpected words are considered as due to distortions of a known structure. Thus, for new well-formed sentences to give rise to new internal representations, a GPN should be able temporarily to switch back to the "restricted propagation" mode. In the planned GPN human–machine architecture of which this parser is a part, a central control unit will be responsible for managing this point through the on-line regulation of the cell parameters. The network would then possibly be completed in the course of processing whenever recognition does not obtain a maximum score.

References

Beaugendre, F., C. d'Alessandro, A. Lacheret & J. Terken 1992. A perceptual study of French intonation. In *International Conference on Spoken Language Processing*, Banff, Alberta, 739–42

Béroule, D. 1988. The never-ending learning. In *Neural computers*, R. Eckmiller & Ch. von der Malsburg (eds), 219–30. Berlin: Springer.

Béroule, D. 1990. Guided propagation: current state of theory and applications. In *Neurocomputing*, F. Fogelman-Soulié and J. Hérault (eds), 241–60. Berlin: Springer.

Jacquemin, C. 1992. Activation diffusion: a connectionist network for robust parsing. In *ECAI '92: 10th European Conference on Artificial Intelligence*, Vienna, 183–7.

Roques, M. 1994. Dynamic grammatical representations in Guided Propagation Networks. In *Grammatical inference and applications*, C. Carrasco & J. Oncina (eds), 189–202. Berlin: Springer.

Roques, M. & D. Béroule 1991. Strategies of unsupervised learning for a parallel parsing architecture. In *International Joint Conference on Neural Networks*, Seattle, Vol. 2, 215–8.

Sabah, G. 1988. *L'intelligence artificielle et le langage: représentation des connaissances*. Paris: Hermès.

Westerlund, P. 1995. *Noise-tolerant parsing with a Guided Propagation Network.* MSc thesis, Department of Speech Communication and Music Acoustics, KTH, Stockholm.

8
Learning semantic relationships and syntactic roles in a simple recurrent network

XINYU WU, MICHAEL MCTEAR
AND PIYUSH OJHA

8.1 Introduction

In recent years there has been growing interest in using connectionist techniques for natural language processing (NLP) (Sharkey 1990, 1992). The most interesting features of connectionist techniques include noise resistance, learning behaviour, neural plausibility, associative retrieval and knowledge integration.

Connectionist models, however, have had some serious problems in representing and applying general knowledge rules that specifically require variables. It has been argued (Fodor & Pylyshyn 1988) that this deficiency strictly limits the usefulness of connectionist networks for modelling high-level cognitive tasks such as language understanding and planning. Therefore, in order to perform sophisticated language processing functions, one will require a hybrid system consisting of a number of simple neural nets controlled by a symbolic processor (Wu et al. 1994a). Such a hybrid system that combines connectionist and symbolic subsystems can be more powerful than systems operating within only one paradigm (Wermter & Lehnert 1989; Hendler 1989; Dyer 1991).

In this paper, we present a simple recurrent network (SRN) which is a part of our hybrid system SYMCON (Wu et al. 1994b) for dealing with the problem of word-sense disambiguation (WSD). Most NLP systems require some knowledge of syntax as a basic prerequisite. Traditionally, much of the research effort in NLP has been concentrated on developing syntactic parsing systems that analyse the languages according to grammars (Winograd 1972; Woods 1970). By contrast, relatively little work has been carried out in developing algorithms that are able to parse sentences by considering both syntactic and semantic information. One major advantage of the connectionist approach to NLP is that the semantic information of the languages may be encoded in the network while the network is being trained using a set of grammatical sentences. This means that the knowledge of syntax and semantics can be integrated in the network.

In the next section, a brief overview of our distributed method for representing the concepts in the network is provided. The subsequent sections describe both the basic structure of the SRN, and the architecture of the recurrent network used in SYMCON. Sections 8.5 and 8.6 present the training procedure and the results, respectively.

8.2 Concept representations in the network

A common method of coping with representation in NLP is to create different input nodes for a particular word at each different absolute position in a sentence. This is inefficient and unable to capture the information of constituency in the input text (Wyard & Nightingale 1990). An improvement strategy of concept representations used in our recurrent network is to encode a set of words (single, pair, triple, etc.) as one concept and store it in one node in the input layer, rather than encode one single word in one node.

Each concept in the network is then represented as a distributed pattern of activation which in this case is a binary vector of ten micro-features. One of the most important improvements of using such a distributed representation is that the network structure can be simplified. On the contrary, for a large system, if the localist representation were used, there could be thousands or hundreds of thousands of separate concepts, and the number of weights could be increased tremendously. This is clearly not an acceptable solution for large networks.

Another important feature of distributed representations is that the concepts may be compared to see how similar or different they are by viewing what micro-features they have or do not have in common (Wu et al. 1993). This indicates that by using distributed representations, the concepts themselves carry some semantic information. This is a basis for learning semantic relationships by the SRN.

In order to understand a language properly, both syntactic and semantic information should be considered. Therefore, each concept is categorized according to the most general term in the hierarchy that describes the concept and its syntactic category. This step abstracts specific concepts to more general terms. Then, these most general thesaurus terms are grouped into ten features describing the basic meaning and the syntactic constraints of a concept. Each feature can be used to describe a different concept, and each concept can have multiple features, which reflect the characteristic of distributed representations. Table 8.1 shows all the features along with some examples used to train our recurrent network.

Table 8.1 Micro-features of the concepts and examples.

Micro-features	Examples
AGENT	*person, police, diver, shark*
ACTION	*eat, give, marry, put*
TRANSFER	*put, throw, move*
PATIENT	*person, ball, diver, shark*
INSTRUMENT	*ball, fork, washing-machine*
LOCATION	*church, washing-machine*
HUMAN	*man, woman, John, diver*
ANIMAL	*shark, cat*
PHY-OBJ	*ball, fork*
EATABLE	*food, cake*

8.3 Simple recurrent network

An SRN was first applied to NLP by Elman (1990). The structure of this type of network is given in Figure 8.1. It is a standard feed-forward network, with an additional set of "context" units. These units store a copy of the activations of the hidden units from the previous time step, which are then used as input at the current time step. The weights from the context units are modified just like any other weights in the network.

The context units serve as a form of memory in which each preceding input item is represented with decreasing precision. As shown in the architecture of the network, the context units remember the previous internal state. Thus, the hidden units have the

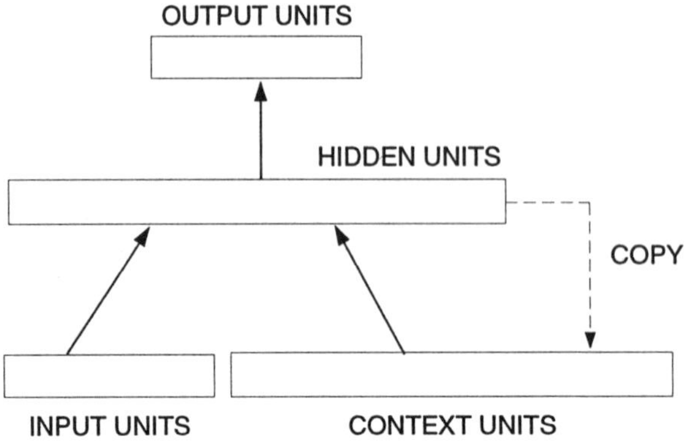

Figure 8.1 *An SRN structure.*

task of mapping both an external input and the previous internal state of some desired output. It is the internal representations developed by the hidden units of the network that mediate the sensitivity of the SRN to the structural properties of sentence-like sequences. Elman (1991) and others (Servan-Schreiber et al. 1991; Reilly 1993) have explored the capacity of these representations primarily from a linguistic point of view, and it is generally agreed that many of the important criticisms made by Fodor & Pylyshyn (1988) of connectionist networks were rebutted by their results.

8.4 Recurrent network in the SYMCON system

The main task of our recurrent network is to learn semantic relationships between concepts, and thus to predict the syntactic role of the next concept in a sentence, given the current concept. The architecture of the network is shown in Figure 8.2. It consists of ten input units which are used to encode the concept nodes in SYMCON as discussed in Section 8.2. The two layers of five hidden units are designed to create a bottleneck at the input and output to encourage the further creation of distributed word representations and also to help reduce the overall connectivity of the network. The context units serve as the temporal memory of the system, and the dashed line represents one-to-one connectivity. The copyback links are not modifiable in our system (the weights in this case are 1.0).

As discussed in Section 8.3, the context units can remember the previous internal state by feeding back the hidden units' activation at the previous time step. Therefore, the information of the previous words can be preserved when parsing the current word, and this is very important for WSD. In order to understand an ambiguous word correctly (i.e. select the best interpretation among alternative inference paths), it is essential to consider all information supplied by the words in the sentence or even the content of the whole context. The context units used in the SRN, together

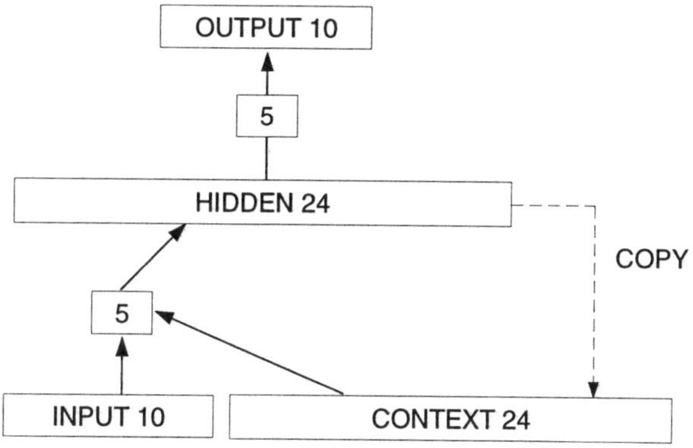

Figure 8.2 *Architecture of the recurrent network.*

with the use of the distributed representations in encoding the concepts, provide a solution to combine various kinds of information contained in the language for parsing a sentence effectively.

8.5 Procedure for training the recurrent network

The above network was trained using a corpus of sentences generated from the nine-rule context-free grammar (CFG) given in (1).

(1) S → NP VP
NP → Det NP2
NP → NP2
NP2 → Noun
NP2 → Adj NP2
NP2 → NP2 PP
VP → Verb
VP → Verb NP
PP → Prep NP

The task of the network is to predict the syntactic role of the next concept in a sentence, given the current concept. For example, if we present (2) to the SRN, a possible fragment of the input and desired output will be as shown in Table 8.2.

(2) John ate the cake with a fork.

The values assigned to each of the microfeatures are chosen arbitrarily, which may affect the training process and lead to undesirable results. In order to make sure that it is the relative values that are assigned to different microfeatures, normalization is adopted in our work.

Table 8.2 A possible fragment of training sequence for example (2).

INPUT				OUTPUT		
John	*ate*	*the cake*	*with a fork*	*ate*	*the cake*	*with a fork*
1.0	0.0	0.2	0.4	0.0	0.2	0.4
0.0	1.0	0.0	0.5	1.0	0.0	0.5
0.0	0.3	0.0	0.0	0.3	0.0	0.0
0.6	0.0	1.0	0.7	0.0	1.0	0.7
0.0	0.0	0.3	1.0	0.0	0.3	1.0
0.0	0.0	0.1	0.0	0.0	0.1	0.0
1.0	1.0	0.0	0.0	1.0	0.0	0.0
0.0	0.8	0.0	0.0	0.8	0.0	0.0
0.0	0.7	1.0	1.0	0.7	1.0	1.0
0.1	1.0	1.0	0.1	1.0	1.0	0.1

After normalization the dot product of each microfeature with itself is equal to a constant (normally 1). This is defined as (3),

$$(3)\quad P_i.P_i = \sum_{k=1}^{n} P_{i_k}^2$$

where P_i represents the ith concept in a given sentence and it has n elements (in this case $n = 10$). P_{i_k} is the kth element of P_i. According to the dot product defined in (3), it is easy to obtain (4).

(4) *John.John* = 1
ate.ate = 1
(*the cake*).(*the cake*) = 1
(*with a fork*).(*with a fork*) = 1

Therefore, after normalization, Table 8.2 will be changed to Table 8.3.

The standard back-propagation learning algorithm (Rumelhart et al. 1986) was used in training the recurrent network. The network was trained on a corpus of 90 simple sentences generated from (1), and another ten unseen sentences which were also generated from the (1) were used as the test sets. The learning rate was set to 0.15 and, as usual with SRNs, a momentum term of 0.075 was used.

In Elman's original specification, the context units were reset at the end of each sentence. This causes a loss of information across sentence boundaries including clausal and sentential information. However, because the information about other

Table 8.3 The training sequence for the example sentence after normalization.

INPUT				OUTPUT		
John	*ate*	*the cake*	*with a fork*	*ate*	*the cake*	*with a fork*
0.65	0.0	0.113	0.234	0.0	0.113	0.234
0.0	0.487	0.0	0.293	0.487	0.0	0.293
0.0	0.146	0.0	0.0	0.146	0.0	0.0
0.39	0.0	0.564	0.41	0.0	0.564	0.41
0.0	0.0	0.169	0.586	0.0	0.169	0.586
0.0	0.0	0.056	0.0	0.0	0.056	0.0
0.65	0.486	0.0	0.0	0.486	0.0	0.0
0.0	0.389	0.564	0.0	0.389	0.564	0.0
0.0	0.341	0.564	0.568	0.341	0.564	0.568
0.064	0.487	1.0	0.059	0.487	1.0	0.059

clauses and sentences is of interest in the network, it was decided not to do the reset to the context units. The result of the training was as good as when the reset was used.

In the previous sections, we have described the distributed connectionist network SRN, which was applied to learning the semantic relationships between the concepts, and thus, anticipating the syntactic role of each concept in a given sentence. The generalization results of the network are discussed in the next section.

8.6 The performance of the network

It is often necessary that during the training process of a network a distinction be made between training and testing material. As mentioned above, 90% of the material generated by the CFG is used as learning material, and the other 10% as test material. The values of the weights in the network including the weights between the context and hidden units are all adjusted according to the error-propagation learning rule. After each learning cycle, the error on learning and testing material is calculated. During the processing of the test material the weights of the network are not adjusted.

In order to judge the performance of the network, not only is the error on the test sets important, but also the difference in performance between learning and test sets: a small difference in performance on learning and testing material is an indication that the network is able to make significant generalizations.

In Figure 8.3 the learning graph of the recurrent network for 900 cycles is given. Average error is plotted against the number of learning and testing cycles.

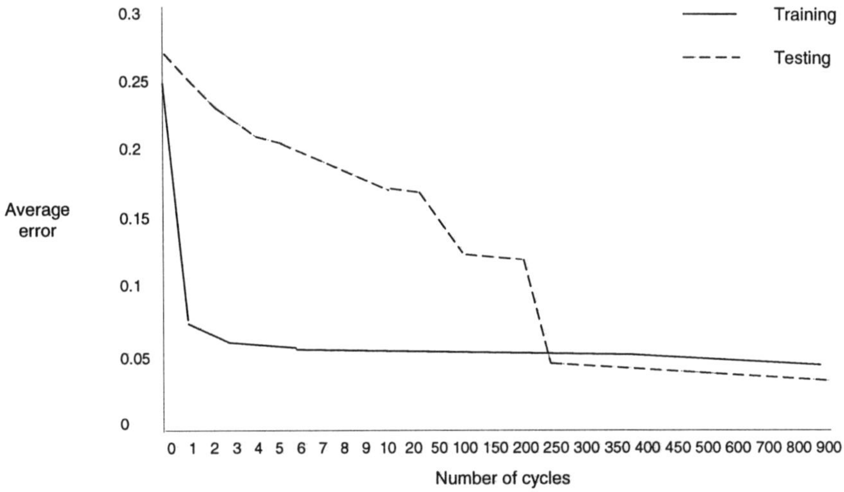

Figure 8.3 *Performance of the recurrent network.*

It is found that after a starting period with rapid improvement, a stage of stabilization sets in, in which the distance between the results of the testing material and those of the learning material remains the same. A straightforward explanation for this phenomenon would be that during the training process, the network initially makes significant generalizations that will also lead to better performance on the test set. The deterioration in the later stage might be ascribed to the fact that the network adapts itself more and more to the peculiarities of the training material. It is usual to cut off the learning process when the results on the test sets begin to deteriorate.

The experiment reflects another very interesting feature of the performance of the recurrent network. From Figure 8.3, it can be seen that the error on the testing material becomes less than that on the training material after a number of cycles, and remains in the stable stage. This indicates that the network has learned to predict the syntactic role of the next concept in a given sentence even when presented with an unseen pattern.

It can also be seen that there is a rapid improvement on the training material during the first 5 cycles and rapid improvement on the testing material during the first 200 cycles. Later on, the improvement on the learning and testing material is minimal. The difference in performance between learning material and testing material is small, and the error on testing material is less than that on learning material after about 220 cycles. After 250 cycles, the decrease in the performance on both the testing material and the learning material is very small, which means the training process of the network can be ended.

8.7 Summary

In this paper, we have presented a distributed connectionist SRN which is applied to learning the semantic relationships between the concepts, and thus, anticipating the syntactic role of each concept in a given sentence. The knowledge learned is used by a hybrid system (SYMCON) as the logical binding constraints. In the hybrid system, the trained recurrent network is integrated with knowledge-based symbolic systems and localist connectionist systems to handle variables and dynamic role-binding, and to further perform the task of high-level inference.

The use of the distributed recurrent network in the hybrid system makes it effective for NLP. The concepts are represented by distributed patterns, and thus carry some semantic information which is an important element in parsing a sentence. The distributed representations are also able to decrease the number of connection weights in the network. The generalization results of the network indicate that it performs the task of syntactic role prediction satisfactorily.

References

Barnden, J. A. & J. B. Pollack (eds) 1991. *Advances in connectionist and neural computation theory, Vol. 1: High level connectionist models.* Norwood, NJ: Ablex.

Dyer, M. G. 1991. Symbolic NeurEngineering for natural language processing: a multilevel research approach. In Barnden & Pollack (1991), 179–212.

Elman, J. L. 1990. Finding structure in time. *Cognitive Science* **4**, 179–211.

Elman, J. L. 1991. Distributed representations, simple recurrent networks, and grammatical structure. *Machine Learning* **7**, 195–225.

Fodor, J. A. & Z. W. Pylyshyn 1988. Connectionism and cognitive architecture: a critical analysis. *Cognition* **28**, 3–71.

Hendler, J. A. 1989. Developing hybrid symbolic/connectionist models. In Barnden & Pollack (1991), 165–79.

Reilly, R. 1993. Boundary effects in the linguistic representations of simple recurrent networks. In *Proceedings of the 15th Annual Conference of the Cognitive Science Society*, Boulder, Colo., 854–9.

Rumelhart, D. E., G. E. Hinton & R. J. Williams 1986. Learning internal representations by error propagation. In *Parallel Distributed Processing, explorations in the microstructure of cognition, Volume 1: Foundations*, D. E. Rumelhart, J. L. McClelland & the PDP Research Group (eds), 318–62. Cambridge, Mass.: MIT Press.

Servan-Schreiber, D., A. Cleeremans & J. McClelland 1991. Graded state machines: the representation of temporal contingencies in simple recurrent networks. *Machine Learning* **7**, 161–93.

Sharkey, N. E. 1990. Connection science and natural language: an emerging discipline. *Connection Science* **2**, 3–5.

Sharkey, N. E. 1992. *Connectionist natural language processing.* Dordrecht: Kluwer.

Wermter, S. & W. G. Lehnert 1989. A hybrid symbolic/connectionist model for noun phrase understanding. *Connection Science* **1**, 255–72.

Winograd, T. 1972. *Understanding natural language.* New York: Academic Press.

Woods, W. 1970. Transition network grammars for natural language analysis. *Communications of the ACM* **13**, 591–606.

Wu, X., M. McTear & P. C. Ojha 1993. Word sense disambiguation by a higher order connectionist net based on distributed representations. In *Proceedings of the IEEE TENCON'93 Conference*, Beijing, 893–8.

Wu, X., M. McTear & P. C. Ojha 1994a. Pronoun disambiguation using a hybrid system. In *Proceedings of the 14th International Conference on AI, KBS, Expert Systems and Natural Language Processing*, Paris, Vol. 3., 67–76.

Wu, X., M. McTear & P. C. Ojha 1994b. *SYMCON: a hybrid symbolic/ connectionist system for word sense disambiguation.* Technical Report, Department of Information Systems, University of Ulster, Newtownabbey, N. Ireland.

Wyard, P. J. & C. Nightingale 1990. A single layer higher order neural net and its application to context free grammar recognition. *Connection Science* **2**, 347–70.

Part III
Corpus-based methods

9 A system for automating concordance line selection

ALEX COLLIER

9.1 Manual abstracting

For several years now, Michael Hoey has been investigating the phenomenon of repeated sequences of lexical items in text and the relationship of these to the core sentences of a text. The phenomenon on which he has focused is known as "lexical cohesion", and is one of the forms of textual cohesion described in Halliday & Hasan (1976). Hoey noticed that the recurrence of certain items across the sentences of a text could be used as an aid to identifying the "key" sentences of that text, where a "key" sentence can be characterized by its centrality to the text and the expressive power which it has in standing in for several other sentences.

In Hoey (1991) the "connection by repetition" is termed a "link", which defines a subset of the relations which Halliday & Hasan termed "ties". Hoey describes several different kinds of repetition, which range in complexity but all contribute to the links present between the sentences of the text. These repetition types can be categorized as follows:

- *Simple (lexical) repetition*: The link exists between two instances of the same word (*dream* ↔ *dream*).

- *Complex lexical repetition*: Here a link is made between members of a lemma, e.g. (*dream* ↔ *dreaming*), which also includes morphologically related antonyms of the *happy* ↔ *unhappy* variety.
- *Mutual substitutability*: This instantiates a link between synonyms or expressions which are coreferential within the text (*clever* ↔ *intelligent*, *John Major* ↔ *the prime minister*).
- *Complex paraphrase*: This covers some cases of repetition by antonym not covered by complex lexical repetition, such as *light* ↔ *dark*.
- *Hyponymy*: Here, superordinates are included as repetitions, e.g. *tulip* ↔ *flower*.
- *Pronominal repetition*: In this case, reference is made to a lexical item by means of a pronoun, and a link is therefore made between the pronoun and the lexical item, e.g. *dream* ↔ *it*.
- *Substitution*: Where a word such as *this* or *the above* is used to refer back to a previous clause, sentence or even larger section of the text, this must also be considered as a link.

On the basis of this analysis Hoey was able to calculate the frequency of recurrent lexical items for each sentence. This information was then used to build up a measure of connectivity between the sentences of the text. This information can be represented in a matrix as in (1), where the number down the left-hand side and the diagonal indicates the sentence number, and the other digits show the number of links between the sentences.

(1) **1**
2 0 **2**
3 2 0 **3**
4 1 0 0 **4**

Thus the matrix shows that there are two links between sentences 1 and 3 and just one link between sentences 1 and 4.

While looking at non-narrative texts, Hoey had noticed that those sentences in a text which had the greatest degree of cohesion could be used to build an abridgement of the text. In order to ascertain the level of cohesion, Hoey introduced an additional measure which he called the "bond", defining it as "a connection which exists between a pair of sentences by virtue of there being an above-average number of links relating them" (Hoey 1991: Glossary). In Hoey's experience the sentences having the greatest bond count tended to cohere together, thus making the abridgement itself seem more like a "text" with internal structure of its own.

The bond strength of a sentence was arrived at by establishing a link threshold, which Hoey set at a minimum of three, whereby any sentence with at least that number of links with another sentence could be said to have one bond with that sentence. Thus, in the matrix above, if we were to set a threshold of two links then sentences 1 and 3 would share one bond, whereas sentence 4 disappears from the equation. This is an important step, since links are always symmetrical; bonds, however, describe a wider relationship between the sentences of a text and enable two sentences which share the same lexical items to obtain differing cohesion scores, thanks to the fact that their links with *other* sentences can be taken into consideration. This can be seen by applying a threshold of just one link: this assigns a score of two bonds to sentence 1 (two links with 3 + one link with 4), but only one bond to sentences 3 and 4, both of which link with 1. Sentence 2, since it has no links at all, fails to register any bonds.

In the course of his research Hoey analysed many texts by this method and in the majority of cases coherent abridgements were created. The link–bond ratio exemplified above is, as stated earlier, far lower than that employed by Hoey and is set at this level for illustrative purposes only.

9.2 Automating the abridgement

In a project at the University of Birmingham carried out in collaboration with British Telecom (see Renouf & Collier 1995) the approach outlined above was developed into a working software suite for the abridgement of electronic text. Within the limits of the project it was only possible to incorporate the two simplest forms of repetition, simple and complex lexical repetition, into the software, as well as offering the user the opportunity of opening a "window" of sentences on to the text whenever a pronoun was encountered in the abridgement; insufficient time was available to us to incorporate the real-world knowledge which would link *John Major* and *prime minister* and the inclusion (manually) of the more simple thesaural links brought only a minor improvement in the results. It may be said that what the software lacked in sophistication it made up for in speed. In a matter of seconds the software created a matrix like the one shown above for a complete newspaper article of 30 to 40 sentences; Hoey's manual approach required many hours of painstaking examination of the text.

Once the matrix has been generated it can be manipulated by selecting a link threshold and calculating the number of bonds for each sentence. Creating an abridgement is then simply a case of setting a *bond* threshold which results in the required number of sentences. Thanks to the fully automated nature of the process, adjusting the link or bond thresholds is a straightforward task, enabling different combinations of parameters to be tried until the optimal result is obtained.

Despite the cruder nature of this method, satisfactory results were produced for a wide range of texts, in that the key sentences identified by the system still tended to reflect a large proportion of the rest of the text.

9.3 The need for automatic selection

In the past decade, the size of corpora has increased significantly. Until relatively recently a typical corpus (based on those such as the LOB (Hofland & Johansson 1982) and the Brown corpus (Kucera & Francis 1967)) amounted to around a million tokens. The task of generating concordances might well have been performed non-interactively, possibly overnight, resulting in a printout representing all the contexts of the type selected, sorted according to the desired criteria. For all but the most frequent types this printout would amount to no more than a few pages, which researchers could easily spread out for inspection and thus gain an overview of the grammatical and collocational behaviour of the word under scrutiny.

There are two main reasons why this approach is not feasible for today's corpora. First, the size of the corpus, which is now measured in tens or hundreds of millions of tokens, has greatly increased the frequency of each type. Second, the working methods of the researchers have evolved to take advantage of the technological benefits now available, such as instant concordance generation and immediate resorting of the concordance lines based on any position relative to the node word. It is now expected that these operations take place on-line at the computer screen.

These factors combine to reduce the overview of a type's behaviour available to the corpus researcher: the amount of data to be presented increases constantly, whereas, paradoxically it may seem, the area in which it can be displayed has shrunk to the size of a computer screen. As corpus size constantly increases the first dimension will continue to increase; by comparison the second dimension, unless we are soon to witness astounding advances in VDU technology, will continue to be a limiting factor to the accessibility of corpus data. This is the point at which the work done on textual abridgement becomes of relevance to the problem.

9.4 Applying lexical cohesion

As the number of concordance lines continues to increase, some method is required which restores the overview of the patterns present. Otherwise, the full benefit will never be reaped from the continued increase in corpus size. The development of a system which automatically selects concordance lines which carry information redolent of the information carried by other lines would be very valuable in combating the problems associated with large corpora. Such a system would in effect extend the notion of centrality from sentences in a text to individual concordance lines within a set of lines. As well as changing in extent, centrality would no longer be defined in terms of propositional or semantic ties but rather in terms of the linguistic ties which exist between members of a concordance set.

The way in which the abridgement methodology can be applied to this problem lies in treating the set of concordance lines for a type as a "text" in which each line is equivalent to a sentence. This is a novel approach for several reasons:

- In Hoey's approach grammatical items were largely excluded from the analysis; here it is essential to include these, since they play a highly significant role in the definition of recurrent patterns.
- We are not dealing with "normal" text, but rather with a composite set of contexts whose only connection, in terms of the way that they are extracted from the corpus, is that they all exemplify the same word.
- A corollary of this is that we cannot expect concordance lines to be cohesive together in the way that the sentences of a text are, yet some relationship clearly does exist between the members of a concordance set. It is this relationship, and the way in which it impinges on the centrality of particular lines, which we wish to define.

From an information retrieval perspective, we could talk of a central line as being one which is informationally rich and useful in providing an "abridgement" of other lines with similar but possibly less "concentrated" features. Put in lexicographical terms, such lines would be candidates for use as examples in a dictionary definition, since they would display some important aspect of the headword that the lexicographer wished to convey to the dictionary user.

The approach which has been taken therefore is to process the set of concordances and build a connectivity matrix by means of the abridgement software. A bond score is then assigned to each concordance line, the hypothesis being that the more central members of the concordance set will score more highly.

There are a number of procedural differences between this approach and that used for creating textual abridgements:

- In the current configuration of the software no lemmatization takes place. Since there are already a large number of variables in place it was felt that lemmatization would add further complexity which might hide important information about the links between individual concordance lines. Naturally, this does not preclude its inclusion at a later stage, once the selection process is better understood.
- Since the underlying system was originally designed to look at *lexical* cohesion, a certain number of grammatical words are automatically disregarded by the system, but the number and nature of these "stopwords" is user-definable when the software is run. One interesting contrast is obtained by comparing the output when first a functionally defined list (e.g. all pronouns, articles and prepositions) and then a frequency-based list (the most frequent 100 words from the corpus) are supplied as stopwords. Of course, this flexibility introduces yet another parameter to the system, which at present offers over a hundred different configurations based on the stopword list, the size of the span and the positional notation employed.

The various parameters involved in the process are described below, but first it may be useful to introduce an example. Figure 9.1 shows a concordance set for the node *kin.*[1]

```
(1) barrier excuses.  As for the "kith and kin" appeal, to quote the Reverend Arth
(2) id. "And I'm sure the cattle's next of kin have been informed but is that quit
(3) ted backing of France for her kith and kin in Algeria and for her Army protec
(4) earted commitment towards our kith and kin overseas." Identity of "race, langu
(5) f they do lecture their white kith and kin rather than the guerrillas, it is p
(6) e a narrow view of who is our kith and kin. Religion very properly tends to em
(7) been seeing to that.  The only next of kin seems to be a cousin in Droitwich.
(8) l kindness toward him, they're not his kin.... That's exactly the feeling. Old
(9) and her property passes to her next of kin under the intestacy rules. That me
```

Figure 9.1 *Concordance set for the node* kin.

If this is provided as input to the system with the links-per-bond threshold set to 1 the output shown in Figure 9.2 is obtained.

```
4 (1) barrier excuses. As for the "kith and kin" appeal, to quote the Reverend Arth
4 (3) ted backing of France for her kith and kin in Algeria and for her Army protec
4 (4) earted commitment towards our kith and kin overseas." Identity of "race, langu
4 (5) f they do lecture their white kith and kin rather than the guerrillas, it is p
4 (6) e a narrow view of who is our kith and kin. Religion very properly tends to em
2 (2) id. "And I'm sure the cattle's next of kin have been informed but is that quit
2 (7) been seeing to that. The only next of kin seems to be a cousin in Droitwich.
2 (9) and her property passes to her next of kin under the intestacy rules. That me
```

Figure 9.2 *Concordance set with links-per-bond threshold set to 1.*

Here the first number on the line indicates the number of bonds that have been identified, whereby any line which fails to bond is omitted. The second number is simply the line number as shown in Figure 9.1. From this simple example the functionality of the system becomes apparent:

- The somewhat atypical line (8) has been dropped because it obtained a bond score of zero and any line failing to form any bonds is excluded from the output.
- The most common pattern of *kith and kin* has been raised to prominence.
- The slightly less common pattern *next of kin* follows closely behind.

As noted earlier, there is one major difference between the central lines in the set of concordances and the central sentences in a conventional text: the central sentences selected by the textual abridgement system are expected to be coherent, i.e. to make sense together; this does not apply in the concordance line scenario, where the expectation is rather that they will have particular linguistic features in common. Naturally, each line in a set of concordances for a given type will contain at least one occurrence of the node word and, not surprisingly, this is actually discarded by the system, since it would introduce one extra link in every line with all other lines. This leads us to the question of what is actually detected as a "feature".

1. Examples are by courtesy of the Birmingham Collection of English Texts (BCET), a corpus of around 20 million tokens of fiction, non-fiction and journalism built at the University of Birmingham in the mid-1980s. See Renouf (1987).

9.5 Lexical cohesion meets collocation

A number of statistical measures have been developed or adapted to rank the collocates of a node word in order of significance (Z-score, MI-score and *t*-score for example) and systems now exist that apply these measures to a set of concordances to produce an overview of the most significant collocates on a position-by-position basis for each slot relative to the node (one to the left, one to the right, two to the left, two to the right, . . .), enabling a picture of the typical environment of the node *in terms of a particular position* to be built up. While there is nothing inherently wrong with these measures, the method by which they are applied to the data tends to tell us little about the more general patterns which occur in concordance lines because they measure the significance of finding a particular word in a particular position. Some attempts have been made to tie the most significant collocates back to the line from which they came, but this tends to become statistically and computationally complex. The method put forward here avoids statistical measures completely and relies upon the raw frequency of occurrence of the recurrent features.

A recurrent feature can be defined in a number of ways depending on the parameters passed to the software:

- *Simple lexical repetition*: This is exemplified in the above example of the *kin* concordances, where the collocate *kith* is identified as occurring somewhere in the context. No attempt is made to pinpoint the location of the collocate relative to the node word.
- *Position relative to the node*: This is a slightly more strict definition of the position of the collocate, in which it is merely specified whether it occurs before or after the node. This would detect features such as phrasal verbs, where the constituent verb and particle do not always maintain a fixed positional relationship.
- *Absolute position*: Here the exact location of the collocate is recorded. In order to count as a link between two lines it must therefore occur in precisely the same location relative to the node in the two lines. By opting for this positional notation and setting a higher link threshold it becomes possible to identify, for example, lines which contain instances of fixed phrases.

9.6 Conclusion

The work described here has grown out of the author's interest in collocational patterns and the concordancing of large corpora. The combination of this interest with work undertaken on the creation of automatic abridgements has led to this attempt to investigate the link between abridgements of real texts and the selection of "central" or "representative" concordance lines. Many different sets of concordances have been processed and the results are, if nothing else, always indicative of the recurrent patterns in the environment of the node word.

To some extent, the correspondence between a line's bond score and its "real" centrality remains a matter of interpretation, for few humans agree on what is a "good" concordance line. On the whole, however, the results accord with linguistic intuitions and blind tests on a group of Birmingham lexicographers demonstrated a high degree of overlap between those lines which scored highly and those considered to be good candidates for inclusion in a dictionary as illustrative citations. It has proved difficult to validate the results at anything beyond this purely intuitive evaluation, since there are no accepted and reliable automatic means of carrying out the analysis described here. It can only be added that output from software tools described earlier, which are designed to point the lexicographer towards the frequently recurring features of a set of concordances, serves to reinforce the centrality of the lines flagged as "central" by this system.

References

Halliday, M. A. K. & R. Hasan 1976. *Cohesion in English.* London: Longman.

Hoey, M. P. 1991. *Patterns of lexis in text.* London: Oxford University Press.

Hofland, K. & S. Johansson 1982. *Word frequencies in British and American English.* Bergen: Norwegian Computing Centre for the Humanities / Harlow, England: Longman.

Kucera, H. & W. N. Francis 1967. *Computational analysis of present day American English*, Providence, RI: Brown University Press.

Renouf, A. J. 1987. Corpus development. In *Looking up*, J. M. Sinclair (ed.), 1–40. London: HarperCollins.

Renouf, A. & A. J. Collier 1995. A system of automatic textual abridgement. In *AI '95: Fifteenth International Conference, Language Engineering '95*, Montpellier, 395–408.

10

A machine learning approach to anaphoric reference

DENNIS CONNOLLY, JOHN D. BURGER
AND DAVID S. DAY

10.1 Introduction

This paper describes research into the application of machine learning techniques to the resolution of anaphoric reference. While a number of theories have been proposed for certain classes of anaphors (e.g. centring: Brennan et al. 1987; Grosz & Sidner 1986), reference resolution remains a difficult problem in the general case and continues to be a major hurdle on the critical path to robust, end-to-end language processing. In this research, we have attempted to cast anaphoric reference as a classification problem for which a classifier can be discovered empirically using traditional learning methods.

One of the goals of this work is to embed reference resolution into the framework of "text understanding in the large", as exemplified by such recent efforts as the Message Understanding Conferences, as well as the current interest in corpus-based approaches to language learning. We are thus interested in determining some empirical performance baselines for the anaphoric reference task. Very little work has been done in this area, except for Walker's (1989) comparison of several algorithms, specifically centring, and the so-called Hobbs algorithm (Hobbs 1976). Though worthwhile, that comparison was not done with automatic methods. Rather, the algorithms in question were executed by hand, presumably with perfect information and fidelity. Thus, the results cannot be compared directly with approaches that operate in the noisy, uncertain world of large-scale, free-text processing.

We believe that our work has demonstrated that an empirical approach can perform on a par with carefully hand-crafted algorithms when it is applied to the output of mechanized free-text parsing. Of equal importance, it has established a baseline for the quantitative evaluation of discourse processing algorithms embedded in real systems. Finally, the learning component of this research has identified issues of import to a more general class of learning problems and has resulted in new classification algorithms that are better suited to such problems than many common alternatives. In particular, this research has led to the development of novel learning techniques designed to address the combination of high dimensionality, sparse data and violated independence assumptions inherent in the reference problem. The pre-eminent role played by these considerations in achieving our current performance leads us to expect even greater improvements with further work along this dimension.

10.2 Resolving anaphoric reference using classifiers

An anaphoric reference such as a pronoun or definite description is a reference to an entity introduced previously in a discourse. For our purposes, these are objects introduced by previous noun phrases in the text. Previous anaphors do not introduce new entities into the discourse since they refer to previously introduced entities. Each unique entity introduced into the text preceding an anaphor is a candidate for resolving that anaphor. Resolving an anaphoric reference requires choosing the best such candidate.

In order to apply machine learning techniques to the selection of the best candidate, we must identify a well-defined problem that is suited to the learning technique. For most learning algorithms, this is a classification problem. Casting our candidate selection problem in terms of classification introduces a number of difficulties, however. The most obvious way to proceed is to define each candidate as a class and to define selection of a best candidate as assignment of the current anaphor to one of these classes. This approach, however, suffers from several severe difficulties. First, the number of classes is very large and varies from problem to problem. Second, it is not clear how to model interactions between candidates.

Another approach, explored in earlier work (Burger & Connolly 1992), uses probabilistic classifiers that determine whether a candidate is a good referent for an anaphor. That is, the classifier is trained on anaphor–candidate pairs grouped into positive and negative examples of correct reference. Since the numeric result of such a classification has well-defined semantics, namely, the probability that the candidate is the correct referent, one can choose the candidate that is assigned the highest confidence by the classifier. This approach, however, assumes high accuracy of the confidence numbers generated by the classifier, and is still unable to model dependencies between candidates.

The approach adopted in the current research is to decompose the candidate selection problem into separate two-class classification problems. Each classification problem is defined on a pair of candidates and an anaphor, where the classes correspond to choosing one of the candidates as a "better" referent for that anaphor. By applying this classifier to successive pairs of candidates, each time retaining the best candidate, we can effectively sort the candidates, thus choosing the best overall. In the absence of the rather strong assumption of transitivity, of course, the selected candidate is not guaranteed to be best, even when classification is perfect, and the procedure is more accurately viewed as a greedy heuristic search.

The classification itself is performed on a discrete-valued feature space. Instances are represented as attribute–value vectors, where attributes describe properties of the anaphor and the two candidates, and relationships between the three. The attributes currently used are described in Figure 10.1. The class attribute is a Boolean identifying which of the two candidates is "better". Training instances are generated by pairing the correct candidate for each anaphor (i.e. the candidate that resolves the anaphor) with every other candidate for that anaphor. Each of these training instances

- **Anaphor-Type**, **Candidate1-Type**, **Candidate2-Type**. Pronoun or definite description.
- **Anaphor-Gram**, **Candidate1-Gram**, **Candidate2-Gram**. Grammatical case: Subject, verb object, prepositional object, other.
- **Recency1**, **Recency2**. Distance from anaphor to each candidate: Zero, one, near, far.[1]
- **More-Recent1**. Whether Candidate 1 is more recent than Candidate 2.
- **Agree-Count1**, **Agree-Count2**. Whether the anaphor and candidate agree in count.
- **Agree-Gender1**, **Agree-Gender2**. Whether the anaphor and candidate agree in gender.[2]
- **Agree-KR1**, **Agree-KR2**. The anaphor's meaning subsumes that of a candidate.[3]

Figure 10.1 *Fifteen features used by pairwise classifiers.*

1. "Zero" means same sentence as the anaphor; "one" means the previous sentence, within the same paragraph; "near" means two or three sentences distant, or the previous sentence, in a different paragraph. All else is "far".
2. Nouns whose meaning indicates a person agree with gendered pronouns such as *he* and *she*, as well as "gender-free" pronouns such as *they*.
3. With respect to the system's lexicon and knowledge representation.

is labelled such that the correct candidate is deemed the better one. In order to avoid teaching the classifier that one position of the pair is to be preferred, each candidate pair is in fact presented twice, with the candidate's positions exchanged (and the class attribute reversed).

Once a classifier has been constructed, it is used by the reference resolution algorithm to select the best candidate using the following strategy. An initial instance is constructed by taking the anaphor and the first two candidates. This instance is given to the classifier, which indicates which candidate is the better one. The "losing" candidate is discarded, and another instance is constructed by pairing the "winner" with the next candidate. The new instance is now given to the classifier, which selects a new winner (which could be the same as the previous winner). This process continues until every candidate has been examined. The last winner is then chosen as the anaphor's referent. In our experiments, candidates are presented to the classifier in linear order, either farthest from the anaphor to closest, or *vice versa.* It turns out that there is very little difference in performance between these two alternatives, and the results we shall present are based upon farthest-to-closest order. That is, the first two candidates in the text form the first pair presented to the classifier.

As an example, consider the following text:

> Last spring [Dupont]$_1$ established [a joint venture in [Shanghai]$_2$ to manufacture [rice herbicides]$_3$]$_4$. Located in [Pudong]$_5$, [a suburb of [Shanghai]$_6$]$_7$ which [the Chinese]$_8$ are trying to promote as [a development zone]$_9$, [the project]$_{10}$ was [the first involving foreign participation in [the area]$_{11}$]$_{12}$.

This fragment contains a total of twelve discourse entities, as identified by the natural language processor. Entities 10 and 11 are anaphors, with the correct referents being 4 and 5, respectively. If training data were being derived from this example, anaphor 10 would have nine possible candidates. Thus eight candidate pairs would be generated as training instances, in which the correct referent, entity 4, would be paired with the eight incorrect candidates:[4]

(4, 1), (4, 2), (4, 3), (4, 5), (4, 6), (4, 7), (4, 8), (4, 9)

Note that this is an extremely naïve algorithm, in that, for each anaphor, *all previously introduced candidates* are examined. This means that, for a reasonable article, the last anaphor may be compared to several hundred candidates. This is patently incorrect, but we have left undisturbed the problem of determining which candidates are to be considered "active" for a given anaphor. Another consequent of this algorithm is that until the real referent is presented to the classifier, it does not matter which candidate the algorithm keeps. In particular, since the correct candidate is likely to be fairly close to the anaphor, most of the decisions made by the classifier are between two incorrect candidates.

4. In fact, for reasons of symmetry noted above, twice as many instances would be generated.

10.3 Experimental methodology

In the experiments discussed in this paper, training and testing sets were drawn from a corpus of 80 news-agency articles (approximately 35 000 words) annotated by hand with reference links. All input features were automatically determined by a natural language understanding system. Thus, there was some noise in the input features in both the training and testing sets.

The training and testing sets were disjoint. Each was composed of 40 articles. This corresponds to approximately 450 anaphoric references in each set, with pronouns and definite descriptions occurring with approximately the same frequency.[5] Because of the naïvety of the resolution algorithm, the average number of candidates per anaphor in the testing set was approximately 80. As discussed above, the training set was actually composed of pairs constructed by grouping the correct candidate for each anaphor with the other potential (but incorrect) candidates. This derived training set constituted approximately 60 000 such pairs.

10.4 Explorations in classification

Having described the classification problem, we must construct a classifier suited to the problem. The major thrust of this work is to explore the construction of these classifiers from empirical data. We have also, however, constructed hand-crafted reference-resolution algorithms in order to validate and better illustrate issues raised by the empirical approach. As we shall see, a major theme throughout this research is the management of dimensionality.

In order to construct a classifier that performs well in a given task, we must choose an appropriate bias. By this we mean a representation that is capable of representing the desired classes and is constrained in some way to avoid overfitting. Different classifiers have different biases. For example, perceptrons represent classes using a single hyperplane in feature space, while decision trees can be thought of as multiple surfaces that are orthogonal to the dimensions of the space.

In our anaphoric reference research, we have explored a number of classifiers and corresponding biases. The performance achieved for reference resolution by each of these classifiers is shown in Table 10.1. In the discussion that follows, we will see that an examination of limitations inherent in the biases of the simpler algorithms accounts for their substandard performance and has motivated new insights that account for the improvements in the more complex classifiers.

---

5. Note that only those pronouns and definite references annotated as anaphoric were processed as such. We thus ignored the problem of determining whether phrases such as *the world* are strictly anaphoric.

Table 10.1 Results of various reference algorithms.

	Percentage correct		
	All references	Definites	Pronouns
Posterior classifier	20.4	7.9	32.7
Bayesian classifier	23.7	11.2	35.9
Hybrid Bayesian	40.0	25.2	52.5
Decision tree	40.6	31.8	49.3
Hybrid decision tree	41.1	30.4	51.6
Neural net	40.6	28.9	52.1
Neural net (subspace trained)	46.4	37.4	55.3
Hand-crafted algorithm	38.7	25.7	51.6

10.4.1 Simple classifiers

Posterior classifier

This is perhaps the simplest classifier. It is constructed by estimating the posterior probability of the classes $\mathrm{P}(class|features)$ directly from relative frequencies observed in the training set and selecting the class with the highest probability. Clearly the abysmal performance reported in Table 10.1 is an indication of the overfitting one would expect when trying to estimate the complete joint distribution of a 16-dimensional space from a sample of mere tens of thousands of instances.

Simple Bayesian classifier

By assuming independence of features and employing Bayes's law, we can address dimensionality by estimating only the likelihood of individual features $\mathrm{P}(F_i|class)$, and priors $\mathrm{P}(class)$ from the data. The posterior probability is computed as (1).

$$(1)\quad \mathrm{P}(class|features) = \alpha \prod_i \mathrm{P}(F_i|class)\mathrm{P}(class)$$

The major weakness here is the assumption of independence that sanctions us to estimate joint probabilities as products of individual probabilities. We believe from knowledge of the domain that this assumption is flawed (e.g. pronouns are more likely to be used when referring to recent mentions) and the results in Table 10.1 seem to bear this out.

C4.5 decision trees

This is Quinlan's (1993) well-known decision tree algorithm, which is essentially the latest version of ID3. The most noteworthy feature of C4.5 for this discussion is that it orders features by an information-theoretic criterion and that pruning is performed on the resulting tree. Paths to leaves in the resulting tree capture joint probabilities of the most informative features. This allows us to address the dimensionality issue without assuming independence.

Neural networks

This is the standard back-propagation algorithm (Rumelhart et al. 1986). As seen in Table 10.1 this approach performs substantially better than some of the other simple approaches. We will have more to say about this later.

10.4.2 Hand-crafted algorithms

The hand-crafted algorithms explored in this research are quite different from the classifiers in that they do not compare pairs of candidates, nor do they examine every candidate. Instead, they take the form of a decision list, each entry of which describes the next anaphor–candidate pair to examine. For example, a very simple decision list is detailed in Figure 10.2. This decision list encodes the following algorithm:

1. Choose the first candidate in the same sentence as the anaphor that agrees in count and gender.
2. **If** there is no such candidate, **then** choose the first one in the same sentence that agrees in count.
3. **Else** choose the first in the *previous* sentence that agrees in count and gender.
4. **Else** choose the first in the previous sentence that agrees in count.
5. **Else** choose the first candidate in the same sentence as the anaphor.
6. **Else** if no candidate meets *any* of the above descriptions, fail.

Recency=Zero,	Agree-Count=Yes,	Agree-Gender=Yes
Recency=Zero,	Agree-Count=Yes	
Recency=One,	Agree-Count=Yes,	Agree-Gender=Yes
Recency=One,	Agree-Count=Yes	
Recency=Zero		

Figure 10.2 *A decision list for reference resolution.*

The decision list in Figure 10.2 has performance near that shown in Table 10.1 *for pronouns only*. In order to achieve even the moderate levels shown in Table 10.1 for all anaphors, a much more complicated decision list was used, with approximately 50 entries.

10.4.3 Hybrid classifiers

When examining the simple classifiers described above, we notice that there is an interplay between dimensionality and independence. By assuming independence, the simple Bayesian classifier addresses the issue of dimensionality, while by explicitly capturing joint probabilities, the posterior classifier and C4.5 address problems where independence does not hold.

We can envision classification problems as residing on a continuum as depicted in Figure 10.3. At one extreme are problems characterized by low dimensionality but exhibiting strong dependencies between features. These are problems that are well suited to the posterior classifier. At the other extreme are problems that have high dimensionality but in which the features are independent. These problems are better suited to the Bayesian classifier.

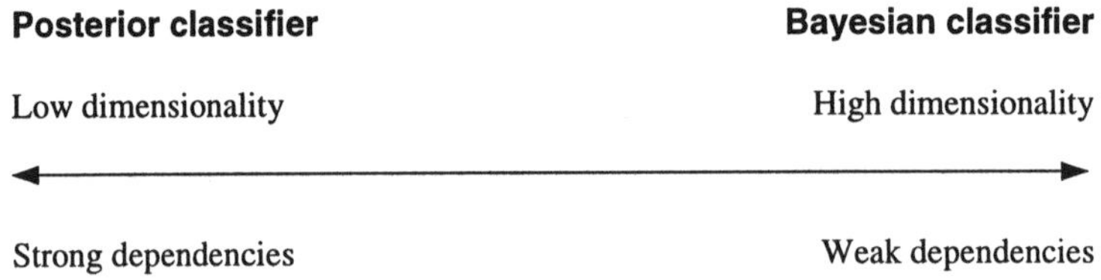

Figure 10.3 *A continuum of classifiers.*

In many real-world problems, however, neither extreme accurately describes the situation. In a large class of problems, there are strong dependencies between some features, but not all. Furthermore, while the dimensionality of the entire feature space may be high, the dimensionality of the subspaces of features that have strong dependencies may be low. In such problems, both classifiers can be expected to perform poorly: the Bayesian classifier because of violated independence assumptions, the posterior classifier because of overfitting. The decision tree goes some way toward addressing this class of problems by explicitly capturing joint probabilities and reducing dimensionality via pruning. This is at the expense of completely discarding features, however.

In order to address these issues, we have been investigating a new class of classifier that attempts to combine important features of both the posterior classifier and the Bayesian classifier. In this model of classifier, we attempt to represent dependencies between features that do exhibit dependence, while exploiting the independence between those features that *are* independent in order to reduce dimensionality. Such classifiers may be viewed as "hybrid" classifiers, which reside in the middle of the continuum in Figure 10.3. We now describe some experiments that we have conducted to explore simple ways of constructing such hybrid classifiers.

The first experiment, referred to as the "hybrid Bayesian" in Table 10.1, attempted to mediate heuristically the trade-off between independence and statistical significance of groups of features. In this experiment, we made use of domain knowledge to partition the features into independent groups. This resulted in a simple partition containing two groups of features. In the first group, we placed all agreement features (e.g. count agreement, gender agreement, etc.). The other group contained all of the remaining features. Alternatively, one could use techniques such as those described in Connolly (1993) to cluster features automatically using a criterion such as mutual information. The important thing is that features in each group are approximately conditionally independent of features in other groups when conditioned upon class. The other component of this heuristic approach is the use of a threshold on observed event counts for features and groups of features to approximate statistical significance. A more principled approach would be to use statistical significance tests.

Putting these elements together, we can construct a simple hybrid classifier as follows. From our training set, we record counts of observed events corresponding to entire feature vectors, individual features (conjoined with class), and groups of dependent features defined by the partition described above. From these, we can compute relative frequencies used to estimate conditional probabilities and examine event counts used to estimate significance. When a new instance is to be classified, we compare the observed event count for the instance with a threshold. If the count exceeds the threshold, we may estimate the posterior probability directly as in the posterior classifier. Otherwise, we compare the counts for the groups of features defined by the partition to the threshold. If these both exceed the threshold, the conditional probability of each group of features conditioned upon class is estimated from recorded frequencies and the results are multiplied together with the prior probability (also estimated from recorded frequencies), yielding (2), an estimate for the posterior probability.

$$(2)\ \mathrm{P}(class|features) = \alpha \prod_k \mathrm{P}(partition_k|class)\mathrm{P}(class)$$

This is essentially the simple Bayesian classifier modified by replacing individual features with composite features defined by the partition. If either of the groups of features is below threshold, the product of the conditional probabilities for the individual features contained in the group are used. If, for example, the *k*th partition containing *j* features does not exceed the threshold, the posterior probability would be (3).

$$(3)\ \mathrm{P}(class|features) = \alpha \prod_j \mathrm{P}(F_j|class) \prod_{k-1} \mathrm{P}(partition_k|class)\mathrm{P}(class)$$

If no partitions exceed threshold, all composite features are replaced by their individual features and the model reduces to the simple Bayesian classifier already seen, (1).

This hybrid classifier then subsumes both the simple posterior classifier and the simple Bayesian classifier. As seen in Table 10.1, even this simple hybrid approach dramatically outperforms both of these simple classifiers when applied to reference resolution.

10.4.4 Hybrid neural networks

As seen in Table 10.1, neural network classifiers perform as well as the hybrid classifiers. This leads us to ask whether neural networks somehow already incorporate some of the ideas described above, or rather benefit from a different set of strengths related to their representational bias. If the latter is the case, it may be possible to enhance their performance further by incorporating some of the insights engendered by the hybrid approach.

A distinguishing feature of the representation found in neural nets is the ability to represent decision surfaces that are not orthogonal to the dimensions of the space. This characteristic can be advantageous in high-dimensional problems since it affords the ability to discover decision surfaces that effectively represent linear combinations of primitive features. This may well account for the relatively higher level of performance exhibited by the neural network on the reference problem. Neural networks are not immune to problems of high dimensionality, however, and are perfectly capable of overfitting data, especially when a large number of hidden units are employed.

In the probabilistic classifiers, including the hybrid classifiers, the primary means of combating dimensionality was by exploiting independence between features. In neural networks it is not immediately obvious how to take advantage of this because of the absence of clear semantics provided by probability theory.

In order to exploit independence in neural networks, let us more closely examine how high dimensionality can cause overfitting in such networks. In the case of the posterior classifier or decision trees, the relationship between high dimensionality and overfitting is clear. Additional features result in smaller cells in feature space and relatively fewer samples in any one cell. By assuming independence we combine the much larger counts in larger cells using multiplication.

The effect of dimensionality on neural networks is a little more subtle. An algorithm such as back-propagation is searching through a space of decision-surface orientations using data to guide the search (i.e. move the decision surface to reduce discrimination error). Higher dimensionality increases the number of degrees of freedom in the movement of these decision surfaces. This allows a few sample points to affect the orientation of a surface in a subspace slice that in a lower dimension would contain more samples.

From this perspective, a handle begins to emerge on how to think about independence in neural networks. Groups of features that are independent should effect the orientation of decision surfaces in their corresponding subspaces independently of the changes of orientation in other subspaces. By searching for orientations in subspaces we can mitigate the effect of the high dimensionality of the containing space.

This then forms the basis of a new classifier, which we refer to as "subspace-trained" (SST) neural network classifiers. Like the hybrid probabilistic classifiers described earlier, these classifiers manage high dimensionality by exploiting independence between features. This is accomplished by training separately in subspaces defined by the independent feature partitions, described earlier. Specifically, new training instances are formed by projecting each original training instance onto these feature partitions and these new instances are presented to the back-propagation regimen. This is essentially equivalent to presenting each original instance once for each feature partition, each time freezing the weights not associated with that partition. Another way of looking at this new training regime is to view training data in a more general way than we have heretofore: training instances play the role of constraints on the search through the space of decision-surface orientations. The results shown in Table 10.1 demonstrate that this approach opens a very promising avenue of research.

10.5 Conclusion

This research has demonstrated that an empirical approach can perform on a par with carefully hand-crafted algorithms when applied to the output of mechanized free-text parsing. Of equal importance, it has established a baseline for the quantitative evaluation of discourse processing algorithms embedded in real systems. Finally, the learning component of this research has identified issues of import to a more general class of learning problems and has resulted in new classification algorithms that are better suited to such problems than are many common alternatives. The pre-eminent role played by these considerations in achieving our current performance leads us to expect even greater improvements with further work along this dimension.

References

Brennan, S. E., M. W. Friedman & C. J. Pollard 1987. A centering approach to pronouns. In *Proceedings of the 25th Annual Meeting of the Association for Computational Linguistics*, 155–62. Stanford, Calif.

Burger, J. D. & D. Connolly 1992. Probabilistic resolution of anaphoric reference. In *Probabilistic Approaches to Natural Language: Papers from the 1992 Fall Symposium*, Menlo Park, Calif., 17–24; also appeared as Technical Report TR FS–92–04, AAAI Press.

Connolly, D. 1993. Constructing hidden variables in bayesian networks via conceptual clustering. In *Proceedings of the Tenth International Workshop on Machine Learning*, 65–72. Amherst, Mass.

Grosz, B. J. & C. L. Sidner 1986. Attention, intentions, and the structure of discourse. *Computational Linguistics* **12**, 175–204.

Hobbs, J. R. 1976. *A computational approach to discourse analysis*. Technical Report 76-2, Department of Computer Science, City University of New York.

Quinlan, J. R. 1993. *C4.5: programs for machine learning*. San Mateo, Calif.: Morgan Kaufmann.

Rumelhart, D., G. Hinton & R. Williams 1986. Learning internal representations by error propagation. In *Parallel distributed processing: explorations in the microstructure of cognition. Vol. 1: Foundations*, D. Rumelhart, J. L. McClelland & the PDP Group (eds), 318–62. Cambridge, Mass.: MIT Press.

Walker, M. A. 1989. Evaluating discourse processing algorithms. In *Proceedings of the 27th Annual Meeting of the Association for Computational Linguistics*, 251–61. Vancouver.

11
Some methods for the extraction of bilingual terminology

ÉRIC GAUSSIER AND JEAN-MARC LANGÉ[1]

11.1 Introduction

Terminology is becoming an essential asset in today's industry, not only because it somehow represents part of the "memory" of a particular company, but also because of its use in different areas, such as the documentation of products. As industrial activities are becoming increasingly international, terminology becomes multilingual.

However, the process of acquisition of terminology is an expert task, which only highly trained specialists can undertake. The process is also very slow, and terminology work is therefore quite expensive.

We want to address here a way to automate partially the process of bilingual terminology acquisition. Our approach is to identify potential terms monolingually in a first step, and then to find equivalences of terms across languages.

Starting with a parallel bilingual (French–English) corpus tagged with parts-of-speech and lemmas, we can extract certain noun phrases which are likely to be terms

1. This work was partially funded under European project EUROTRA ET-10/63.

in both French and English. The main lines of this extraction process are given in Section 11.2. We then address the problem of translating terms with the help of statistical measures which are described in Section 11.3. Finally, an evaluation of the different measures is given in Section 11.4.

11.2 Preliminary work: using linguistics to extract monolingual candidate terms

One obvious characteristic of terms in a technical text is the fact that they are often composed of several words (for example, *receiving antenna* or *diskette unit*). Moreover, the vast majority of terms are noun phrases, and as such they obey precise rules of morphosyntactic combination (for example, the two terms above follow the pattern N+N). One can therefore use relevant linguistic patterns in order to look for monolingual terms in a technical corpus: these patterns define the structure of multi-word units (MWUs) which are likely to be terms. We define the length of an MWU as the number of *main items* (nouns, adjectives, verbs or adverbs) it contains. Terms of length 1 correspond to words connected with either a hyphen or an apostrophe, and are easy to identify, or to single words (e.g. *telematics*) the identification of which is a different problem which we have not addressed. The study of MWUs of length 3 and more shows that most of them are built from MWUs of length 2 by either composition ([*side lobe*] *regrowth*), modification (*interfering* [*earth station*]), or coordination (*packet assembly/disassembly*). We thus focused our efforts on MWUs of length 2 which we will refer to as "base MWUs". Examples of patterns retained for the base MWUs are N+prep+N (*antenne de réception*) or N+Adj (*station terrienne*) in French, and N+N (*telecommunication satellite*) or Adj+N (*parabolic antenna*) in English. Details of this extraction of monolingual candidates can be found in Daille (1993) and Daille et al. (1994).

From a translational point of view, correspondences between base MWU patterns across languages do not follow precise rules. We can, however, pick up general trends, such as French base MWUs of structure N1+*de*+(det)+N2 regularly translate into English base MWUs of structure N2+N1 (*distance de séparation*↔*separation distance*); and, similarly, French base MWUs of structure N+Adj regularly translate into English base MWUs of structure Adj+N (*cornet pyramidal*↔*pyramidal horn*). But irregularities in pattern alignment do exist. These are of two types: the use of an alternative form (abbreviations, ellipsis) implying a break in the syntactic structure of the MWU on the one hand, and pattern switching as in (1), as opposed to the regularities pointed out above.

(1) [N1+*de*+N2] émetteur de Terre↔[Adj+N] terrestrial transmitter

We have not addressed the problem raised by abbreviations and ellipsis, which requires a specific independent treatment.

Given these linguistic specifications, we implemented a finite-state machine which allows the extraction of base MWU candidates in the form of lemma pairs. It has to be noted that these candidates are not always "good" terms but simply noun phrases (or parts of noun phrases) corresponding to specific linguistic patterns that are known to be term-productive. We thus obtain a list of about 4000 candidates for each language, from a 200 000-word bilingual corpus.

11.3 Candidate term translation

Since we want to extract bilingual terminology, the problem is now one of finding correspondences between candidates across languages (i.e. between English and French).

We make the following general assumptions:

(a) The translation of a source candidate belongs to the set of target candidates.

(b) We should be able to find the translation of a source term in texts which are translations of one another.

(c) We can restrict the preceding point, noting that if a source term appears in a sentence of the source text, then its translation is likely to appear in the corresponding sentence of the target text.

Therefore, we start from a parallel corpus, aligned at sentence level (Brown et al. 1991; Gale & Church 1993; Simard et al. 1992). Each pair (source sentence, target sentence) is called a "region". In a sentence, we only take into consideration candidate terms extracted by the above method. Typically, in a technical text, a pair of sentences, each of them containing about 20 words, contains 3 such terms monolingually.

If we have s candidates in the source sentence and t in the target, then we have $s \times t$ possibilities for finding term equivalence. The idea is to enumerate all possible pairs of candidate terms for all pairs of sentences in our corpus. One can hope that in the total corpus, strong associations such as (*receiving antenna*↔*antenne de réception*) will emerge.

In fact, we followed two methods to address this problem. In the first one, we proceeded as outlined above, counting all bilingual pairs of candidate terms found in aligned sentences. Nevertheless, we have experimental information about pattern transformations in the bilingual process, and thus introduce it in our model. In the second method, we first look for bilingual associations of single words, in the same way as we do for candidate terms. For a given pair of candidate terms, we then derive a measure from the scores of the single words composing the candidates.

11.3.1 First method

One of our goals was to test and evaluate the different statistical measures one can find in the literature. From both a mathematical study and monolingual tests, of fifteen measures we retain four that are relevant to our problem. These measures are: mutual information, ϕ^2 (Church & Hanks 1990), Fager and McGowan's coefficient (Clifford & Stephenson 1975) and the likelihood ratio test used in Dunning (1993), which we will call "Loglike". Most of these measures are the ones generally used in the field of computational linguistics, and are usually derived from contingency tables.

For each pair (source candidate term, target candidate term), we thus constructed a two-by-two contingency table, as in Church & Hanks (1990), and then computed the four scores obtained. The evaluation and comparison of these scores is given in the next subsection.

Nevertheless, we can try to improve this method by taking advantage of available linguistic information, namely the correspondences across languages between the part-of-speech patterns of the candidates (discussed above). Given a source–target pair of candidates, we use the term "pattern affinity" for the probability that the pattern of the source candidate gets translated into the pattern of the target candidates.

Using pattern affinities

In the preceding measures, each time a source–target pair is found in a region, its count is incremented by 1. But, when dealing with pattern affinities, the increment has to be weighted. It is not straightforward to build a measure relying on both pattern affinities and contingency tables. Fortunately, mutual information can be derived without contingency tables, as described in Brown et al. (1988). We used this latter computation to deal with pattern affinities.

In this computation of mutual information, when a source–target pair is found in a region of the text, its "count" is incremented by *1/Nbcand*, where *Nbcand* is the number of possible target candidates in the given region. This formula gives one way of estimating the probability of aligning the source item with a target item in a region of the text. We just rewrite this probability in order to take the patterns of MWUs into account, and derive a new increment for the "count" of the source–target pair.

Let s be the source item, t the target item, p_s and p_t the patterns for s and t. Since p_t and p_s are completely determined by t and s, we can write the probability P of t and s as in (2):

$$(2)\ P(t,s) = P(t,p_t,p_s,s)$$

which can be rewritten as in (3):

$$(3)\ P(t,s) = P(t|p_t,p_s,s) \times P(p_t|p_s,s) \times P(p_s|s) \times P(s)$$

We thus make the assumption that aligning t with s amounts to producing p_s knowing that we have s, then aligning p_t with p_s, and lastly producing t knowing p_t, motivated by the fact that our prior knowledge only consists of pattern affinities. Thus, the probability of aligning s with t in a region of the text can be approximated by (4).

$$(4)\ P(t|s) \simeq P(p_s|s) \times P(p_t|p_s) \times P(t|p_t)$$

Of course, $P(p_s|s) = 1$. In a region, the probability of producing t knowing p_t can be estimated by $C(t)/C(p_t)$, where $C(p_t)$ is the number of target items in the region that have pattern p_t and $C(t)$ is the number of times t is encountered in the region. The formula thus becomes (5).

$$(5)\ P(t|s) \simeq P(p_t|p_s) \times \frac{C(t)}{C(p_t)}$$

We estimated *a priori* pattern-alignment probabilities on a sample consisting of 10% of the candidate terms. But these probabilities do not deal with which region of text we are in. We therefore computed the pattern-alignment probabilities in the region following the maximum likelihood approach, and weighted these probabilities with the *a priori* probabilities. This yields the formula (6),

$$(6)\ P(p_t|p_s) = \frac{P_{ap}(p_t|p_s)}{\sum\limits_x P_{ap}(p_x|p_s)} \times \frac{C(p_t)}{C(p_x)}$$

where P_{ap} is the *a priori* probability. We finally obtain (7),

$$(7)\ P(t|s) = \frac{P_{ap}(p_t|p_s)}{\sum\limits_x P_{ap}(p_x|p_s)} \times \frac{C(t)}{C(p_x)}$$

a value that will be used to increment the score of the pair (s,t). It has to be noted that the above formulation verifies (8).

$$(8)\ \sum_{t \in \text{region}} P(t|s) = 1$$

11.3.2 Second method

When we look at a pair of terms such as *earth station↔station terrienne*, we intuitively feel that *earth* has a relation with *terrienne* and *station* with *station*. The question is: could we make use of single-word alignment to extract multi-word alignment?

The second method consists essentially of aligning terms using bilingual associations of single words that have previously been computed by statistical methods (as in Brown et al. 1988). The score used here is mutual information, which we refined to take the distance between words into account.

Let e_1 and e_2 denote the two words composing a given English candidate and, similarly, f_1 and f_2 those for a given French candidate. We make the assumption that if two candidates are translations of one another, then f_1 is likely to be the translation of either e_1 or e_2, and so is f_2. We also make the assumption that e_1 and e_2 are independent variables (and so are f_1 and f_2). This assumption seems reasonable for candidates which are not terms but is no more valid for candidates which are terms. Anyway, it has the advantage of simplicity and appeared to work well in practice.

Let $I(e; f)$ denote mutual information between the English word e and the French word f. We use the notations defined in Gallagher (1968). We have (9):

$$(9)\ I(e_1, e_2; f_1, f_2) = \log\left(\frac{P(e_1e_2|f_1f_2)}{P(e_1e_2)}\right)$$

As a result of our second assumption, we can write (10):

$$(10)\ \frac{P(e_1e_2|f_1f_2)}{P(e_1e_2)} \simeq \frac{P(e_1|f_1f_2) \times P(e_2|f_1f_2)}{P(e_1) \times P(e_2)}$$

and, thus (11):

$$(11)\ I(e_1, e_2; f_1, f_2) \simeq I(e_1; f_1, f_2) + I(e_2; f_1, f_2)$$

Finally, the same reasoning leads us to the measure in (12), which will be referred to as "double-assoc".

$$(12)\ I(e_1, e_2; f_1, f_2) \simeq I(e_1; f_1) + I(e_1; f_2) + I(e_2; f_1) + I(e_2; f_2)$$

11.3.3 Conclusion

We finally derived seven measures of associations between French and English candidate terms: mutual information computed from contingency tables, ϕ^2, Fager and McGowan's coefficient, a likelihood ratio test (referred to as "Loglike"), mutual information computed as in Brown et al. (1988) (referred to below as MI_{Brown}), this latter measure with pattern affinities (MI_{patt}), and "double-assoc".

11.4 Results

In order to perform an automatic evaluation of the output of the bilingual statistics programs, we built a reference list which contains source–target pairs of base MWUs. This list was constructed from an existing list established by terminologists in the field of telecommunications (as is our corpus). To ensure a high coverage of our candidates, we complemented, with the help of some colleagues, the existing list with the good pairs extracted from our corpus. The evaluation then consists in (automatically) comparing our candidate list with the reference list. For any list of candidate-pair alignments, we compute *precision*, defined as the ratio of the number of hits in the reference list to the total number of candidates tested (which shows the proportion of good candidates in our candidate list), and *recall*, defined as the ratio of the number of hits to the total number of reference items in the reference list (which indicates the completeness of our result).

Of course, precision and recall are quite dependent on the quality of the reference list. Since we do not claim to have built an exhaustive reference list, our results in terms of precision and recall will have to be taken relatively. This was the price we had to pay in order to have the possibility of performing fast cheap evaluation of different approaches.

On the other hand, our final goal is to provide terminologists with lists of terms and their translations; we know beforehand that no automated process can be perfect in that field, and that human post-editing is a necessity where high accuracy is required. Since our results will be of lower quality for low scores, we can improve the overall satisfaction of the human post-editor by setting thresholds in order to discard the less relevant candidates. Therefore, in our list of candidates sorted according to the particular score being evaluated, we will compute precision and recall for the first 100 elements, the first 200, and so on till the end.

We ran the bilingual statistics programs against the lists of monolingual base MWU candidates with a frequency of at least 2. We then applied the selection criterion described in Gaussier et al. (1992) to keep only the most relevant candidates. For each measure, we sorted the list of bilingual correspondences with decreasing scores and then evaluated precision and recall for this measure.

We will give here only the results for "Loglike", MI_{Brown}, MI_{patt} and "double-assoc". These measures clearly behave better than the others.

Table 11.1 summarizes the comparison of these measures. It shows for each measure the evolution of precision and recall with the number of candidates considered.

This brings us to the following observations.

11.4.1 Involving pattern affinities or not

If we compare the MI_{Brown} and MI_{patt} columns, we see that taking pattern affinities into account does not significantly improve the results, although for the top 100 elements precision increases from 90% to 94%, which is an appreciable gain. We believe that the slight difference between the results comes from the reliability of alignment counts, which are sufficient to leave all other parameters in the background. However, when the length of the lists increases, the scores of association decrease and so do the counts of the elements; then the difference between the two methods grows, in favour of the one involving pattern affinities.

11.4.2 The different measures of the first method

When we do not take pattern affinities into account, we observe that the measures give quite identical results for the topmost candidates. Anyway, the results obtained with "Loglike" degrade rapidly with the number of candidates. In fact, there is no ideal measure which is the best in the whole range of the candidates. For most of the measures we used, rare events are privileged. From this point of view "Loglike" is surely the most relevant in so far as it is able to deal realistically with rare events.

Table 11.1 Comparison of the measures.

Number of elements	First method						Second method	
	Without pattern				With pattern			
	"Loglike"		MI_{Brown}		MI_{patt}		"Double-assoc"	
	Precision	Recall	Precision	Recall	Precision	Recall	Precision	Recall
100	88.0	7.1	90.0	7.2	94.0	7.6	89.6	7.0
200	87.0	14.1	88.5	14.2	87.5	14.1	88.6	13.8
300	83.3	20.2	82.6	20.0	84.0	20.3	87.0	25.0
400	78.5	25.4	80.5	26.0	81.0	26.2	86.0	26.0
600	71.0	34.4	77.5	37.5	78.3	37.9	79.9	43.6
800	62.9	40.6	73.2	47.3	74.6	48.2	77.8	52.1
900	57.1	41.5	71.6	52.1	72.7	52.9	75.2	59.3
1000	52.5	42.4	66.2	53.4	70.4	56.8	73.0	61.0
1200	54.0	52.3	59.5	57.6	61.7	59.8	71.0	74.3
1500							65.9	84.6
1900							60.1	93.7

Nevertheless, most of the measures do not provide a simple way of dealing with pattern affinities, except MI_{Brown} of course. That is the reason why our preference goes to this latter measure.

11.4.3 First method vs. second method

The second method ("double-assoc") yielded more associations than the other. It behaves better for candidates of rank 1000 and more, but worse for the first 100 best candidates. In fact, the two methods emphasize quite different associations. If we consider the first 100 candidates obtained by each method, only 6 term pairs are common. Of course this could be because of the restriction to the very best candidates; but, suspecting that there is more to it, we combined the candidates from both methods: we obtained an improvement of precision in the whole range of candidates, which makes this mixed-blood approach the best one up till now.

11.5 Conclusion

The results we obtained are quite interesting: if we filter the topmost 500 candidates, we extract 80% of "good term associations". The methods we developed can thus provide efficient tools to which to submit lists of potential terms to terminologists.

It has to be noted that these methods involve statistical scores and linguistic information, which confirms the relevance of mixing statistics and linguistics in NLP. Furthermore, the methods involve prior steps that also make use of statistical methods: part-of-speech tagging and bilingual sentence alignment.

Of course, there is still a lot of work to be done. For example, we can no longer restrict ourselves to MWUs of length 2. We now have to extend the methods to candidates of length 3 or more, and to bilingual candidates of different lengths.

References

Brown, P. F., J. Cocke, S. A. DellaPietra, V. J. DellaPietra, F. Jelinek, R. L. Mercer & P. S. Roossin 1988. A statistical approach to language translation. In *COLING BUDAPEST: Proceedings of the 12th International Conference on Computational Linguistics*, Budapest, 71–6.

Brown, P. F., J. C. Lai & R. L. Mercer 1991. Aligning sentences in parallel corpora. In *Proceedings of the 29th Annual Meeting of the Association for Computational Linguistics*, Berkeley, Calif., 169–76.

Church, K. W. & P. Hanks 1990. Word association norms, mutual information, and lexicography. *Computational Linguistics* **16**, 22–9.

Clifford, H. T. & W. Stephenson 1975. *An introduction to numerical classification.* London: Academic Press.

Daille, B. 1993. Extraction automatique de terminologie monolingue. In *Colloque Informatique et Langue Naturelle*, Nantes, 81–101.

Daille, B., É. Gaussier & J.-M. Langé 1994. Towards automatic extraction of monolingual and bilingual terminology. In *COLING 94: The 15th International Conference on Computational Linguistics*, Kyoto, Japan, 515–21.

Dunning, T. 1993. Accurate methods for the statistics of surprise and coincidence. *Computational Linguistics* **19**, 61–74.

Gale, W. A. & K. W. Church 1993. A program for aligning sentences in bilingual corpora. *Computational Linguistics* **19**, 75–102.

Gallager, R. G. 1968. *Information theory and reliable communication.* New York: John Wiley.

Gaussier, É., J.-M. Langé & F. Meunier 1992. Towards bilingual terminology. In *Proceedings of the Joint ALLC/ACH Conference*, Oxford, 121–4.

Simard, M., G. F. Foster & P. Isabelle 1992. Using cognates to align sentences in bilingual corpora. In *Fourth International Conference on Theoretical and Methodological Issues in Machine Translation: TMI-92*, Montreal, 67–81.

12
Probabilistic part-of-speech tagging using decision trees

HELMUT SCHMID

12.1 Introduction

Word forms are often ambiguous in their part-of-speech (POS). The English word form *store*, for example, can be either a noun, a finite verb or an infinitive. In an utterance, this ambiguity is normally resolved by the context of a word: e.g. in (1), *store* can only be an infinitive. The predictability of the POS from the context is used by automatic POS taggers.

(1) The 1977 PCs could store two pages of data.

Several methods have been proposed to annotate words automatically with POS tags. Some researchers have been using rule-based systems (Greene & Rubin 1971; Brill 1993). Others implemented probabilistic methods, e.g. Bahl & Mercer (1976), Church (1988), Cutting et al. (1992), DeRose (1988), Kempe (1993). Finally, neural network models have also been tested in POS tagging (Federici & Pirrelli 1994; Schmid 1994) and the related problem of POS prediction (Nakamura et al. 1990).

All probabilistic methods cited above are based on first-order or second-order Markov models. Because of the large number of parameters (particularly in the case of trigrams), these methods have difficulties in estimating small probabilities accurately from limited amounts of training data.

In this paper, a new technique, the TreeTagger, is presented which avoids this sparse-data problem by using a decision tree to obtain reliable estimates of transition probabilities. The decision tree automatically determines the appropriate size of the context which is used to estimate the transition probabilities. Possible contexts are not only trigrams, bigrams and unigrams, but also other kinds of contexts as in (2).

(2) tag_{-1} = ADJ and tag_{-2} ≠ADJ and tag_{-2} ≠DET

12.2 Probabilistic tagging

The TreeTagger has much in common with a conventional *n*-gram tagger (Church 1988; Kempe 1993). Both of them model the probability of a tagged sequence of words (in the case of a second-order Markov model) recursively as in (3).

$$(3)\quad P(w_1 w_2 \ldots w_n, t_1 t_2 \ldots t_n) := P(t_n | t_{n-2} t_{n-1}) \times P(w_n | t_n) \times P(w_1 w_2 \ldots w_{n-1}, t_1 t_2 \ldots t_{n-1})$$

The methods differ, however, in the way the transition probability $P(t_n | t_{n-2} t_{n-1})$ is estimated. Often, *n*-gram taggers estimate the probability using equation (4) based on the *maximum likelihood estimation* (MLE) principle.

$$(4)\quad P(t_n | t_{n-2} t_{n-1}) = \frac{F(t_{n-2} t_{n-1} t_n)}{F(t_{n-2} t_{n-1})}$$

where *F(xyz)* is the number of occurrences of the trigram *xyz* in the corpus and *F(xy)* is the number of occurrences of the bigram *xy*.

This estimation method is problematic since many frequencies are so small that the corresponding probabilities cannot be estimated reliably. Particular difficulties are posed by zero frequencies: it is difficult to decide whether the corresponding trigram is syntactically incorrect (in which case the probability is 0) or just rare (in which case the probability has a small positive value). Another point is that a robust tagger should be able to cope with ungrammaticalities in the input. Otherwise, ungrammaticalities would lead to the assignment of a zero probability to a whole utterance, independent of the sequence of tags. This should be avoided.

Therefore, (4) is often modified by replacing zero frequencies with a small value (for a comparison of some of the methods, see Kempe 1993). A proper choice of the replacement value is essential for the quality of the tagging result.

12.3 The TreeTagger

In contrast to an *n*-gram tagger, the TreeTagger estimates transition probabilities with a binary decision tree. Figure 12.1 shows a sample decision tree. The probability of a given trigram is determined by following the corresponding path through the tree until a leaf is reached. If we look, for example, for the probability $P(\mathrm{NN}|\mathrm{DET}, \mathrm{ADJ})$ of a noun which is preceded by a determiner and an adjective, we must first answer the test at the root node. Since the tag of the previous word is ADJ, we follow the "yes" path. The next test (tag_{-2} = DET) is true as well and we end up at a leaf node. Now, we just have to look for the probability of the tag NN in the table which is attached to this node.

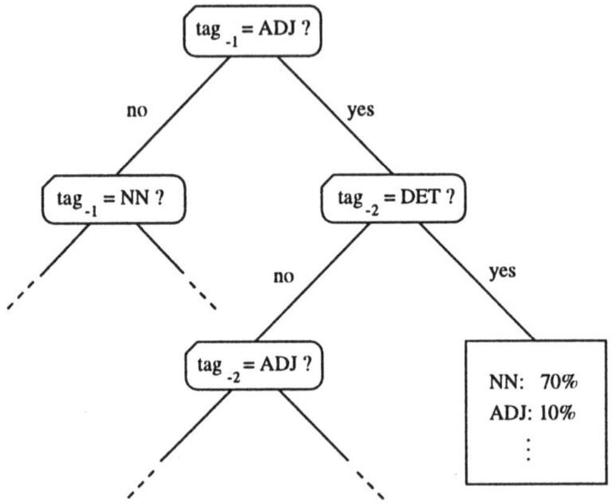

Figure 12.1 *A sample decision tree (incompletely drawn).*[1]

12.3.1 Construction of the decision tree

The decision tree is built recursively from a training set of trigrams using a modified version of the ID3 algorithm (Quinlan 1983). In each recursion step, a test is created which divides the set of trigram samples into two subsets with maximal distinctness regarding the probability distribution of the third, predicted tag. The test examines one of the two preceding tags and checks whether it is identical to some tag t. Such a test has the form (5),

(5) $\mathrm{tag}_{-i} = t; \quad i \in \{1,2\}; \; t \in T$

where T is the tagset.

At each recursion step, all possible tests are compared and the best one yielding most information is attached to the current node of the decision tree. This node is then expanded recursively on each of the two subsets of the training set which are defined by the test. The resulting subtrees are attached to the current node as the "yes"- and "no"-subtrees.

The criterion which is used to compare all possible tests q is the amount of information which is gained about the third tag by making each test. Maximizing the information gain is equivalent to minimizing the average amount of information I_q which is still needed to identify the third tag after the result of test q is known, (6).

1. This is not a realistic example. It is just for illustration.

$$(6)\quad I_q = P(c_+|c).J_+ + P(c_-|c).J_-$$
$$J_\alpha = \sum_{t \in T} P(t|c_\alpha) \log_2 P(t|c_\alpha)$$

Here, c is the context which corresponds to the current node, and c_+ and c_- are equal to c plus the condition that test q succeeds or fails respectively. $P(c_\alpha|c)$ is the probability that test q succeeds or fails (depending on the sign of α), and similarly $P(t|c_\alpha)$ is the probability of the third tag t if the test succeeded or failed. These probabilities are estimated from frequencies with MLE, (7)–(8):

$$(7)\quad P(c_\alpha|c) = \frac{F(c_\alpha)}{F(c)}$$
$$(8)\quad P(t|c_\alpha) = \frac{F(t, c_\alpha)}{F(c_\alpha)}$$

where $F(c)$ is the number of trigrams in the current training set, $F(c_\alpha)$ is the number of trigrams which do (do not) pass the test, and $F(t, c_\alpha)$ is the number of trigrams which do (do not) pass the test and whose third tag is t.

The recursive expansion of the decision tree stops if the next test would generate at least one subset of trigrams whose size is below some predefined threshold, e.g. 2 (i.e. $F(c_\alpha) < 2$). Tag probabilities $P(t|c)$ for the third tag are then estimated from all trigrams which have been passed to this recursion step and they are stored at the current node, (9).

$$(9)\quad P(t|c) = \frac{F(t, c)}{F(c)}$$

12.3.2 Pruning the decision tree

After the initial version of the decision tree has been built, the tree is pruned. If both subnodes of a node are leaves, and the *weighted information gain* at the node is below some threshold, the subnodes are removed and the node itself becomes a leaf. The weighted information gain G is defined as (10),

$$(10)\quad G = F(c)(I^0 - I_q)$$
$$I^0 = \sum_{t \in T} P(t|c) \log_2 P(t|c)$$

where I^0 is the amount of information which is needed to disambiguate at the current node and I_q, as above, is the amount of information which is still needed after the result of test q is known. This information gain criterion should not be used during the construction of the decision tree, because it is possible that a node might fail to meet it, even when all that node's subnodes did. So, this part of the tree would not be constructed if the information gain criterion were used at first.

As other probabilistic taggers do, the TreeTagger determines the best tag sequence for a given sequence of words with the Viterbi algorithm (Viterbi 1967).

12.4 The lexicon

The lexicon contains the *a priori* tag probabilities for each word and is similar to the lexicon which was used by Cutting et al. (1992). It has three parts: a *full-form* lexicon, a *suffix* lexicon and a *default* entry.

During the lookup of a word in the lexicon of the TreeTagger, the full-form lexicon is searched first. If the word is found there, the corresponding tag probability vector is returned. Otherwise, the upper-case letters of the word are turned to lower-case, and the search in the full-form lexicon is repeated. If it fails again, the suffix lexicon is searched next. If none of the previous steps has been successful, the default entry of the lexicon is returned.

The full-form lexicon was created from a tagged training corpus (some 2 million words of the Penn Treebank Corpus, Marcus et al. 1993). The number of occurrences of each word–tag pair was counted and those tags of each word with a relative frequency of less than 1% were removed since they were in most cases the result of tagging errors in the original corpus.

The second part of the lexicon, the suffix lexicon, is organized as a tree. Each node of the tree (except the root node) is labelled with a character. At the leaf nodes, tag probability vectors are attached. During a lookup, the suffix tree is searched starting at the root node. In each step, the branch that is labelled with the next character from the end of the word suffix is followed.

Assume, for example, that we want to look for the word *tagging* in the suffix lexicon which is shown in Figure 12.2. We start at the root (labelled "#") and follow the branch which leads to the node labelled "g". From there, we move to the node labelled "n", and finally we end up in the node labelled "i". This node is a leaf and the attached tag probability vector (which is not shown in Fig. 12.2) is returned.

The suffix lexicon was automatically built from the training corpus. A *suffix tree* was constructed from the suffixes of length 5 of all words that were annotated with an open-class POS[2] and tag frequencies were counted for all suffixes and stored at the corresponding tree nodes. Then an information measure $I(s)$ was calculated for each node of the tree, (11):

$$(11)\quad I(s) = -\sum_t P(t|s)\log_2 P(t|s)$$

2. Open-class POSs are those which are possible POSs of newly created words (e.g. noun, verb, adjective).

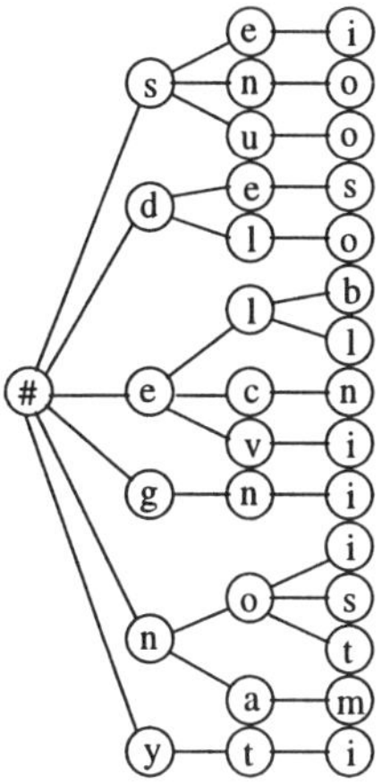

Figure 12.2 *A sample suffix tree of length 3.*

where s is the suffix that corresponds to the current node and $P(t|s)$ is the probability of POS tag t, given a word with suffix s.

Using this information measure, the suffix tree has been pruned. For each leaf, the weighted information gain $G(s_{\text{cur}})$ was calculated with (12):

(12) $G(s_{\text{cur}}) = F(s_{\text{cur}})(I(s_{\text{par}}) - I(s_{\text{cur}}))$

where s_{par} is the suffix of the parent node, s_{cur} is the suffix of the current node and $F(s_{\text{cur}})$ is the frequency of suffix s_{cur}.

If the information gain at some leaf of the suffix tree is below a given threshold,[3] the leaf is removed. The tag frequencies of all deleted subnodes of a parent node are collected at the *default node* of the parent node. If the default node is the only remaining subnode, it too is deleted. In this case, the parent node becomes a leaf and it is also checked to see whether it is deletable.

To illustrate this process consider the example where *-ess* is the suffix of the parent node, *-less* is the suffix of one child node and *-ness* is the suffix of the other child node. Sample tag frequencies of the nodes are given in Table 12.1.

Table 12.1 Sample tag frequencies at a tree node and its two child nodes.

Tag	Suffix *-ess*	Suffix *-ness*	Suffix *-less*
JJ	86	1	85
NN	10	2	8
NP	45	45	0
RB	2	0	2
Total	143	48	95

3. We used a gain threshold of 10.

The information measure for the parent node is (13).

$$(13)\quad I(ess) = -\frac{86}{143}\log_2\frac{86}{143} - \frac{10}{143}\log_2\frac{10}{143} - \ldots \approx 1.32$$

The corresponding values for the child nodes are 0.39 for *-ness* and 0.56 for *-less*. Now, we can determine the weighted information gain at each of the child nodes. We get (14) and (15).

$$(14)\quad G(ness) = 48(1.32 - 0.39) = 44.64$$
$$(15)\quad G(less) = 95(1.32 - 0.56) = 72.20$$

Both values are well above our threshold of 10, and therefore neither of them should be deleted.

As explained before, the suffix tree is searched during a lookup along the path where the nodes are annotated with the letters of the word suffix in reverse order. If a leaf is reached at the end of the path, the corresponding tag probability vector is returned. If no matching subnode is found at some node on the path, the default node is followed if it exists. If no default node exists, the search in the suffix lexicon fails and the default entry is returned.

The *default entry* is constructed by subtracting the tag frequencies at all leaves of the pruned suffix tree from the tag frequencies at the root node and normalizing the resulting frequencies. In this way, relative frequencies are obtained which sum to 1.

12.5 Tests

The performance of the TreeTagger was tested on data from the Penn Treebank corpus. Some 2 million words were used for training and 100 000 words from a different part of the Penn Treebank corpus for testing.

The TreeTagger was compared to a trigram tagger (Kempe 1993) which was trained and tested on the same data. In contrast to the TreeTagger, the trigram tagger does not use a suffix lexicon. Instead, its full-form lexicon was augmented by about 170 000 additional entries which were created from a word list with a morphological analyser.

Two versions of the TreeTagger were tested. In the first version, zero frequencies are replaced by 0.1 – which was found to be optimal – before the tag probabilities at the leaves of the decision tree were calculated. In the second version, zero frequencies were replaced by a very small value,[4] namely 10^{-10}, to see how strong is the influence of the choice of this parameter on the tagging accuracy. In another test, how much the tagging accuracy depends on the size of the training corpus was

4. Transition probabilities are not allowed to be equal to 0, because this would mean that the whole tagging process breaks down if this particular context appears in the input.

examined. A bigram version and a quadgram version of the TreeTagger were tested as well. Finally, the influence of the pruning threshold on the accuracy of the trigram and quadgram versions of the TreeTagger were examined.

Training of the TreeTagger as well as tagging itself was very fast. Training with trigrams on 2 million tokens took only about 6 minutes on a SPARC10 workstation and about 10 000 words were tagged per second.

12.6 Results

As Table 12.2 shows, the trigram version of the TreeTagger achieved an accuracy which is about 0.3% better than that of the standard trigram tagger. It is also about 0.6% better than the bigram version of the TreeTagger. Increasing the context to quadgrams still results in a very small improvement of the accuracy. This shows that the TreeTagger is able to trim the context effectively, where this is necessary to get reliable estimates. Changing the replacement value for zero frequencies in the decision tree from a very small value to 0.1 resulted in a small improvement of the accuracy. So, in contrast to more standard Markov-model taggers, a proper setting of this parameter is not important.

Table 12.2 Comparison of accuracy of different taggers.

Method	Context	Accuracy (%)
Kempe's tagger	trigram	96.06
TreeTagger	bigram	95.78
TreeTagger (0.1)	trigram	96.34
TreeTagger	quadgram	96.36
TreeTagger (10^{-10})	trigram	96.32

Figure 12.3 shows the influence of the size of the training corpus on the tagging quality. In contrast to the trigram tagger, the accuracy of the TreeTagger deteriorates slowly, as the size of the training corpus shrinks. Further, the difference between the bigram version of the TreeTagger and the trigram version is small for very small sizes of the training corpus. This shows that the TreeTagger is much more robust than the standard trigram tagger with regard to the size of the training corpus.

Figure 12.4 shows that the influence of the pruning threshold on the accuracy is small (below 0.03% for the trigram version and below 0.12% for the quadgram version). The best results are obtained with thresholds between 40 and 50. The diagram shows also that the quadgram version of the TreeTagger is consistently better than the trigram version for thresholds above 15.

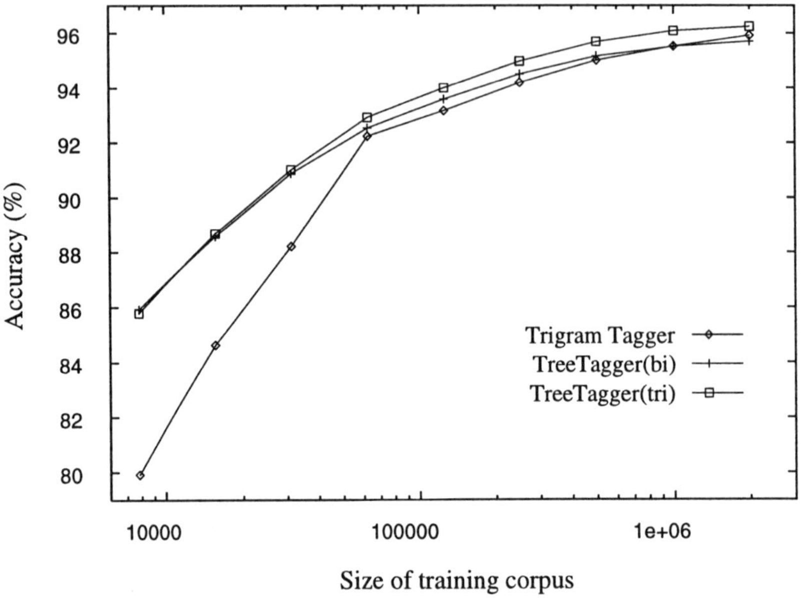

Figure 12.3 *Accuracy for varying sizes of the training corpus.*

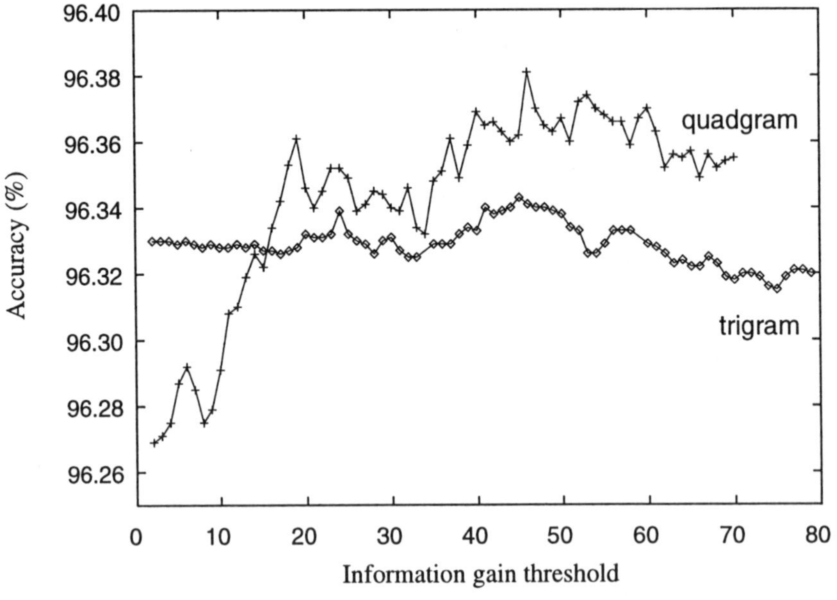

Figure 12.4 *Accuracy for different pruning thresholds.*

Table 12.3 compares the number of possible *n*-gram contexts against the number of leaf nodes and thereby the number of contexts that the TreeTagger distinguishes. In the case of bigrams, all possible contexts are used by the TreeTagger, in the case of trigrams the number of leaves is about a third of the number of possible contexts, and in the case of quadgrams only about 2% of all possible contexts are distinguished.

Table 12.3 Number of contexts distinguished by taggers.

Context	Number of contexts	Number of leaves	Depth
bigram	47	47	47
trigram	2209	710	62
quadgram	103823	2251	67

12.7 Summary

A new tagging method, the TreeTagger, has been presented. It differs from other probabilistic taggers in the way the transition probabilities are estimated, namely with a decision tree. A method for the construction of a decision tree was presented and it was demonstrated that the resulting tagger achieves higher accuracy than a standard trigram tagger. Further, it was shown that the TreeTagger is robust with respect to the size of the training corpus. Small training corpora did not result in a sharp degradation of the accuracy, as was observed for trigram taggers. The TreeTagger trims the size of the context where this is necessary to obtain reliable probability estimates. Hence, it was possible to improve the accuracy of the tagger by using a quadgram context. The tagger is able to tag up to 10 000 tokens per second on a SPARC10 workstation. Thus, the TreeTagger is a fast and high-quality tool for the annotation of corpora with POS information.

References

Bahl, L. R. & R. L. Mercer 1976. Part-of-speech assignment by a statistical decision algorithm. In *IEEE International Symposium on Information Theory*, Amherst, Mass. 88–9.

Brill, E. 1993. *A corpus-based approach to language learning*. PhD thesis, University of Pennsylvania, Philadelphia, Pa.

Church, K. W. 1988. A stochastic parts program and noun phrase parser for unrestricted text. In *Proceedings of the Second Conference on Applied Natural Language Processing*, Austin, Tex., 136–43.

Cutting, D., J. Kupiec, J. Pedersen & P. Sibun 1992. A practical part-of-speech tagger. In *Proceedings of the Third Conference on Applied Natural Language Processing*, Trento, Italy, 133–40.

DeRose, S. J. 1988. Grammatical category disambiguation by statistical optimization. *Computational Linguistics* **14**, 31–9.

Federici, S. & V. Pirrelli 1994. Context-sensitivity and linguistic structure in analogy-based parallel networks. In *Current Issues in Mathematical Linguistics*, C. Martin-Vide (ed.), 353–62. Amsterdam: North-Holland.

Greene, B. & G. Rubin 1971. *Automatic grammatical tagging of English*. Technical Report, Department of Linguistics, Brown University, Providence, RI.

Kempe, A. 1993. *A probabilistic tagger and an analysis of tagging errors*. Technical Report, Institut für maschinelle Sprachverarbeitung, Universität Stuttgart.

Marcus, M. P., B. Santorini & M. A. Marcinkiewicz 1993. Building a large annotated corpus of English: the Penn Treebank. *Computational Linguistics* **19**, 313–30.

Nakamura, M., K. Maruyama, T. Kawabata & K. Shikano 1990. Neural network approach to word category prediction for English texts. In *COLING-90: Papers presented to the 13th International Conference on Computational Linguistics*, Helsinki, Vol. 3, 213–18.

Quinlan, J. R. 1983. Learning efficient classification procedures and their application to chess end games. In *Machine learning: an artificial intelligence approach*, R. Michalski, J, Carbonell & T. Mitchell (eds), 463–82. San Mateo, Calif.: Morgan Kaufmann.

Schmid, H. 1994. Part-of-speech tagging with neural networks. In *COLING 94: The 15th International Conference on Computational Linguistics*, Kyoto, Japan, 172–6.

Viterbi, A. J. 1967. Error bounds for convolutional codes and an asymptotically optimal decoding algorithm. *IEEE Transactions on Information Theory* **13**, 260–69.

13
A new direction for sublanguage NLP

SATOSHI SEKINE[1]

13.1 Introduction

There have been a number of theoretical studies devoted to the notion of sublanguage. Some of them claim that the notion is important in processing natural language text, owing to lexical, syntactic, or semantic restrictions. A number of these studies have examined actual texts in order to verify the claim (Kittredge & Lehrberger 1982; Grishman & Kittredge 1986; Slocum 1986; Biber 1993).

Furthermore, there are some successful natural language processing (NLP) systems that have explicitly or implicitly addressed the sublanguage restrictions. For example, TAUM-Météo (Isabelle 1984) is a machine translation (MT) system that deals only with sentences in the weather forecast domain, and it works remarkably well.

1. The work reported here was supported by the Advanced Research Projects Agency under contract DABT63-93-C-0058 from the Department of the Army. I should like to thank BBN for providing the data. Also, I should like to thank my colleagues at NYU, in particular Professor Grishman, whose comments have been very useful. A part of the research described in this chapter has been previously reported in the *Jōhō Shori Gakkai Journal of Natural Language Processing* (Sekine 1995).

However, there remain two major unsolved problems for the utilization of the sublanguage notion:

- automatic definition of a sublanguage and dynamic identification of a text to it;
- automatic linguistic knowledge acquisition for a sublanguage.

Thanks to the appearance of large machine-readable corpora, there are now new opportunities to address these issues. The explosion of large corpora has led to a flowering of research on linguistic knowledge acquisition from corpora (Armstrong-Warwick 1993). Several studies have mentioned the importance of the sublanguage notion (Grishman & Sterling 1992; Sekine et al. 1992). Although these are still small experiments in terms of accuracy and coverage, they address the second problem listed above, and could lead to a breakthrough for future NLP systems by reducing the costly and error-prone task of linguistic knowledge encoding by human linguists.

The first problem has not received so much attention. In previous sublanguage NLP systems, the domain of the system was defined manually. For example, the sublanguages of "weather forecasts", "medical reports" or "computer manuals" are artificially or intuitively defined by a human. This is certainly one method of defining the sublanguage of the text, and, in a sense, it seems to work well. However, it is not always possible and sometimes it may be wrong. For example, in a large-vocabulary speech recognition system, which may have to handle a variety of domains, it is impossible to tune to a sublanguage in advance. Also, if we take the "computer manual domain" as a sublanguage, the domain contains a mixture of linguistic phenomena. The "computer manual domain" ranges from a "word-processor manual for novices" to an "operating-system reference manual", and their linguistic usages are different. In short, a new step to expand sublanguage research is long overdue.

13.2 Two definitions of "sublanguage"

The notion of sublanguage has been much discussed in the last decade or two. We can find two kinds of definitions, although the difference has not received serious attention up to now. One definition can be inferable from Zellig Harris: "Certain proper subsets of the sentences of a language may be closed under some or all of the operations defined in the language, and thus constitute a sublanguage of it" (1968: 152). From this definition, we can infer that a sublanguage can be defined empirically by observing language behaviour. The other type of definition is exemplified by the following sentence in Bross et al. : "Informally, we can define a sublanguage as the language used by a particular community of speakers, say, those concerned with a particular subject matter or those engaged in a specialized occupation" (1972: 1303).

In this paper, the former definition will be called an "inductive definition", since a sublanguage can be defined by observation of data. The second definition, on the other hand, will be called a "deductive definition", since it is based on the principle that a particular subject matter would define a sublanguage.

Many practical projects have been using the deductive definition intentionally or unintentionally. For example, the TAUM project took two subject domains for its MT applications: one was weather forecasts and the other aircraft maintenance manuals. This is a deductive definition of sublanguage, because they took a particular subject as their target. However, the deductive definition is not always possible and sometimes it may be wrong, as discussed above.

13.3 Benefits from large corpora

Recently, a number of large corpora have become available in machine-readable form. The appearance of large corpora is of benefit to sublanguage study. In particular, it can be useful for the inductive definition of sublanguage. Although Harris's notion was mainly concerned with operations on sentences, there are several other factors that are related to the sublanguage notion, for example, lexical, syntactic and semantic restrictions, a high frequency of certain constructions, and use of special symbols (these factors are borrowed from Lehrberger 1982). These can be useful for the inductive definition of sublanguage, as well as themselves being characteristics of sublanguage. In other words, we may be able to find sublanguages by observing texts in terms of similarities of these characteristics. The other factors in Lehrberger's list of sublanguage characteristics – limited subject matter, deviant rules of grammar and text structure – are harder to utilize for the inductive definition of sublanguage.

The strategy for inductive definition of a sublanguage using corpora is to analyse the corpora in terms of lexical, syntactic or semantic characteristics, and then make clusters in which the values of the factors are similar. However, in practice, it is still difficult to analyse a sentence correctly in terms of syntax and semantics, so the preliminary experiment in this paper employs only the lexical factor to build up a sublanguage as an initial attempt.

13.4 Sublanguage definition

Our experiments can be divided into two parts: the definition of sublanguage and the identification of the sublanguage of a new text. We will consider an experiment in sublanguage definition in this section, and then in the next section, we consider some experiments in sublanguage identification.

We use a newspaper (7.5 MB of the *San Jose Mercury*, 2147 articles) in our experiments. Each article in the newspaper is regarded as a unit of data, and a sublanguage will be formed by gathering similar units in terms of word appearance.

This is almost identical to the text clustering technique which has been well studied in the field of information retrieval (Willett 1988). However, the aim of that study is slightly different from ours. Willett tries to make clusters that are useful for human information-retrieval purposes, so the linguistic features of the clusters are not so important. In contrast, our purpose is to find a sublanguage that is useful for NLP systems, so we are very interested in the linguistic features of clusters.

One of the problems in making clusters is how to define the number and size of clusters. The number of clusters can range from one, with all the articles in the cluster, to the number of articles, each cluster containing just one article. The problem here is that we have no objective means of deciding the number and the size. This problem is crucial for automatic sublanguage definition, because otherwise we need manual intervention or artificial thresholds. In order to explore this problem, we introduce the following statistics.

13.4.1 Perplexity and expected perplexity

"Perplexity", or more precisely "unigram perplexity", as used in this paper, is a notion from information theory. The formal definition of perplexity P, (1), uses unigram entropy H, (2),

(1) $P = 2^H$

(2) $H = -\sum_{w} p(w) \log_2 (p(w))$

where $p(w)$ is the probability of a token w being in the source. This probability may be estimated from a text by dividing the number of occurrences of the tokens by the total number of tokens in the text. From this estimated probability, we can get an estimated entropy and perplexity. Roughly speaking, perplexity indicates the amount of information in the source. On condition that the sizes of two texts are the same in terms of number of tokens, then we can roughly say that the text with the larger perplexity has the greater variety of tokens.

We can also calculate perplexity for a set of texts, treating the set as a single text. If two texts have a large number of overlapping tokens, which means the two texts are similar in terms of the words that appear in them, the perplexity for the combined text will be smaller than that of a text that has tokens chosen at random from the entire corpus. In short, if the perplexity for a text set is small in comparison with perplexity for a random text, we may say that the set has sublanguage tendency.

In order to observe perplexities of texts, clusters were made based on similarities of articles. Clusters are grown from one initial article by adding similar articles in the order of their similarity to the initial article. The similarity measurement was borrowed from information retrieval research. It uses basically "log of inverse document frequency" with the cut at 200 (tokens that occur more than 200 times in the corpora are not taken into account), minimum of two occurrences (only the tokens that occur two or more times in the article are considered) and minimum of two co-occurrences (relationships are established if the two articles have two or more tokens in common). These numbers were established experimentally. A cluster was grown in this way around each article in the corpus.

In order to make an objective measurement, one has to compare these estimated perplexity values with the perplexity of random text. Because the estimated perplexity depends on the size of the sample text, the need is to compare the cluster with a sample text of the same size obtained by selecting tokens at random from the entire corpus. The expected perplexity used in the experiment was the average of three of these trials.

Figure 13.1 shows some examples of the relationship between the number of tokens in a cluster and the ratio of its perplexity to that of random estimation. The points in the graph starting from the left-hand side indicate data for the first article, the first article and the closest article combined, and so on.

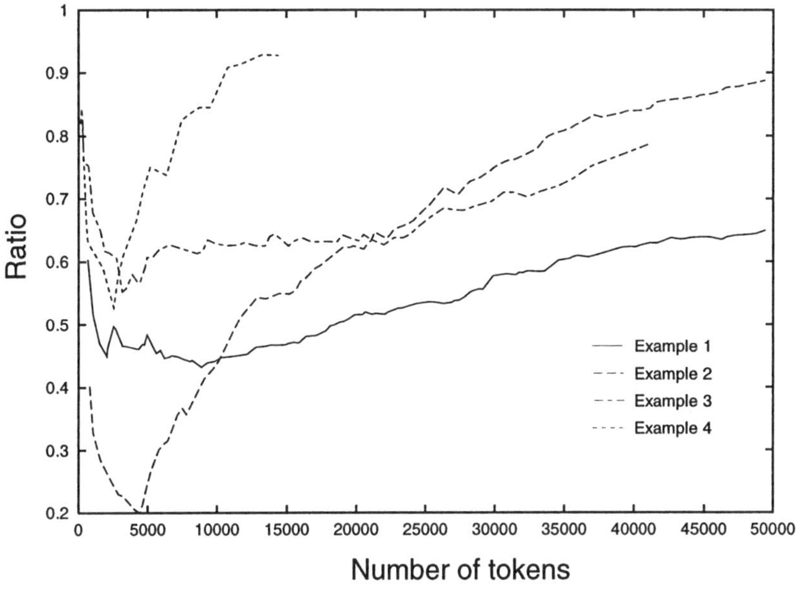

Figure 13.1 *Ratio of perplexities to random estimation.*

13.4.2 Observations regarding Figure 13.1

It is natural that the ratio moves toward 1.0 as the number of tokens becomes bigger, because the cluster is approaching the set of all articles combined. However, we can see that in all four examples there is a minimum point at a small number of tokens. This could happen if the combining texts have a larger number of overlapping words than expected. Now, this minimum point appears to suggest one of the definitions of sublanguage in terms of word appearance. This phenomenon was observed not only in the four examples shown, but also for many of the other clusters. The articles involved were examined and a promising pattern was found. In Example 2, all nine articles from the beginning until the minimum point were obituaries, while the next three were real-estate articles. In Example 1, the first article and 54% of the articles up to the minimum point were about college basketball. The rest were either about high-school or professional basketball (24% and 8%, respectively), hockey (8%) or football (4%). On the other hand, only 16% of the next 25 articles and 6% of the rest of the articles up to the 185th were about college basketball. These examples intuitively support the claim that the minimum point of each line on the graph would be an objective indicator of the size of a text cluster or a sublanguage.

13.4.3 Sublanguage clusters

We may take the articles from the beginning to the minimum point as representing a sublanguage. These clusters are used in the next experiment, identification of the sublanguage of a new text. As there are 2147 articles in the corpus, the same number of (not necessarily distinct) clusters exist. The number of articles in a cluster ranges from 1 to 31, and the average number is 4.26 articles.

13.5 Sublanguage identification for a new text

The next stage took 244 new test articles from the *San Jose Mercury* which had not been used in the sublanguage definition experiment described above. In this section, the method of identifying the closest cluster for each test article is described.

For each test article, similarity measures to all the clusters were calculated to find the closest one. Basically, the similarity measure was the same as the one in the previous experiment. The similarity between a test article and a cluster was set equal to the maximum similarity between the test article and any of the articles in the cluster. If there was a tie, the cluster that contained the smallest number of articles won. This calculation was not expensive, because there were a limited number of words that had to be taken into account in the calculation. The number was normally much less than the number of tokens in the test articles. Also, the number of clusters to be examined for each word was less than the cut-off number (50 in the experiment), so this calculation is almost linear in the number of words in the test article, if there is enough space to store the word index.

In this experiment, the parameters for the similarity calculation were set slightly different from the ones in the definition experiment. The cut-off number was 50, minimum occurrence was 1 and minimum co-occurrence was set to 3, based on empirical adjustments.

13.5.1 Results of the identification experiment

The result of the identification experiment will be described. The evaluation measure was based on how many tokens in the test article also exist in the closest cluster, i.e. the number of tokens that overlap between the test article and the closest cluster. A straightforward measurement is its coverage, which is how many tokens are overlapping against the total number of tokens in the article. This figure could be useful in deciding how useful this method is, but it might still be difficult to make an objective decision. So the number of overlapping tokens was compared with an expected number of overlapping tokens. This was computed by taking two sets randomly that have the same number of tokens as the test article and the selected cluster, then calculating the average number of overlapping tokens between them. This expected number (*E*) was calculated by the formula in (3),

$$(3)\quad E = \sum_{w} \frac{N_t f_w}{N}\left(1 - \left(1 - \frac{N_c}{N}\right)^{f_w}\right)$$

where N_t is the number of tokens in the test article, N_c is the number of tokens in the cluster, N is the number of tokens in the entire corpus, and f_w is the frequency of word w. The expected number of overlapping tokens can be classified into certain frequency ranges, applying the variables f_w and N_t to the range.

It is well known that high-frequency words like *the* or *of* are relatively common regardless of the topic or sublanguage. On the other hand, low-frequency words, which are often regarded as indicating the topic, are expected to occur together in the same articles. So we can anticipate in this evaluation that low-frequency words will overlap between test articles and the closest clusters more than the expected values. (Note that, because words with $|f_w| < 50$ are used in the similarity calculation, those words must be specially treated in the evaluation. To observe such details, we classified the results based on document frequency of words in the entire corpus. Table 13.1 shows an example of the results. In this example, the number of tokens in the article was 129, the number of tokens in the cluster 1265, and the cluster consisted of five articles.

The first column shows the frequency range of tokens. The second and third columns show the expected and actual numbers of tokens. For example, the expected number of tokens whose frequency ranges from 100 to 199 is 12.0, but actually 25 were found in the article. These two figures show the balance of the word frequency distribution in the article, and we can see that most of them were well balanced.

The fourth and fifth columns show the corresponding information about overlapping tokens. For example, 95 tokens out of 129 in the entire article were overlapping to the closest cluster, compared to 67.6 expected.

The sixth column shows the coverage of overlapping tokens in the test article. We can see that the entire overall coverage was 73.6% in this sample.

The total in the final column indicates that tokens in the article were overlapping 1.23 times the expected value. Also, 6.01 and 2.40 times the expected number

Table 13.1 An example of the results.

Frequency	Number of tokens		Overlap		Coverage	Ratio
	Expected	Found	Expected	Found	(%)	
0	4.6	0				
1-49	34.9	20	1.0	6	30.0	6.01
50-99	11.6	11	2.1	5	45.5	2.40
100-199	12.0	25	8.2	15	60.0	1.82
200-299	6.9	10	5.7	9	90.0	1.57
300-499	7.1	10	7.5	7	70.0	0.94
500-999	16.9	12	11.7	12	100.0	1.03
1000-	35.1	41	41.0	41	100.0	1.00
Total	129.0	129	67.6	95	73.6	1.23

of overlapping tokens were found in the article in the frequency ranges 1–49 and 50–99, respectively. As mentioned above, the result for words whose frequency ranges between 1 and 49 cannot be evaluated directly. As the method to find the closest cluster is like the single linkage technique, so the words in the closest article are used in the cluster search. The number of tokens overlapping between the test article and the closest article in the frequency range 1–49, i.e. number of tokens used in the similarity calculation, is three for this sample (not shown in the table). This means that out of five overlapping tokens between the test article and the closest cluster, three tokens are found in the closest article and the other two tokens are found in the rest of the articles in the cluster. So these figures show the benefit of clustering in increasing the overlapping tokens.

The average of the coverage and the ratio throughout the 236 test articles is given in Table 13.2. Note that for eight articles, no closest cluster could be found because of the thresholds.

The second column of the table shows the percentage of overlapping tokens in the test articles, and the third shows the average ratio of overlapping tokens to expected overlapping tokens. From the figures in Table 13.2, we can observe the success of the method. For example, tokens in the frequency range 50–99 are found with 1.94 times the expected value in the closest cluster. Also the ratio in the range 100–199 is 1.90, i.e. almost double the expected number. These figures can be explained by saying that lower-frequency words co-occur together more than expected. This is the very fact that we had expected and proves the existence of a sublanguage. On the other hand, the ratios at the higher frequencies are about 1. This means that the distribution of these words is almost just as expected. This is understandable, because many high-frequency words are closed-class words and these words can

Table 13.2 Average coverage and ratio.

Frequency	Coverage (%)	Ratio
1-49	16.7	7.98
50-99	26.4	1.94
100-199	34.5	1.90
200-299	45.9	1.03
300-499	57.7	1.19
500-999	76.6	1.00
1000-	95.8	0.98
Total	51.1	1.18

occur in any of the articles. So the expected number of overlapping words is about the same as the number of tokens, as can be seen in Table 13.1. Actually, almost all the words whose frequency is more than 1000 are closed-class words, like *the*, *of* or *it*, and occur in many of the articles.[2]

13.6 Experiment with the first two sentences

For some NLP applications, it may be impossible to see all the sentences of a text in advance of the processing. For example, spontaneous speech recognition systems have to process each utterance as it occurs. The algorithm described above cannot be applied to these applications directly, because the system cannot pre-scan the material before the processing. Therefore an experiment was conducted using the first two sentences in the test articles, instead of all the sentences in the articles, to find the closest cluster. This process can be called "dynamic sublanguage identification", because it utilizes knowledge that is acquired during the process. If it can find a good cluster (i.e. sublanguage) that is useful for the rest of the article, we can say the dynamic sublanguage identification performed well. Table 13.3 shows the results of this experiment.

Surprisingly, the result is almost the same as the previous one. Actually, 72.5% of the test articles (177 out of 244 articles) had the same cluster selected as was selected in the previous experiment. This result is intuitively understandable, because the first sentences in a newspaper article normally indicate its topic and the sentences could be helpful in identifying its sublanguage. This result indicates that this method can be applicable to speech recognition systems or other scenarios where it is impossible to pre-scan all the sentences before processing.

2. There are only 68 words that have frequencies over 1000. The total number of words is 39 217.

Table 13.3 Average coverage and ratio for experiment with the first two sentences.

Frequency	Coverage (%)	Ratio
1-49	17.2	6.40
50-99	26.7	1.67
100-199	34.9	1.90
200-299	47.7	0.95
300-499	56.8	1.16
500-999	75.4	0.96
1000-	95.6	0.98
Total	51.2	1.18

13.7 Application

In this section, we consider a preliminary experiment that aims to observe the possibilities of applying the technique to speech recognition systems. As contiguous speech recognition has not yet been perfected, all speech recognition systems are liable to make misrecognitions. Sometimes words that are related to the topic of the article are replaced by words that are irrelevant to the topic. To rectify this kind of mistake was the objective of this application. BBN's speech recognizer was used, and the *North American Business News* (published by LDC) was the source of sublanguage sets. The relative unigram perplexities were calculated for the sentences produced by the recognizer and the correct transcriptions. Two kinds of perplexity were calculated, based on the whole corpus and on an interpolated model. The interpolated model was constructed by the probabilities of words in the sublanguage set, the cache model and the whole corpus, in proportions of 0.18, 0.02 and 0.8. Here, cache model probability is the probability of words in the preceding sentences of the article.

We will see how it works by means of an example. In the fourth sentence in one article concerning an Arabian prince, the system misrecognized *prince* as *France*. As the previous sentences of the article contained words like *prince* and *royal*, the sublanguage technique could extract such articles and form a sublanguage set from them. Table 13.4 shows the probabilities of words *prince* and *France* in its sublanguage set, the cache, the whole corpus and the interpolated model. The figures are shown as percentages.

As the probability of *prince* in the whole corpus is much less than that of *France*, the relative perplexity of the recognized sentence is smaller than that of the correct one. However, the probability of *prince* in the interpolated model is greater than that of *France*. Because of high probabilities in the sublanguage and the cache, the relative perplexity of the correct sentence is smaller than that of the recognized

Table 13.4 Probabilities of the words.

Word	Sublanguage	Cache	Corpus	Interpolated
prince	0.2889	2.6866	0.0036	0.1345
France	0.0421	0	0.0139	0.0187

one. This shows an improvement derived from the sublanguage model. In a test set consisting of 310 sentences, the model was able to make 17 such improvements, i.e. the perplexity of the correct sentence was smaller than that of the recognized sentences in the whole-corpus model, but greater in the interpolated model. In six cases, the model got it wrong, i.e. preferred an incorrect interpretation since the perplexity of the correct sentence was deemed greater than for the whole corpus.

As the improvement is heavily dependent on the recognizer, it is not easy to evaluate the result. However, it must be worthwhile to continue this line of trial, because of the positive indication. A more complete experiment is reported in Sekine et al. (1995).

13.8 Discussion

We have proposed "inductive definition of sublanguage" and "dynamic sublanguage identification". In doing so, we do not deny the metric of the conventional approach to sublanguage definition. Obviously, the domain of a text is one of the most important keys of sublanguage definition. However, the inductive definition could be useful in situations where the domain name is not available or the domain definition is too vague. Our results suggest that the perplexity measurement can play a significant role in automating the definition process.

The result of sublanguage identification using the first two sentences suggests the possibility of practical applications of this method. For example, we can construct an adaptable MT system, which can take inputs from any kinds of subject domain or sublanguage. The system would find which sublanguage the input belongs to in its initial process, and adapt knowledge of the sublanguage to analyse the following sentences. Intuitively, this procedure looks very similar to what a human does.

As is easily inferable from the sublanguage literature, the definition of "sublanguage" may differ depending on its objective or usage. In this experiment, the sublanguage notion is aimed at utilizing language restrictions (word usage), so the inductive definition based on lexical appearance is suitable. In the future, we could probably extend this technique by using other sublanguage characteristics, i.e. syntactic and semantic restrictions. A recent corpus observation by Gale et al. (1992) supports the usefulness of semantic restrictions. Furthermore, we could seek a hybrid concept of the two, deductive and inductive sublanguage definitions, in order to maximize the gains from the idea of sublanguage.

We can identify several directions for future study. One is, of course, to refine the algorithm and to make larger experiments. With regard to applications, as we saw in the previous section, speech recognition is one of the most interesting applications. Also, this technique can be applicable for MT or other NLP systems, by utilizing sublanguage knowledge for disambiguation or generation. The results of this sort of experiment may tell us much more about the value of this approach. The way in which it is applied may depend heavily on the features of the application system. However, we believe that the sublanguage concept is common to many kinds of NLP systems.

13.9 Conclusion

It appears that the inductive definition of sublanguage could become realistic by using large-scale corpora. This would be very beneficial for NLP since the evaluation results show that automatically identified sublanguage knowledge is useful in processing a new text. The second experiment described proves that the method is applicable not only for static applications which can pre-scan the material before its actual processing, but also for applications that process the sentence sequentially, such as a speech recognition system. The preliminary experiment for speech recognition shows the potential of the technique.

References

Armstrong-Warwick, S. (ed.) 1993. Special Issue on Using Large Corpora. *Computational Linguistics* **19**(1–2).

Biber, D. 1993. Using register-diversified corpora for general language studies. *Computational Linguistics* **19**, 219–41.

Bross, I. D. J., P. A. Shapiro & B. B. Anderson 1972. How information is carried in scientific sub-languages. *Science* **176**, 1303–7.

Gale, W., K. Church & D. Yarowsky 1992. One sense per discourse. In *Proceedings, 4th [DARPA] Speech and Natural Language Workshop*, Harriman, NY, 233–7.

Grishman, R. & R. Kittredge 1986. *Analyzing language in restricted domains*. Hillsdale, NJ: Lawrence Erlbaum Associates.

Grishman, R. & J. Sterling 1992. Acquisition of selectional patterns. In *Proceedings of the fifteenth International Conference on Computational Linguistics, COLING-92*, Nantes, 658–64.

Harris, Z. 1968. *Mathematical structures in language*. New York: John Wiley.

Isabelle, P. 1984. Machine translation at the TAUM group. In *Machine translation today*, M. King (ed.), 247–77. Edinburgh: Edinburgh University Press.

Kittredge, R. & J. Lehrberger (eds) 1982. *Sublanguage: studies of language in restricted semantic domains*. Berlin: de Gruyter.
Lehrberger, J. 1982. Automatic translation and the concept of sublanguage. In Kittredge & Lehrberger (1982), 19–38.
Sekine, S. 1995. A new direction for sublanguage N.L.P. *Jōhō Shori Gakkai Journal of Natural Language Processing* **2**, 75–87.
Sekine, S., S. Ananiadou, J. Carroll & J. Tsujii 1992. Linguistic knowledge generator. In *Proceedings of the fifteenth International Conference on Computational Linguistics, COLING-92*, Nantes, 560–6.
Sekine, S., J. Sterling & R. Grishman 1995. NYU/BBN 1994 CSR evaluation. In *Spoken Language Technology Workshop*, Austin, Tex., 148–55.
Slocum, J. 1986. How one might automatically identify and adapt to a sublanguage. in Grishman & Kittredge (1986), 195–210.
Willett, P. 1988. Recent trends in hierarchic document clustering: a critical review. *Information Processing and Management* **24**, 577–97.

14

Efficient disambiguation by means of stochastic tree-substitution grammars

KHALIL SIMA'AN[1]

14.1 Motivation

Natural language grammars often assign many syntactic structures to the same sentence. Most of these structures are perceived as implausible by a human language user. At present, many natural language models employ statistical information about natural language use in order to approach this human ability. Some models assume a context-free grammar (CFG) in which each rule receives an unconditional application probability, e.g. Fujisaki et al. (1989), Jelinek et al. (1990). Needless to say, "context-free"[2] probabilities are not sufficient for natural language syntactic disambiguation that is "context-sensitive" in its nature. In contrast, other

1. I am grateful to Rens Bod, Steven Krauwer and Remco Scha for the discussions and suggestions concerning data-oriented parsing and natural language processing. I thank Rens again for reading and correcting previous versions of the paper. I also thank Yoad Winter for suggestions concerning the notation.

2. The "context" of a CFG rule is any syntactic tree in which it appears. A tree is viewed as the result of the constraints that the lexical items (i.e. frontier nodes) impose on the structure a sentence can be assigned.

models (Schabes 1992) employ "mildly" context-sensitive grammars at the cost of computational efficiency. Somewhere in between one finds those models that parse only the context-free languages but still assume context-sensitive application probabilities, e.g. Magerman & Weir (1992), Bod (1992), Carroll & Briscoe (1992).

"Data-oriented parsing" (DOP), proposed in Scha (1990) and developed in Bod (1992, 1993a), distinguishes itself from other statistical models in that it omits the step of inferring a grammar from the corpus. Instead, the corpus is employed as if it were a stochastic grammar. At present DOP takes a manually annotated corpus of parse trees for a stochastic tree-substitution grammar (STSG): an input string is parsed by combining "subtrees"[3] of parse trees from the corpus by means of substitution. As a consequence, one parse tree of the input sentence can be constructed by *exponentially* many different sequences of substitutions each called a "derivation" of that parse. The probability of any subtree is extracted directly from the corpus; it is the ratio of the number of its occurrences in the corpus to the number of all the occurrences of subtrees that have the same root nonterminal. While the probability of a derivation is the product of the probabilities of all subtrees that participate in it, the probability of a parse is the sum of the probabilities of all its derivations. Clearly, the most probable parse (MPP) for an input sentence is not necessarily generated by its most probable derivation (MPD) (Bod 1993a). Previous experiments with DOP on the Penn Treebank (Marcus et al. 1993), using Monte Carlo techniques, yield 96% test set *parsing accuracy* as against only 65% *derivation accuracy*[4] (Bod 1993a). These MPP accuracy figures suggest that DOP does not suffer from undergeneration. However, DOP does suffer from overgeneration and Monte Carlo parsing (on its own) does not provide an efficient solution for disambiguation (although it has provided a useful verification tool).

STSGs are a limited form of stochastic tree-adjoining grammars (STAGs) (Resnik 1992) where only substitution is allowed. Polynomial parsing of TAGs has been considered in Vijay-Shanker & Weir (1993), and studies of STAGs and limited forms of them (e.g. Schabes 1992; Schabes & Waters 1993) lead to polynomial algorithms for computing both the MPD and the probability of a sentence. However, as far as I know, there exist neither polynomial algorithms for computing the probability of a given parse nor for finding the MPP of an input sentence. Moreover, there are no optimizations of the exponential algorithms for finding the MPP.

In this paper we study the efficiency aspect of natural language disambiguation by means of STSGs under the DOP model. First, we consider a polynomial algorithm ($\mathcal{O}(n)$) for computing the probability of a given parse of a sentence of n words. Secondly we consider polynomial algorithms for computing the probability of an

3. A subtree *st* of a tree *t* is a connected subgraph of *t* such that every node in *st* fulfils the following condition: if it has any children then these are equal to the children of its corresponding node in *t*. Thus, DOP considers the set of all subtrees of the trees of the corpus to be the set of elementary trees of an STSG.

4. The notions of "parsing accuracy" and "derivation accuracy" are defined as the percentage of the test sentences for which the MPP and the parse generated by the MPD respectively are identical to the test-set parse in the Treebank.

input sentence and its MPD. And finally we discuss a useful optimization technique for the exponential search algorithm for the MPP.

A major concern in designing the present algorithms has been the size of the grammar. In the case of DOP, the expected STSG size has a greater impact on execution time than the input sentence length has. A precompilation step, discussed in Section 14.3, significantly reduces the effect of the grammar size on the execution time of the present algorithms. The achieved time complexity of these algorithms, for DOP natural language STSGs, is approximately $\mathcal{O}(|A|n^3)$.

14.2 Definitions and conventions

An **STSG** is a quintuple (V_N, V_T, S, $\mathcal{C}$, PT), where V_N and V_T denote respectively the (finite) set of nonterminal and the set of terminal symbols, S denotes the start nonterminal, $\mathcal{C}$ is a set of elementary trees (of arbitrary depth ≥1) and PT is a function that assigns a value $0 < PT(t) \leq 1$ (probability) to each elementary tree t such that

$$\sum_{root(t)=N}^{t\in\mathcal{C}} PT(t) = 1$$

(where $root(t)$ denotes the root of tree t). An elementary tree in $\mathcal{C}$ has only nonterminals as internal nodes but may have both terminals and nonterminals on its frontier. A frontier nonterminal is called an "open tree". The quadruple (V_N, V_T, S, $\mathcal{C}$) of a given STSG (V_N, V_T, S, $\mathcal{C}$, PT) is called the TSG underlying the STSG.

Substitution: If the left-most open tree N of tree t is equal to the root of tree t_1 then $t \circ t_1$ denotes the tree obtained by substituting t_1 for N in t. The partial function $\circ$ is called "left-most substitution". Notice that the value $PT(t)$ for elementary tree t with root N is the probability of substituting t for any open tree N in any elementary tree in $\mathcal{C}$.

A **left-most derivation** (*lmd*) is any sequence of left-most substitutions

$$lmd = (\ldots(t_1 \circ t_2) \circ \ldots) \circ t_n$$

where $t_1, \ldots, t_n \in \mathcal{C}$, $root(t_1) = S$ and the frontier of *lmd* consists only of terminals. The probability $P(lmd)$ is defined as

$$P(lmd) = PT(t_1) \times \ldots \times PT(t_n)$$

For convenience, we will use the term "derivation" for left-most derivation.

A **parse** is any tree that is the result of a derivation. A parse can have various derivations. The probability of a parse is defined as the sum of the probabilities of all its derivations.

A **finitely ambiguous grammar** is any grammar that does not derive a finite string in an infinite number of left-most derivations.

A **proper grammar** has only such nonterminals whose further rewriting eventually results in terminal strings.

An STSG is in **extended CNF** (ECNF) if in each elementary tree each nonterminal node has *one nonterminal* child, *two nonterminal* children or only *one terminal* child (the last two constitute the Chomsky Normal Form (CNF)).[5]

Notation:

A, B, C, N denote nonterminal symbols.

w denotes a terminal symbol.

α, β denote strings of zero or more symbols that are either terminals or nonterminals.

z denotes strings of one or more terminal symbols.

Attaching subscripts to the above symbols does not change their type.

CFG *lmds* of zero or more, exactly one, and at least one step(s) are denoted respectively by $\rightsquigarrow$, $\rightarrow$, $\overset{+}{\rightsquigarrow}$. Note that $\rightarrow$ is also used in declarations of functions.

Definition: A context-free rule (CF rule) $R = A \rightarrow A_1, \ldots, A_n$ is said to "appear" in a tree $t \in \mathcal{C}$ if one of the following is true:

- A is the root of t and $A_1, \ldots, A_n$ are its direct children (in this order from left to right).
- R appears in the (sub)tree under one of the children of the root of t.

Definition: $(V_N, V_T, S, \mathcal{R})$ is the CFG underlying the TSG $(V_N, V_T, S, \mathcal{C})$ *iff* $\mathcal{R}$ is the set $\{R \mid \text{rule } R \text{ appears in a tree in } (V_N, V_T, S, \mathcal{C})\}$. An *item* of a CFG is any of its rules of which the right-hand side (rhs) contains a dot.[6] *ITEMS* denotes the set of all items of a CFG.

Global assumption: We deal only with STSGs for which the underlying CFG is proper, finitely ambiguous and in ECNF.

14.3 Rule-based STSGs

As is always the case with algorithms, efficiency requirements constrain the range of the data structures they can employ. In our case this expresses the need to compile the STSG into another form more suitable for the efficient computations we intend to study.

5. Each STSG can be transformed into this form without disturbing the probabilistic model. Moreover, a reverse transformation of any result obtained in the ECNF is easy and valid.

6. Items serve as notation for bottom-up parsing. The dot serves as a marker; the part to its left is the part already recognized, while to its right lies the part yet to be recognized.

14.3.1 Granularity of parsing units

As a starting point we assume tabular parsing methods, e.g. CKY (Younger 1967) and Earley (1970), simply because they enable the efficient parsing of all CFGs and because they construct a useful table, also called a "parse forest", of the input sentence. For an STSG, a parse forest may be constructed by using either elementary trees or CF-rules as basic parsing units. However, we have two reasons to prefer CF-rules above trees as basic parsing units. First, the employment of too coarse parsing units usually means the lack of information necessary for the execution of certain tasks. For example, employing trees disables the distinction between derivations that result in different parses (since two trees that fit in the same contexts might have different internal structure). And, secondly, since the grammar size affects the efficiency of parsing, it is worthwhile considering how to reduce this effect by using basic knowledge about natural language. In our case, it is clear that the number of possible natural language CF-rules is usually much smaller than the number of possible trees. Later on we show that this justifies our preference for rules over trees. Thus, we choose to employ a suitable CF-rule-based representation of STSGs that captures their (limited) context-sensitivity.

14.3.2 Intuition

Assume we assign to each nonfrontier nonterminal in each elementary tree in C a unique code from a code domain Π (say, the integers), and consider the parse generated by an STSG derivation. The code sequence obtained by collecting (in e.g. Node-Left-Right order[7]) the codes from this tree correspond to the particular derivation at hand. Moreover, no other derivation has an equal code sequence. However, not all such sequences correspond to STSG derivations. A closer study of an STSG derivation reveals the following properties:

- The code of its start nonterminal S corresponds to the root of an elementary tree.
- For any two nonterminals N and N_j, which are a parent and its jth child ($j \in \{1,2\}$) in the derivation, one of the following holds:
  - — N's code is parent of N_j's code in an elementary tree.
  - — N's code appears in an elementary tree with N_j as its open-tree child, and N_j's code is the code of the root of an elementary tree.

Therefore, the derivations of an STSG are simply parses of its underlying CFG decorated with codes in a way that fulfils the constraint embedded in this property. Next we use this observation to infer the rule-based STSG (RB-STSG) where this property is captured in the "viability" relation.

7. The function NLR is defined recursively as follows. If t is a terminal then NLR(t) is the empty code sequence. Else NLR($t[t_1 \ldots t_n]$) is the code sequence that starts with the code of t followed by the sequence #[NLR(t_1)# . . . #NLR(t_n)], where # delimits codes in code sequences.

14.3.3 The RB-STSG

Given an STSG in which the nonfrontier nodes of all its elementary trees are coded uniquely with values from Π (e.g. the integers), infer three predicates from it:

- *Parent?*(c, c', j) denotes the proposition "c and c' are respectively the codes of a parent and its jth child in a tree in $\mathcal{C}$".
- *Root?*(c) denotes the proposition "c is the code of the root of a tree in $\mathcal{C}$".
- *OT?*(c, j) denotes the proposition "child j (enumeration always from left to right) of the node with code c is an open tree".

The seven-tuple (V_N, V_T, S, $\mathcal{R}$, $\mathcal{A}$, *Viable?*, P) is the RB-STSG representation of the STSG (V_N, V_T, S, $\mathcal{C}$, PT), where:

- (V_N, V_T, S, $\mathcal{R}$) is the CFG underlying STSG,
- *Viable?*(c, c_j, j) = *Parent?*(c, c_j, j) **or** (*OT?*(c,j) **and** *Root?*(c_j)),
- $\mathcal{A} = \{\mathcal{A}(R) | R \in \mathcal{R}\}$, where
  $\mathcal{A}(R = N \rightarrow \alpha) = \{c \mid c$ is code of N for an appearance of R in $\mathcal{C}\}$.
- P: $\Pi \rightarrow (\Pi \times \{1, 2\}) \rightarrow [0\ .\ .\ 1]\}$

$$P(c)(c', j) = \begin{cases} PT(t) & \textbf{if } c \text{ is code of the root of some } t \in \mathcal{C} \\ 1 & \textbf{else if } Viable?(c', c, j) \\ 0 & \textbf{otherwise} \end{cases}$$

where c, $c' \in \Pi$ and and $j \in \{1,2\}$.

The set $\mathcal{A}(R)$ in this definition denotes the set of all "appearances" of a rule $R \in \mathcal{R}$ in the tree set. In any decorated parse tree in which c decorates a node, the term $P(c)$ denotes the probability of c as a function of the code of its parent c' and its child number j (from left to right).[8] It expresses the fact that, in an STSG, the probability of a CF-rule of its underlying CFG is "context-sensitive"; the probability of a given rule is a function of its particular appearance (code) in the tree set.

Thus, the RB-STSG models the STSG as a grammar of two components, the syntactic and the statistical components, where the second is applied as a selection rule on top of the first. Therefore, the algorithms presented below are two-phase algorithms: initially the parse forest is constructed, using the CFG underlying the STSG at hand, and consequently the statistical relations are calculated on this parse forest.

An RB-STSG derivation is a decorated parse, of the underlying CFG, in which the viability relation holds between any two codes that are parent and child, and of which the root is decorated with a code of a root of a tree from $\mathcal{C}$.[9]

8. Given a tree t from $\mathcal{C}$, the function P assigns to the root of t the value $PT(t)$ and to all other internal nodes of t the probability 1. This way the probability of an elementary tree computed from those of its parts is equal to $PT(t)$. On the other hand, the probability of any other tree *not* in $\mathcal{C}$, which consists of branches from different trees (non-whole trees), is equal to 0. For this reason, the notation we employ for functions in the sequel is as follows: by definition, any real number p can be applied to any tuple (as if being a function), and the result is the real number itself. A function that has two parameters P:$\Pi \rightarrow \Pi \rightarrow \mathcal{R}$ may be applied to a first parameter $c \in \Pi$ to become a function of the second parameter $P(c)$:$\Pi \rightarrow \mathcal{R}$.

9. For some parses of the CFG the only decoration that fulfils these conditions results in empty sets. For such parses there are no corresponding STSG parses.

14.3.4 Derivation forests of parses

The main problem is how to represent an STSG parse in the RB-STSG in a way that bypasses the exponential number of derivations a parse can have. The answer is that a parse can be represented as a "derivation forest" in which node-sharing enables polynomial-time decoration (and probability computation) of that parse. A derivation forest of a parse is a decoration of each nonterminal node in the parse with a code set. The code set decorating a node contains only those codes that start a subderivation[10] of the subparse under that node. The decoration function *DF* below computes the derivation forest for a given parse of the CFG underlying the RB-STSG. It does so in two passes which can be categorized respectively as bottom-up and top-down.[11] During the bottom-up phase (henceforth function $\mathcal{D}$) *DF* decorates a parse *Par* with sets of codes that are in the viability relation with some of their children. During the top-down pass all codes in each decorating set that are not in the viability relation with any of their parents are eliminated. For the definition of *DF(Par)* we assume that two functions are given: *Parent* and *Child#*. Given a subparse *Sub*, *Parent(Sub)* denotes the smallest subparse of *Par* of which *Sub* is a subparse.[12] In that case, *Child#(Sub)* denotes the child-number of the root of *Sub* with respect to the root of *Parent(Sub)*.

Algorithm 1. Computing the derivation forest for *Par*, and for each of its subparses *Sub*:

$$DF(Par) = \{c \in \mathcal{D}(Par) | Root?(c)\}$$

$$DF(sub) = Eliminate(DF(Parent(Sub)), \mathcal{D}(Sub), Child\#(Sub))$$

Algorithm 2. *Eliminate* eliminates from a decoration set *S*2 all codes that have no viable parent in decoration set *S*1. We assume that *S*2 decorates the *i*th child of the node decorated with *S*1 in a parse.

$$Eliminate(S1, S2, i) = \{c2 \in S2 | \exists c1 \in S1 \text{ such that } Viable?(c1, c2, i)\}$$

Algorithm 3. Computing the derivation forest $\mathcal{D}(Par)$ for a given RB-STSG subparse *Par* of length[13] $l \geq 1$:

$l = 1$: Assume *Par* is derived from rule $R = N \rightarrow u$ then $\mathcal{D}(Par) := \mathcal{A}(R)$.

$l > 1$: Let $Par = N \rightarrow N_1 \ldots N_i \rightsquigarrow z_1 \ldots z_i$, where $i \in \{1,2\}$. Let also for each $1 \leq j \leq i$, the following denote the subparse of *Par* under N_j (of length $l_j < l$),

$$Par_j = N_j \rightarrow \alpha_j \rightsquigarrow z_j$$

10. A subderivation of the STSG is a generalization of the notion of a derivation where its root nonterminal is not necessarily *S*, and the code of that root is not necessarily equal to that of a root of an elementary tree.

11. The two phases resemble the two phases of the CKY algorithm in which in the first phase, bottom-up, the table is constructed and items are added, and in the second phase, top-down, the items that do not participate in parses of the input sentence are eliminated (i.e. the pruning phase).

12. Only in case *Sub* = *Par* the equality *Parent(Sub)* = *Sub* holds.

13. The number of CF-rule applications in the left-most derivation of its underlying CFG-subparse.

and denote with R the rule $N \rightarrow N_1 \ldots N_i$.

$$\mathcal{D}(Par) = \left\{ c \in A(R) \mid \begin{array}{c} \forall 1 \leq j \leq i: \\ \exists c_j \in \mathcal{D}(Par_j) \text{ such that } Viable?(c, c_j, j) \end{array} \right\}$$

Algorithm $\mathcal{D}$ (also *DF*) decorates a parse of length l in time $\mathcal{O}(|\mathcal{A}(R)|^2 l)$, where $|\mathcal{A}(R)| = \max\{|\mathcal{A}(R)| \, | R \in \mathcal{R}\}$ (i.e. the size of the decorating sets). However, a time complexity of $\mathcal{O}(|\mathcal{A}(R)| l)$ can be achieved by exploiting a property of the viability relation discussed below. For finitely ambiguous grammars (the STSG is proper and finitely ambiguous *iff* its RB-STSG is also so), l is polynomial $\mathcal{O}(n)$ in the length n of the sentence (i.e. the frontier of the parse).

The property of the viability relation mentioned above (denoted *property*†) is the following. Let *Par*, Par_j, R and j be as in Algorithm 3. The set $\mathcal{A}(R)$ is partitioned at position j into two complementary subsets. The first subset, denoted *OT*(R, j) contains those codes that have an open-tree child at position j, where substitution can take place. The other subset, denoted $I(R, j)$, contains all codes of which child j is an internal node in an elementary tree.

$$OT(R, j) = \{c \in \mathcal{A}(R) | OT?(c, j)\}$$

$$I(R, j) = \{c \in \mathcal{A}(R) | \exists c', Parent?(c, c', j)\}$$

The codes of *OT*(R, j) are either all in $\mathcal{D}(Par)$ or none of them is. Moreover, it is enough to do the computations on $\mathcal{D}(Par_j)$ (e.g. computing the MPD or the total probability) only for one of these codes and copy the result to the rest. This is simply because all codes in *OT*(R, j) allow the same substitutions to take place at position j. As for the codes in $I(R, j)$, each of these has one unique code child that must be searched for in $\mathcal{D}(Par_j)$; however, it is possible to maintain a function that computes, in $\mathcal{O}(1)$, for each code the position of its unique child.[14] In all cases, for each code in $\mathcal{D}(Par)$ the computations that must be carried out are of complexity $\mathcal{O}(1)$. We note here that this applies not only for the algorithms above but also for the remaining algorithms in this and the next section.

14.3.5 The probability of a parse

The derivation forest constructed above enables the use of the following property of real numbers:

$$a \times b_1 + \ldots + a \times b_m = a \times (b_1 + \ldots + b_m)$$

This property holds for the total probability of all subderivations, of a subparse *Par*, that start with a code a (in the equation, the probability of a is represented by a itself). The code b_i, for all $1 \leq i \leq m$, should be in the decorating set of the jth child of *Par*'s root. Moreover, for all $1 \leq i \leq m$ the relation $Viable?(a, b_i, j)$ must hold. Thus, it is possible to maintain one single probability value for all the derivations of a parse that start with the same code. The following algorithm P computes the probability

14. There is one and only one rule R_k such that child code c' is in $\mathcal{A}(R_k)$. If c' is given position l in $\mathcal{A}(R_k)$ (implemented as an ordered list) then the function should return position $\langle k, l \rangle$.

of a parse.[15] It employs the algorithm *Pp* to compute for each code *c*, which starts some of the derivations of *Par*, the total probability of these derivations.[16]

Algorithm 4. Computing the probability of a given parse *Par*:

$$P(Par) = \begin{cases} \sum_{c \in DF(Par)} Pp(c) & \textbf{if } DF(Par) \neq \emptyset \\ 0 & \textbf{otherwise} \end{cases}$$

Algorithm 5. The function *Pp* computes for a given code *c* the total probability of all derivations that start with it. The computation is inductive over *l*, the length of *Par*:

$l = 1$: $Pp(c) = P(c)$

$l > 1$: Assume $Par = N \rightarrow N_1 \ldots N_i \rightsquigarrow z_1 \ldots z_i$, $i \in \{1,2\}$. And that for each $1 \leq j \leq i$, $Par_j = N_j \rightarrow \alpha_j \rightsquigarrow z_j$ is the subparse of *Par* under N_j (of length $l_j < l$).

$$Pp(c) = P(c) \times \sum_{c_1 \in DF(Par_1)} \cdots \sum_{c_i \in DF(Par_i)} Pp(c_1)(c,1) \times \ldots \times Pp(c_i)(c,i)$$

Since function *Pp* is recursive in such a way that the probability of a child is computed before that of its parent then these probabilities shall be functions of the parent and child-number. The term $Pp(c_i)(c,i)$ expresses the instantiation of the probability of the child c_i as soon as its (possible) parent *c* and its child-number *i* are at hand.

14.4 Parsing an input sentence

In this section we use the algorithms discussed in the previous section to deal with input sentences. Instead of one parse, we have to deal with many. A suitable representation of the CFG parses of an input sentence is a parse forest constructed by the CKY algorithm. For the RB-STSG, such a parse forest can be constructed on the basis of the CFG underlying it. However, it is again necessary to construct the derivation forest for such a parse forest. The derivation forest of an input sentence serves as the basis for the algorithms for computing the probability of the sentence and its MPD in polynomial time. The problem of finding the MPP is discussed in Section 14.5.

---

15. This algorithm assigns probability 0 to each parse of the CFG that is not a parse of the STSG. However, in real-life implementations such parses can be eliminated beforehand by function *DF* and the CKY algorithm.

16. Notice that the distributivity property $a \times b_1 \oplus \ldots \oplus a \times b_m = a \times (b_1 \oplus \ldots \oplus b_m)$ holds for many operators $\oplus$ on reals, e.g. $+$, *min*, *max*, where *min* and *max* compute the minimum and maximum respectively of two reals. In particular, if instead of $\oplus$ we choose the operator *max*, then we obtain the algorithm for computing the most probable derivation for the given parse. The main necessary change in the algorithm is then to exchange each Σ with *max* on sets of reals.

14.4.1 Parse forest

A well-known and widely used algorithm for constructing parse forests for CFGs in polynomial time is the CKY (Younger 1967). It parses an input sentence $w_0^n = w_1 \ldots w_n$ and constructs a parse forest $\mathbb{C}$. Such a parse forest is a table of $n \times n$ entries, each representing a set of "items". For a specification of this algorithm see the Appendix. For the algorithm itself the reader is referred to Aho & Ullman (1972) and Jelinek et al. (1990). For convenience, in what follows, we say that *item* = $A \rightarrow \alpha \bullet \beta$ parses w_i^j *iff* $Par = A \rightarrow \alpha\beta \rightsquigarrow w_i^j \beta$. In that case, we also say that *Par* is a parse of w_i^j from *item.*

14.4.2 The derivation forest

The derivation forest is a generalization of Algorithm 5, i.e. it is also a decoration two-pass function *DF*. For lack of space, we only consider the bottom-up pass (function $\mathcal{D}$). Roughly speaking, $\mathcal{D}(item, i, j)$ is the set of all codes that start any of the (sub)derivations of the (sub)parses of w_i^j from *item.* Therefore, $\mathcal{D}(item, i, j)$ should be the union of all decorations of the parses of w_i^j from *item.* For the algorithm and its polynomiality see the Appendix.

14.4.3 Probability of an input sentence

The computation of the total probability of an input sentence (parse forest) is a generalization of that for a given parse. $P(w_0^n)$ denotes the probability of the sentence w_0^n and *Pp*: $\Pi \times ITEMS \times [0,n] \rightarrow [0,n]$ is the generalization of the former function *Pp* (it computes the sum of the probabilities of all derivations that start with code *c* for a given item in an entry of the CKY table).

Algorithm 6. $$P(w_0^n) = \sum_{\substack{S \rightarrow \alpha\bullet \in \mathbb{C}[0,n] \\ c \in DF(S \rightarrow \alpha\bullet, 0, n)}} Pp(c, S \rightarrow \alpha\bullet, 0, n)$$

$Pp(c, item, i, j) =$ **Case** *item* **of**

$$A \rightarrow w_{i+1}\bullet : P(c)$$

$$A \rightarrow B\bullet : P(c) \times \sum_{\alpha} \sum_{c1 \in DF(B \rightarrow \alpha\bullet, i, j)} Pp(c1, B \rightarrow \alpha\bullet, i, j)(c, 1)$$

$$A \rightarrow B \bullet C : \sum_{\alpha} \sum_{c1 \in DF(B \rightarrow \alpha\bullet, i, j)} Pp(c1, B \rightarrow \alpha\bullet, i, j)(c, 1)$$

$$A \rightarrow BC\bullet : P(c) \times \sum_{\alpha, (i<j<k)} \sum_{c2 \in DF(C \rightarrow \alpha\bullet, k, j)} Pp(c, A \rightarrow B \bullet C, i, j) \times Pp(c2, C \rightarrow \alpha\bullet, k, j)(c, 2)$$

Algorithm 6 can be adapted to finding the MPD for a sentence if every Σ is exchanged with the operator *max* on sets of reals. The polynomiality of its computation follows from that of the CKY and from the fact that the sets DF are all bounded in size by a constant.

Algorithm 6 shows great similarity to the algorithm of Schabes & Waters (1993) for stochastic lexicalised CFGs. The main difference is in our RB-STSG representation which results in the derivation forest discussed above. This reduces the effect of the grammar size on execution time as shown below. Moreover, such a forest is essential for the algorithms and optimizations discussed in the next section.

Constructing the parse forest for $(V_N, V_T, S, \mathcal{R}, \mathcal{A}, Viable?, P)$ using the CKY is of time-complexity $\mathcal{O}(|\mathcal{R}|n^3)$, where $|\mathcal{R}|$ denotes the number of CF-rules. Computing the derivation forest and the MPD (or sentence probability) has time-complexity $\mathcal{O}(|\mathcal{A}||\mathcal{R}|n^3)$, where $|\mathcal{A}|$ is the number of internal nodes of all trees in $\mathcal{C}$ (there are at most $|\mathcal{R}|$ different items in each of the n^2 entries of the CKY table, for each of these items an average of $|\mathcal{A}|/|\mathcal{R}|$ codes should be computed for each of the $n|\mathcal{R}|$ children nodes of that item.[17] Therefore, in total this algorithm has time-complexity given by the term $\mathcal{O}(|\mathcal{R}|n^3) + \mathcal{O}(|\mathcal{A}||\mathcal{R}|n^3)$. For sufficiently small values of $|\mathcal{R}|/|\mathcal{A}|$ this algorithm has time-complexity $\mathcal{O}(|\mathcal{A}|n^3)$. We have good reasons to believe that the "real-world" STSGs that DOP assumes are in the set of STSGs for which this is indeed the case (see also Section 14.6). In comparison, the algorithm presented in Schabes & Waters (1993) can be tailored for STSGs to achieve time-complexity $\mathcal{O}(|\mathcal{A}|^2 n^3)$.

14.5 The most probable parse

In this section we study the problem of finding the MPP for an input sentence in RB-STSGs. Probabilities of subderivations and subparses in RB-STSGs are context-sensitive since CF-rules receive probabilities that depend on the trees they appear in (reflected by the viability relation). This context-sensitive probability adds a dimension to the MPP problem that is absent in SCFGs. Some comparable models are the CFG with context-sensitive probability (Magerman & Weir 1992), SLCFG (Schabes 1992; Schabes & Waters 1993) and Unification-based CFG (Carroll & Briscoe 1992). While Schabes & Waters (1993) do not consider the MPP problem, Carroll & Briscoe (1992) estimate the MPP by selecting, at each shared node, the most probable of all partial parses. In Magerman & Weir (1992), new emerging nodes are added to the parse table only if they are admitted by a special "probabilistic predictor". Thus none of these approaches guarantees a polynomial (exact) solution such as the Viterbi (Fujisaki et al. 1989) for SCFGs. This should not be surprising: because of their context-sensitive probabilities it is harder to predict with certainty that some subparses will result in less probable parses. This early "prediction" is our aim in this section, where we present a technique to discover some of the subparses

17. Remember that the same property † of the viability relation, discussed in Section 14.3, holds here and enables computation in $\mathcal{O}(1)$ per code.

that surely do not lead to the MPP. This technique is a generalization of the adaptation of the Viterbi to STSGs (RB-STSGs). Unfortunately, even this generalization does not guarantee polynomial search for the MPP for STSGs.

14.5.1 A Viterbi-like optimization

For SCFGs it is possible to use the so-called "Viterbi elimination" (Fujisaki et al. 1989) which guarantees that the maximum number of parses at each step of CKY is bounded by a constant.[18] A similar elimination mechanism for RB-STSGs does not exist yet. However, an optimization based on the same idea is possible. It might reduce the amount of work but does not guarantee that the number of parses at each step of the search will be bounded by a constant.

The following lemma states two conditions that a pair of subparses of the same part of the sentence must fulfil in order to eliminate one of them. It demands that the first "fits (at least) in the same contexts" as the second which in its turn must be "less probable". It then states that the second may be eliminated. The requirement "fit in the same contexts" in this case goes beyond the equality of the root nonterminals of both subparses as in the Viterbi. In the RB-STSG, the range of contexts of a subparse is also affected by the viability relation between the codes of the context and the codes of the subparse. Therefore, the requirement is that for each subderivation of the second subparse there are subderivations of the first that start with the same codes.

The second requirement, "less probable", is also influenced by the context-sensitivity of probabilities. We cannot simply sum up the probabilities of the subderivations because this sum implies nothing about how much each of them will be influenced by the context (the rest of the sentence). Therefore, it is necessary to compare the probabilities of the respective subderivations.

For the statement of this lemma it is necessary to define the function *Psucc*. As noted in earlier sections, the function $P{:}\Pi \rightarrow (\Pi \times \{1,2\}) \rightarrow [0,1]$ is defined for codes $c \in \Pi$ to be a function of the code of the parent and the child-number of c. Such is the case with probabilities of codes that decorate subparses, given by function *Pp*. The function *Psucc* instantiates a given function $Pp(c_j)$ to any c and j that fulfil $Viable?(c, c_j, j)$, in case $Root?(c_j)$ does *not* hold. And otherwise $Psucc(Pp(c_j))$ is simply $Pp(c_j)$.

Lemma 1. Let $Par1 = N \overset{+}{\rightsquigarrow} \alpha \overset{+}{\rightsquigarrow} z$ and $Par2 = N \overset{+}{\rightsquigarrow} \beta \overset{+}{\rightsquigarrow} z$ be two (partial) parses of the CFG underlying the RB-STSG, encountered while parsing the string $xzv \in V_T{}^+$, where $\alpha \neq \beta$. Moreover, let Pp_{Par1} and Pp_{Par2} be the two instances of function *Pp* (as defined in Algorithm 6) computed for *Par*1 and *Par*2 respectively. It is possible to eliminate *Par*2 if the following conditions hold:

- $DF(Par2) \subseteq DF(Par1)$
- $\forall a \in DF(Par2) : Psucc(Pp_{Par1}(a)) \geq Psucc(Pp_{Par2}(a))$

18. The idea behind Viterbi is that two different parses of the same part of the sentence having the same root can both be developed (if at all) to parses of the whole sentence in the same ways (i.e. if one appears in a parse then it can be replaced by the other). Therefore, if one of these two (sub)parses has lower probability then it can be eliminated even before it becomes a parse of the whole sentence.

The proof can be seen as the Viterbi applied for each of $a \in DF(Par2)$. Intuitively speaking, if there is any parse *Parse*2 of the whole input sentence of which *Par*2 is part, then there is another parse *Parse*1 which can be obtained from *Parse*2 by exchanging *Par*2 with *Par*1. This is true because $\mathcal{D}(Par2) \subseteq \mathcal{D}(Par1)$. Therefore, $P(Parse1) \geq P(Parse2)$ holds, provided that the second condition of the lemma also holds.

The conditions of this lemma are more restrictive than those stated by the SCFG's Viterbi. Moreover they are quite costly to check. However, if SCFGs are viewed as STSGs of which the trees are of depth 1, then this lemma reduces to the SCFG's Viterbi.

14.5.2 A more general optimization

A clear weakness of the aforementioned Viterbi-like optimization is that its requirements are very restrictive. This stems from not knowing beforehand what contexts influence the probability of a given subparse. This can be (partially) dealt with if an upper and a lower bound are given on the probabilities of the parses in which the subparse at hand participates. To compute such upper and lower bounds, however, it is necessary to have upper and lower bounds on the "outside probability" of each subderivation of the subparse at hand. An optimization technique based on this observation is presented below. It generalizes the Viterbi-like optimization in that it is applicable at least as often. Moreover, in most cases, checking its requirements is less time-consuming.

Assume for the rest of this section that *Par* and *Sub* denote respectively a parse of w_0^n and its subparse that derives w_i^j, for some $0 \leq i < j \leq n$.

For convenience, we first explain the idea on SCFGs. For SCFGs, the "outside probability" of subparse *Sub* w.r.t. a given parse *Par* is defined as the ratio between the probability of *Par* and that of *Sub* (see Fig. 14.1).

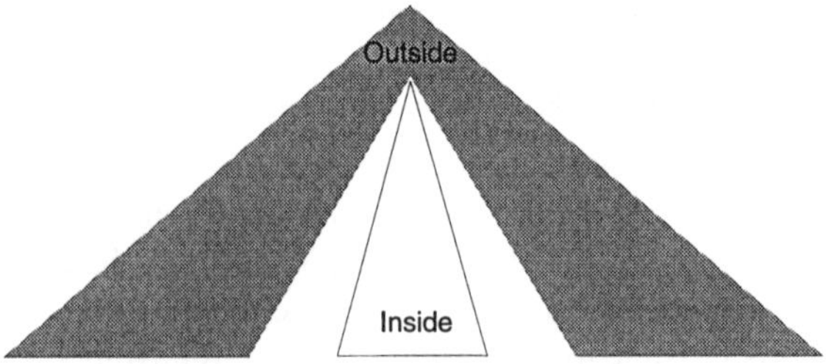

Figure 14.1 *The outside of a subparse.*

Given the sentence w_0^n and its $\mathbb{C}$ table, an upper bound on the outside probabilities (UBO) of all those (sub)parses of w_i^j that share the same root non-terminal *N* is defined as follows. It is the maximum of all outside probabilities each computed for a subparse *Sub* that has root *N* w.r.t. a parse *Par* (of which *Sub* is a subparse as assumed above).[19]. A lower bound on the outside probability (LBO) is computed by taking the minimum instead.

Now, given such bounds on outside probabilities (for each item or nonterminal in entry $\mathbb{C}[i, j]$), the original Viterbi can be modified to compare not only subparses that have the same root but also subparses that have different root nonterminals. For each subparse *Sub*, encountered while searching for the MPP, an upper (lower) bound on the probability of a parse *Par* (related to *Sub* as assumed above) is computed by multiplying the probability of *Sub* by the suitable UBO (LBO) probability appearing in entry $\mathbb{C}[i, j]$.[20] If the *lower* bound of one subparse that derives w_i^j is higher than the *upper* bound of another subparse of w_i^j, then clearly the last subparse can be eliminated. To cover also all Viterbi cases then we may also state that when both subparses have the same root nonterminal, it is sufficient that the upper bound of the first be higher than that of the second to eliminate the second. Although such an optimization is redundant for SCFGs, it can be useful for RB-STSGs.

In what follows, we assume also that *Der* is a derivation of *Par* and that *SubDer* is a subderivation of it deriving w_i^j (i.e. is also a derivation of *Sub*).

For RB-STSGs, the outside probability of a subparse w.r.t. a given parse cannot be defined as the ratio mentioned above for SCFGs, since the probability of an RB-STSG parse, in general, is not simply a series of multiplications. However, the outside probability of a subderivation *SubDer* w.r.t. a derivation *Der* may be defined as the ratio between the probability of *Der* and that of *SubDer*. The outside probability of *SubDer* w.r.t. parse *Par* is then defined as the sum of all the outside probabilities of *SubDer* w.r.t. each derivation *Der* (of which *SubDer* is a subderivation, of course, as just assumed).[21] For lack of space, we only describe here what these UBO and LBO values are for each shared node in the derivation forest of a sentence.[22]

Given an input sentence w_0^n and its derivation forest (Algorithm 8), for each code in the derivation forest we compute the UBO and LBO probabilities as follows. The UBO (LBO) probability for code *c*, from the decorating set of an item *item* in entry $\mathbb{C}[i, j]$, is the maximum (minimum) on all outside probabilities of any subderivation *SubDer* (from *item*) starting with code *c* w.r.t. any parse *Par*. Now we have a derivation forest in which the UBO and LBO probabilities decorate each of its edges. As mentioned earlier, any subparse *Sub* is in fact a set of codes *DF(Sub)* (which is the set decorating its root in its derivation forest). An upper bound UB

19. Of course, this definition is only a declaration of intentions. A polynomial algorithm is achieved by simple adaptation of the CKY algorithm.

20. The UBO probability is attached to the item from which *Sub* is a parse of w_i^j in the sense defined in Section 14.4.1.

21. Clearly the probability of any derivation *Der* is the product of the outside probability of *SubDer* w.r.t. it with the probability of *SubDer*. The sum of the probabilities of *Der* is then equal to the product of the probability of *SubDer* with the sum of all its outside probabilities each w.r.t. a derivation *Der*.

22. The algorithm computes these values by employing another algorithm that computes upper and lower bounds on *inside* probabilities (UBI and LBI) for each shared node in the derivation forest. The UBI (LBI) is obtained from Algorithm 6 by exchanging each left-most Σ into *max* (*min*) on sets of reals in function *Pp*. The computation of the UBO and LBO then proceeds top-down starting from entry $\mathbb{C}[0,n]$.

(lower bound LB) on the probability of any parse *Par* of which *Sub* is a subparse is achieved as the sum of products of the UBO (LBO) of a c in *DF*(*Sub*) with the sum of the probabilities of all derivations of *Sub* that start with c.[23] The optimization technique then states the following. For any two subparses of w_i^j encountered during the search for the MPP, if the UB of the one is smaller than the LB of the other then the first can be eliminated. Moreover, to cover all Viterbi cases also, if both subparses fulfil the first condition of Lemma 1 then it is sufficient that the UB of the first be larger than the UB of the second in order to eliminate the second.

The computation of the UBO and LBO values on the derivation forest of a given sentence is accomplished in polynomial time. The above UB (LB) value is indeed an upper (lower) bound simply because it is an over- (under-) estimation[24] of the probability of any possible parse *Par* that can be obtained from *Sub*. Moreover, the values UB and LB obtained for subparse *Sub* converge to the probability of *Par* as $j-i$ becomes closer to n. This implies that as the number of parses grows during bottom-up search for the MPP, the estimations of UB and LB become better and thus the elimination of subparses becomes more frequent. However, it is easy to show that this optimization does not necessarily result in polynomial algorithms for finding the MPP.

14.5.3 Finding the most probable parse

It is probable that a polynomial algorithm for finding the MPP for STSGs is not feasible. A proof of this is necessary, however. An alternative, for natural language disambiguation, is a potentially exponential algorithm that employs the present optimization together with a method of choosing a fixed number from among the remaining subparses at each shared node by, for example, heuristic, probabilistic prediction or Monte Carlo. At this stage of the research it is more likely that non-biased methods offer a better choice. Therefore, the Monte Carlo technique (Bod 1993a) (biased only towards larger numbers of sampling) seems more attractive. Moreover, it is explicitly tunable towards a better trade-off between accuracy and performance.

14.6 A first experiment under the DOP model

The present algorithms have been developed for general STSGs. A subclass of the STSGs is the STSGs of which the set of elementary trees is inferred from a treebank under DOP (Bod 1993b). DOP takes the set of all subtrees, of arbitrary maximal depth,[25] of all trees in a given treebank to represent an STSG elementary tree set.

23. Computed as *Pp*(c) as in Section 14.4.3.

24. It is an over- (under-) estimation because the probability of each subderivation of *Sub* is multiplied by the maximum (minimum) outside probability on all parses it participates in.

25. Longest path from the root to a leaf-node.

The probability of any subtree t is computed as the ratio between the number of appearances of t in the treebank and the total number of appearances of all subtrees (in the treebank) that have the same root-nonterminal as t.

Previous experiments with DOP (e.g. Bod 1993a), have employed Monte Carlo techniques to estimate the MPD and MPP of an input sentence (no estimations were given of sentence probability). Monte Carlo enabled the verification of DOP's disambiguation accuracy, given a treebank representative for its domain (the ATIS corpus as annotated in the Penn Treebank). Although the accuracy results of these experiments have acknowledged DOP's faithfulness as a performance model of natural language, these experiments were overshadowed by the time-expensive computations that Monte Carlo requires for achieving good estimations.

Preliminary evaluation of the efficiency of the present MPD (and sentence probability) algorithm was tried by reconstructing parts of an experiment described in Bod (1993a). The experiment was applied on the ATIS treebank by taking all subtrees of maximal depth 4. The number of different subtrees of maximal depth 4 (i.e. $|\mathcal{C}|$) was 74 450. The number of different CF-rules these subtrees contain (i.e. $|\mathcal{R}|$) was 870.[26] The number of different internal nodes (i.e. $|\mathcal{A}|$) was 436 831. The length of the sentences used for the experiment varied between 5 and 17 words (in fact these were the POS tags and not the lexical morphemes). These figures give a ratio $|\mathcal{R}|/|\mathcal{A}|$ of less than 0.002, which justifies the claim that the algorithm's time-complexity is $\mathcal{O}(|\mathcal{A}|n^3)$. The execution time obtained is on average about 30 times smaller than the time required by Monte Carlo. Only a small fraction (less than 5%) of the execution time was spent on parse-forest generation (the rest of the time was spent on disambiguation). However, further experiments for a better evaluation of the present algorithms and optimization techniques, and the accuracy they achieve, are certainly necessary.

14.7 Conclusions and future work

We may conjecture that the parsing approach and optimization technique for finding the MPP for a given input sentence discussed in the last section can be generalized to all TAGs. Among the future activities the following are directly related to this work. First, a thorough evaluation of the present algorithms on various corpora is necessary. Secondly, the development of either a polynomial algorithm for the MPP, if that is feasible, or methods for good *estimations* of the MPP for STSGs in polynomial time. Finally, the development of further directions for reducing the effect of the corpus size on the execution time of the algorithms presented in this paper.

---

26. Of which 48, 10 and 812 had respectively a terminal, one nonterminal and two nonterminals on their right-hand sides.

Appendix

The CKY algorithm

The CKY algorithm constructs a table $\mathbb{C}$ for a given input sentence w_0^n and a CFG. Each entry $\mathbb{C}[i, j]$ is a set of items. An item $A \rightarrow \alpha \bullet \beta$ is in $\mathbb{C}[i, j]$ *iff* α derives w_i^j as subparse Par_i^j, and there is a parse of the whole sentence of which Par_i^j is a subparse. Formally speaking, for all $0 \leq i < j \leq n$, *item* is in $\mathbb{C}[i,j]$ *iff*:

If (i=0 and j=n)
Then *item* = $A \rightarrow \alpha\bullet$, where α is either $a \in V_T$, $B \in V_N$ or $BC \in V_N \times V_N$, and $S \leadsto A \rightarrow \alpha \leadsto w_0^n$
Otherwise:

$$item = A \rightarrow w_{i+1}\bullet : j = i+1 \text{ and } S \leadsto w_0^i A\gamma \rightarrow w_0^i w_{i+1}\gamma \leadsto w_0^n$$

$$item = A \rightarrow B\bullet : S \leadsto w_0^i A\gamma \rightarrow w_0^i B\gamma \leadsto w_0^j \leadsto w_0^n$$

$$item = A \rightarrow B\bullet C : S \leadsto w_0^i A\gamma \rightarrow w_0^i BC\gamma \leadsto w_0^j C\gamma \leadsto w_0^n$$

The derivation forest of an input sentence

The function $\mathcal{D}$ below constructs the derivation forest of a given input sentence (it constitutes the bottom-up phase while the other, top-down, phase is not shown here). In the definition of $\mathcal{D}$ we employ the function *Elim* which is very similar to *Eliminate* from Algorithm 2.

Algorithm 7. The function *Elim* eliminates from a decoration set $S2$ all codes that have no viable child in decoration set $S1$. $S1$, $S2$ and i are as in Algorithm 2.
$Elim(S1, S2, i) = \{\mathrm{c2} \in S2 | \exists \mathrm{c1} \in S1 \text{ such that } Viable?(\mathrm{c2}, \mathrm{c1}, \mathrm{i})\}$

Algorithm 8. Computing the derivation forest of an input sentence.
For $1 \leq j \leq n$ **Do**
For $j \leq i \leq 0$ **Do**
For each *item* in $\mathbb{C}[i,j]\$$ **Do**
$\mathcal{D}(item,i,j)$ = **Case** *item* **Of**

$$A \rightarrow w_{i+1}\bullet \ : \ \mathcal{A}(A \rightarrow w_{i+1});$$

$$A \rightarrow B\bullet \ : \ \bigcup_{\alpha} Elim(\mathcal{D}(B \rightarrow \alpha\bullet, i, j), \mathcal{A}(A \rightarrow B), 1);$$

$$A \rightarrow B \bullet C \ : \ \bigcup_{\alpha} Elim(\mathcal{D}(B \rightarrow \alpha\bullet, i, j), \mathcal{A}(A \rightarrow BC), 1);$$

$$A \rightarrow BC \ : \ \bigcup_{\substack{\alpha \\ (i<k<j)}} Elim(\mathcal{D}(C \rightarrow \alpha\bullet, k, j), \mathcal{D}(A \rightarrow B \bullet C, i, k), 2)$$

Since for any item $A \rightarrow \alpha \bullet \beta$ the result of the union in the algorithm is always a subset of $\mathcal{A}(A \rightarrow \alpha\beta)$, then $\mathcal{D}$ always computes a set of codes limited in size to the constant $|\mathcal{A}|/|\mathcal{R}|$. Therefore, the whole computation (based on the CKY algorithm) is accomplished in polynomial time, i.e. $\mathcal{O}(n^3)$.

References

Aho, A. & J. Ullman 1972. *The theory of parsing, translation and compiling.* Englewood Cliffs, NJ: Prentice-Hall.

Bod, R. 1992. A computational model of language performance: data oriented parsing. In *Proceedings of the fifteenth International Conference on Computational Linguistics: COLING-92*, Nantes, 855–9.

Bod, R. 1993a. Monte Carlo parsing. In *Proceedings of the Third International Workshop on Parsing Technologies*, Tilburg, 1–11.

Bod, R. 1993b. Using an annotated corpus as a stochastic grammar. In *Sixth Conference of the European Chapter of the Association for Computational Linguistics*, Utrecht, 37–44.

Carroll, J. & T. Briscoe 1992. Probabilistic normalization and unpacking of packed parse forests for unification-based grammars. In *AAAI Fall Symposium Series: Probabilistic Approaches to Natural Language*, Cambridge, Mass., 33–8.

Earley, J. 1970. An efficient context-free parsing algorithm. *Communications of the ACM* **13**, 94–102.

Fujisaki, T., F. Jelinek, J. Cocke, E. Black & T. Nishino 1989. A probabilistic method for sentence disambiguation. In *Proceedings of the First International Workshop on Parsing Technologies*, Pittsburgh, 139–51.

Jelinek, F., J. Lafferty & R. Mercer 1990. *Basic methods of probabilistic context free grammars.* Technical Report RC16374 (#72684). IBM, Yorktown Heights, NY.

Magerman, D. M. & C. Weir 1992. Efficiency, robustness and accuracy in $\mathcal{P}$icky chart parsing. In *30th Annual Meeting of the Association for Computational Linguistics*, Newark, Del., 40–7.

Marcus, M. P., B. Santorini & M. A. Marcinkiewicz 1993. Building a large annotated corpus of English: the Penn Treebank. *Computational Linguistics* **19**, 313–30.

Resnik, P. 1992. Probabilistic tree-adjoining grammar as a framework for statistical natural language processing. In *Proceedings of the fifteenth International Conference on Computational Linguistics: COLING-92*, Nantes, 418–24.

Scha, R. 1990. Taaltheorie en taaltechnologie: competence en performance. In *Computertoepassingen in de Neerlandistiek*, Q. de Kort & G. Leerdam (eds), 7–21. Almere: Landelijke Vereniging van Neerlandici.

Schabes, Y. 1992. Stochastic lexicalized tree-adjoining grammars. In *Proceedings of the fifteenth International Conference on Computational Linguistics: COLING-92*, Nantes, 426–32.

Schabes, Y. & R. Waters 1993. Stochastic lexicalized context-free grammar. In *Proceedings of the Third International Workshop on Parsing Technologies*, Tilburg, 257–65.

Vijay-Shanker, K. & D. J. Weir 1993. Parsing some constrained grammar formalisms. *Computational Linguistics* **19**, 591–636.

Younger, D. 1967. Recognition and parsing of context-free languages in time n^3. *Information and Control* **10**, 189–208.

Part IV
Example-based Machine Translation

15
Towards automatically aligning German compounds with English word groups

DANIEL JONES AND MELINA ALEXA

15.1 Introduction

The work of various research groups over the last few years (e.g. Brown et al. 1990; Catizone et al. 1989; Gale & Church 1993; Kay & Röscheisen 1993) illustrates a desire to demonstrate the effectiveness of processing natural language without the need for human intervention, particularly with respect to Machine Translation (MT). This is a very attractive idea as it means that much time can be saved in creating lexical and grammatical information before the system can begin translating. In contrast, purely sub-symbolic processing simply entails presenting a system with sufficient bilingual material from which the system can induce the information necessary to translate source language input.

15.2 Motivation

The research reported here[1] is directly motivated by a need to produce alignment data for a sub-symbolic example-based MT system. The MEG system (Multilingual Example-based Generation) aims to allow (monolingual) users to produce translations of a sublanguage text they are composing. As the the source text is being composed in real time (and in conjunction with the translation system) and has not been written before being presented to the translation system as is usually the case, this form of translation has been referred to as "translation without a source text" (Somers et al. 1990).

MEG aims to be as sub-symbolic as possible in the way it carries out the translation process, that is, the information it uses to produce a translation should be produced without any human intervention, i.e. knowledge in the form of human-produced grammars (monolingual and transfer) and lexicons should not be used or relied upon for maintenance reasons. As much information should be extracted from the bilingual corpora as possible so that the bootstrapping process for the incorporation of new languages and the extension of translation capability should be achieved as quickly and as cleanly as possible.

The system architecture (at its simplest level) incorporates processes for matching input text with translation examples in the bilingual corpus and a recombination process that recombines elements of high-scoring matches extracted from the corpus. As the recombination process deals with source and target language translation fragments of various sizes, the recombinator will be greatly facilitated if it has some confidence in how the translation units align with each other. The motivation for producing static (produced off-line) and dynamic (produced at run time) alignment data is then clear.

15.3 Methodology

The bilingual corpus used in the experiments was a manually extended sententially aligned English–German version of the Avalanche Bulletin material obtained from ISSCO in Geneva (Bouillon et al. 1992). The exploratory initial experiments were performed on a small subset of this English–German material. As the requirement for sentential alignment had already been satisfied there was no need to align the sentences using techniques such as those described by Gale & Church (1993).

Kay and Röscheisen (1993) have demonstrated interesting results in the area of word alignment. The results they report for word alignment, i.e. the probability that source word *S* is a translation of target word *T*, appear encouraging. From their first 50 word alignments they claim (approximately) an 84% success rate.

1. This research was sponsored by the Science and Engineering Research Council, grant number GR/G43546.

The procedures involved in this form of word alignment can be expressed generally as follows:

1. Make word lists for each of the separate language corpora.
2. Pair two words from the source and target language lists. As this is a statistical procedure no *a priori* judgements are made regarding which source words align with which target words, so this pairing is random.
3. Locate sentences in source and target corpora that contain these words.
4. Seek justification for the current word pairing being an actual alignment. The more times this pair of words occurs in aligned sentences the greater the probability they are translations of one another. Also, the frequency each word in the pair occurs across the corpus as a whole adds weight to the probability of alignment. For example, if a word only occurs once throughout the entire source corpus, the possibility of its producing spurious data is greater.

15.4 Experiments in word alignment

A relatively small subset of the parallel sententially aligned English–German corpus was used for the initial word-alignment experiments (approximately 40 bulletins). The raw corpus sizes were 2 543 English words and 1 898 German words. These corpora yielded 290 and 369 unique English and German lexical items respectively.

The algorithm described above was applied to a section of the avalanche corpus. Additionally, as in Kay & Röscheisen's work, Dice's coefficient (van Rijsbergen 1979) was used in order to calculate the alignment probabilities (1),

$$(1)\ P = \frac{2c}{N_S(s) + N_T(t)}$$

where c denotes the number of pairs of sentences in which the proposed aligned words occur, $N_X(x)$ the number of times word x occurs in text X. For example, if the words *the* and *das* occur in a text 23 and 27 times respectively, and they both occur in the same sentences 50 times, the probability that they are in alignment is 1. This seems logical as this distributional behaviour suggests that whenever these two words appear in the text they always occur in the same sentence. By the same token if a source and target word are paired but they never occur in the same sentences, it would be unreasonable to predict that they are in any kind of translation relation.

Generally, the accuracy rate was 35–40% on a single-source-word to single-target-word basis. It was observed that one of the main reasons for this relatively poor performance is the fact that German compounds are used very frequently in the corpus. It is interesting though that this program matches the individual English words that constitute the translation of a particular German compound with only that compound word, providing, however, different probability scores, as shown in Table 15.1.

Table 15.1 Probability scores for individual word alignments between *risk*, *of* and *avalanche*, and *Schneebrettgefahr*.

English	German	Score
risk	Schneebrettgefahr	0.691 589
of	Schneebrettgefahr	0.391 892
avalanche	Schneebrettgefahr	0.638 298

In the similar case of a type of set phrase, only one word of this phrase is matched with both or all the English equivalents. So for the phrase *to be approached with caution* (*vorsichtig zu beurteilen*) we get the alignment shown in Table 15.2.

Table 15.2 Probability scores for individual word alignments between *approached* and *caution*, and *beurteilen*.

English	German	Score
approached	beurteilen	0.857 143
caution	beurteilen	0.857 143

In addition, it is not only German but English compounds that are problematic, as is the case with *as well as* (Table 15.3).

Table 15.3 Probability score for individual word alignment between *well* and *sowie*.

English	German	Score
well	sowie	0.926 829

The problem of compounding with respect to this approach is clear. The "fertility" (Brown et al. 1990) of words in an aligned English–German sentence containing compounds is much greater than sentences where no compounding occurs. Figure 15.1, for example, shows that the single German lexical item *Schneebrettgefahr* actually aligns with four individual English lexical items. The system as it stands will never be able to align compounds with their translation equivalents unless either the compounds are identified or a different method for hypothesizing word groupings is used.

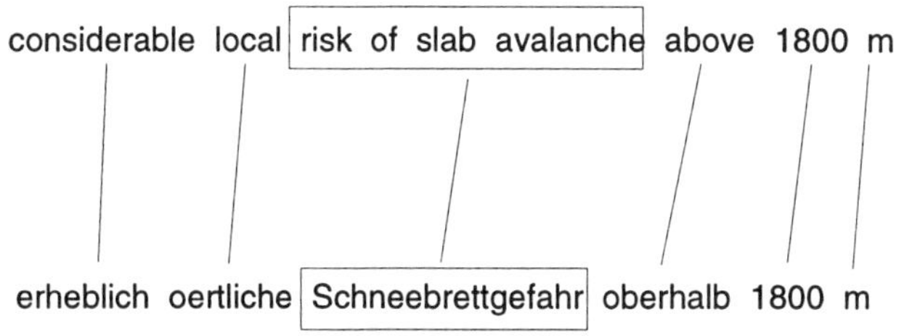

Figure 15.1 *The German–English compound alignment problem.*

Kay & Röscheisen recognize this problem:

The present algorithm rests on being able to identify one-to-one associations between certain words. It is clear . . . that very few correspondences are noticed among everyday words . . . The most interesting further developments would be in the direction of loosening up this dependence on one-to-one associations . . . There are two obvious kinds of looser associations . . . One would consist of connections between a single vocabulary item in one language and two or more in the other, or even between several items in one language and several in the other. (Kay & Röscheisen 1993: 141)

15.5 *n*-gram associations

Loosening up the dependence on one-to-one word relations can be done by increasing the size of the "words" used in the alignment processing. Rather than define a word as a set of characters, a word can be regarded as an *n*-gram.

For these experiments, word lists containing "words" of varying sizes were generated from both the German and English corpora. The aim of the experiments was to establish whether trying to pair different-sized "words" would capture the lexical fertility differences between the two languages.

A set of "words" for aligning was produced by moving a sliding window of varying size (n) across the sentences of the corpus. For example, a sentence can be represented as a set of words (w_i, w_{i+1}, w_{i+2}, . . . , w_N), where $1 \le i \le N-n$.

If the window is to contain three words at a time (n = 3), the first pass will have words i, i+1, and i+2 and in subsequent passes i+1, i+2, i+3 and so on. A range of results was generated by producing *n*-grams where n was as large as 7. Not surprisingly, the results showed most promise when the sizes of the source and target *n*-grams were around the same, i.e. when "word" units only differed by a maximum of three or four actual words. Alignments of 1–6 or 1–5 (source–target) were not very fruitful.

The results of these experiments showed a distinct ability to capture the relations between compounds and non-compounded expressions. For example, in an experiment where alignments were attempted between all possible linear groupings of three

English words and two German words, it was discovered that German compounds and their corresponding English translations were indeed being linked.

15.5.1 German compound identification

Table 15.4 shows sample high-scoring alignments for three English words to two German words. Of course, this is just part of the data produced where the size of "word" used in the alignments varies from 1 to some reasonable number, e.g. 5 or 6. Such a range of data can be used to identify German compounds.

Table 15.4 3–2 alignments.

Three English words	Two German words	Score
section danger levels	Section Gefahrenstufen	1
slab avalanche above	Schneebrettgefahr über	0.444 444
alpine slopes in	Alpennordhang im	0.769 231
the rest of	im übrigen	0.551 724
steep slopes as	Steilhängen sowie	1
drift accumulations as	Triebschneeansammlungen sowie	1
to be approached	zu beurteilen	0.857 143
m there is	m besteht	0.666 667
is a temporary	sind kurzfristig	1
Alpine ridges northern	Alpenhauptkamm nördliches	1
of Valais and	Wallis und	1
this is restricted	diese beschränkt	1
the entire Swiss	ganzen schweizerischen	1
Swiss alpine region	schweizerischen Alpengebiet	0.800 000
Upper Engadine including	Oberengadinin schliesslich	1
and southern Ticino	und Südtessin	1
low avalanche risk	geringe Lawinengefahr	1
safety measures should	Sicherungsmassnahmen sollten	1
with a further	bei zusätzlicher	1
exposed connecting roads	exponierte Verbindungswege	1
on the remaining	am übrigen	1

The method is quite straightforward in that for each set of data, i.e. 1–1, 2–3, 4–2, etc., the highest-scoring alignment from each group is selected. These highest-scoring examples are then compared. For example, if the highest-scoring associations for the input German compound *Schneebrettgefahr* are extracted for each *n*-gram dataset, the associations with English word groups shown in Table 15.5 are revealed.

Table 15.5 Identification of German compound *Schneebrettgefahr*.

N–M	Highest-scoring English alignment	Score
1–1	slab	1.00
2–1	moderate local	0.50
3–1	risk of slab	0.40
4–1	risk of slab avalanche	0.53
5–1	local risk of slab avalanche	0.50

Ignoring for the moment the initial unary word value of 1 for *slab*, the highest value[2] is given to the correct translation, i.e. *risk of slab avalanche*. The influence of *slab*, although scoring 1, should be ignored as it is subsumed by the larger *n*-grams. If a compound is correctly aligned with its word-group translation then it makes sense that individual words from that grouping should also score highly according to Dice's coefficient as their distributional behaviour will be the same. It should be expected that the largest of the *n*-grams should subsume a majority of the smaller *n*-gram groupings. By the same token, words that do not display compounding behaviour will *not* demonstrate such signs of subsumption, e.g. *und* as in Table 15.6.

Table 15.6 Identification of German non-compound *und*.

N–M	Highest-scoring English alignment	Score
1–1	and	1.00
2–1	in the	0.33
3–1	are to be	0.21
4–1	risk of slab avalanche	0.15
5–1	local risk of slab avalanche	0.12

Note that, in this case, there is only one case of subsumption, i.e. 4–1/5–1, and there is a gradual reduction in the score as the unit size of the *n*-gram equivalents increases. This would seem to indicate that the word *und* is not part of a compound.

15.6 Observations and conclusions

The results reported here go some way towards demonstrating the feasibility of at least alleviating the problem of German compounding when bootstrapping a

2. Calculated in the same way with single word–word comparisons, i.e. by using Dice's coefficient.

statistically-based MT system. Being able to identify this type of cross-language lexical fertility is important for establishing potential translation units for the recombinatorial stage (Jones 1996) of the example-based translation process.

The limitations of the experiments so far have to a large extent been caused by the relatively small amount of data used. However, even when, for example, the 1–1 alignment is technically wrong, the highest alignment scored is usually contextually closely associated with what should have been the correct alignment.

Further experimentation will involve increasing the size of the bilingual data. It is assumed that results will improve as spurious distributional data will be eliminated.

References

Bouillon, P., K. Boesefeldt & G. Russell 1992. Compound nouns in a unification-based MT system. In *Proceedings of the Third Conference on Applied Natural Language Processing*, Trento, 209–15.

Brown, P. F., J. Cocke, S. A. Della Pietra, V. J. Della Pietra, F. Jelinek, J. D. Lafferty, R. L. Mercer & P. S. Roossin 1990. A statistical approach to Machine Translation. *Computational Linguistics* **16**, 79–85.

Catizone, R. G. Russell & S. Warwick 1989. Deriving translation data from bilingual texts. In *Proceedings of the First International Lexicon Acquisition Workshop*, Detroit.

Gale, W. A. & K. W. Church 1993. A program for aligning sentences in bilingual corpora. *Computational Linguistics* **19**, 75–103.

Jones, D. 1996. *Analogical natural language processing*. London: UCL Press.

Kay, M. & M. Röscheisen 1993. Text–translation alignment. *Computational Linguistics* **19**, 121–43.

Somers, H., J. Tsujii & D. Jones 1990. Machine Translation without a source text. In *COLING–90: Paper presented to the 13th International Conference on Computational Linguistics*, Helsinki, Vol. 3, 271–6.

van Rijsbergen, C. J. 1979. *Information retrieval*. London: Butterworth.

16
Corpus-based acquisition of transfer functions using psycholinguistic principles

PATRICK JUOLA

16.1 Introduction

The development of symbolic machine translation (MT) systems is difficult and expensive, but the development of non-symbolic MT systems is typically not much easier or less expensive. An ideal MT system would be able to identify the structure of the source and target languages without the assistance of human engineers, but at the same time be easily understood, corrected and updated to reflect new information and situations. For the second, a symbolic approach is almost a necessity, as sub-symbolic or completely automatic inference systems tend to produce nearly opaque sets of numbers as their outputs. However, the process of describing human languages in symbolic terms is difficult and knowledge-intensive. A prototype system, METLA, is described which derives linguistically plausible and understandable transfer functions from paired corpora without the necessity of human intervention or pre-analysis.

16.2 Background

The major engineering bottleneck in MT, in general, is the development of the knowledge base, such as the linguistic analysis tools and the bilingual dictionary. The costs of developing dictionaries or linguistically sophisticated parsers are comparable to the cost of developing an expert system. Many researchers have looked for tools that could be used to automatically develop an analyser for the source language (or a generator for the target language) from samples, or for that matter, a method of developing a bilingual dictionary from samples.

Nagao (1984) proposed just such an analytical method with his proposal of what would become known as "example-based machine translation" (EBMT). Instead of encoding explicit transfer rules, translation systems would store a collection of translation examples that would provide coverage *in context* for the input. A novel sentence would then be compared against the sentences most similar to it in the database, and the similar components would be combined into a translation. Although the notions of "similar" and "component" still require a fair amount of human engineering, systems have been built (e.g. Sumita et al. 1990; Sato 1991) that show good results without an explicit dictionary.

Another approach (Brown et al. 1990) that avoids the knowledge acquisition bottleneck uses a huge bilingual corpus to attempt to solve the translation problem as a mapping between Markov chains. The researchers treat every sentence as generated by a Markov process and then consider every sentence to be a possible translation of every other sentence. The "translation" is simply the most probable translation of a given source sentence. Although this approach avoids the knowledge acquisition problem and can achieve good results, the grammar and analysis techniques are psychologically implausible.

16.3 Self-organizing automatic translation

The present work rests largely on the work of Green (1979) and others (Morgan et al. 1989; Mori & Moeser 1983) and their results on the psycholinguistics of language learning and the inherent structure of natural language. In particular, their research indicates that grammatical constructions are typically marked at surface level by the appearance of a closed-class word or morpheme. A transparent example of this can be seen in Japanese. The basic sentence structure of Japanese is SOV. However, the noun phrase that fills the subject role is specifically *marked* by the appearance of a particle such as *wa* or *ga* immediately following. The object noun phrase is also specifically marked by the particle *o*. Similarly, in English, a noun phrase is typically structured as a determiner or quantifier, a possible set of modifiers, and then the head noun itself. The determiner strongly signals the beginning of a complete noun phrase. If a prepositional phrase follows, it is marked by the appearance of a preposition, and then another noun phrase with its attendant structure. Such markers have not only been attested cross-linguistically, but have been shown in psychological experiments to help language learning greatly. This set of observations together constitute the "Marker Hypothesis".

This hypothesis may provide a way to cast translation problems into a form solvable by standard multivariate optimization techniques. If languages are assumed to be largely compositional and grammatically structured, most of the preliminary work in translation is to identify the grammatical structures and corresponding structures in the target language as well as to find the appropriate expression of those structures. These marker constructions can provide powerful cues to these structures. Using a rewrite-rule formalism defined below, one can define the translation problem as the problem of simultaneous identification of:

- the grammatical organization of the source language;
- the changes necessary to convert the grammar of the source language into that of the target language (which in a context-free language can be done by permutation operations);
- the "dictionary": a table lookup expressing the most appropriate translation for each grammatical element in the source language.

The input to this system is simply a set of paired sentences in the source and target languages. The only preprocessing done is the compilation of a list of the tokens appearing in the input data, to simplify the construction of a source–target dictionary. Unlike Sumita et al. (1990) and others, there is no extensive semantic processing, so the development of a new dataset for a new language pair requires only data entry from an existing body of translated text. The output of this learning, of course, is a description of the translation algorithm as defined above.

16.3.1 The formalism

Juola (1994) demonstrates the existence of a normal form for context-free grammars (CFGs) that incorporates some of the properties of the Marker Hypothesis as described above. Specifically, grammars in "marker-normal form" have all rules in one of the forms shown in (1), and therefore all nonterminal constituents are marked by a terminal symbol.

(1) a. $A \rightarrow \epsilon$
b. $A \rightarrow a$
c. $A \rightarrow bBcCdD \ldots$

This template thus gives a skeletal grammar scheme that can be used to describe large classes of grammars in terms of a relatively small number of parameters (how many rules there are, what terminal symbol appears at position i of rule j, what nonterminal symbol appears at position i+1 of rule j, and so forth).

Given a filled set of these parameters, a closely related grammar can be used to partition sentences into their constituents. In (1c), the initial A-phrase would be partitioned into the "phrases" (bB) (cC) (dD) . . . and each phrase would be recursively parsed using additional rules or sets of rules.

Any phrase (typically a single-word phrase) that cannot be further broken down by this procedure will be treated as a unit for purposes of translation. Such lexicalized units can simply be looked up in a dictionary and replaced by a corresponding target word, most often a direct translation. These translations are used as the basic blocks for constructing the target sentence. The entire process can be learned and run without human intervention, but is understandable enough to permit human analysis and correction if necessary.

16.3.2 The learning algorithm

If there is such a thing as a "most general" problem in computer science, one candidate is certainly nonlinear multivariate optimization. Almost any task of interest can be described as an equation or a set of equations over some complex mathematical space. The reduction of Boolean logic to algebra is well known, and symbolic (discrete) tasks can be easily converted to continuous search spaces by incorporation of an additional term that adds large amounts of error to a system when the parameters are "distant from" the desired discrete numbers. Because of this simple reduction, any semi-mathematical learning situation can be easily cast as a task of simultaneous parameter estimation.

Within this learning framework, it is easy to turn the individual components of the translation system described into semi-numerical optimization tasks. For example, most of a dictionary is a simple word-to-word mapping. With some gross simplifying assumptions, one can simply guess the entire dictionary mapping and then tune the guess, one entry at a time, to reflect the actual contents of the dictionary. Words with multiple definitions (for example, *you* can be translated into French as *tu* or *toi* depending upon its grammatical role) can be handled by simply learning a large number of mappings to be used in the "appropriate" contexts. One-to-many and many-to-one translations (for example, *not* to *ne . . . pas*) can be handled by accepting the null string as a potential word, and thus insertions and deletions can be done in certain specific contexts.

As has been stated above, the task of restructuring the source parse tree to reflect target structure can be performed by a simple permutation of the daughters at a given node. The task of learning a specific minimal-cost permutation has been well studied in optimization theory as the "travelling salesman problem". This can also be solved by a guess-and-tune algorithm where two cities (or constituents) are swapped at each iteration and compared against the desired results. Although in theory each rule of the source grammar will have a permutation to learn, there are few constituents per rule and the problem should still be tractable.

The hardest subproblem to cast into this optimization framework is the acquisition of the grammar. As has been discussed above, the existence of marker words makes the task much easier. If every constituent is marked by the appearance of a closed-class word, then by identifying the relevant marker words, one can segment the sentence into its constituents and parse recursively. Some work (Smith & Witten 1993) has been done on sophisticated methods for identifying such words, but for the present prototype system, the input vocabulary was small enough that the system could simply acquire the marker-word set and all words are therefore potential marker words. The acquisition proceeds as follows: for each rule in the grammar, one must identify the subset of marker words that are relevant to that rule (for example, determiners are relevant to noun phrases) and the classes of the constituents themselves (for example, $S \rightarrow \bar{N}\ \bar{V}$). Guess-and-tune will obviously serve for subset selection (each marker word is either in or out of the relevant set and can be changed individually), and can be made to serve for class identification by enumerating all potential nonterminal symbols and allowing the system to select among them for every symbol on the right-hand side of a skeletal grammar. Given this grammar, the system can use it to parse and translate selected sentences from the training set.

Once the numerical framework is in place, one has a free hand in selecting the learning algorithm itself; the work described below uses a simple variant of simulated annealing. Originally a model of crystal growth, simulated annealing has the advantage of being well known, well studied, and relatively uncontroversial as an optimization technique. This technique is a modified version of a simple random walk through the dataspace of interest. The system starts out at some location in the dataspace (the guess) and makes modifications, at random, to the parameter set. At each stage, the new parameter set is measured against the old parameter set, and if it results in improved performance, the old parameter set is discarded and replaced (the tuning). Even if the new set results in reduced performance, the old set may be discarded and replaced if the reduction is not too bad. As the tuning progresses, the notion of "too bad" is gradually tightened until the system accepts only improving changes and will eventually find the global optimum. Despite the simplicity of this algorithm –

> It guesses some random grammar and then looks to see if it works well enough. If not, it randomly changes something to see if that makes it better. (James Martin, personal communication)

– simulated annealing is actually a relatively powerful and efficient technique for nonlinear optimizations. Other experiments are in progress using other optimization techniques such as genetic algorithms, but the results have been largely similar to the work presented here and so are omitted for brevity. For interim evaluation, as required for error measurement, the system uses an edit-graph formalism (Myers 1986) (`diff`, to UNIX programmers) as an approximate measure of the amount of work that would be necessary to convert the results of the translation into the actual target sentences from the example database.

16.3.3 The translation algorithm

Once a skeletal transfer function has been generated, and particularly at the conclusion of the learning phase, the system should have a list of numerical parameters that describe the actual transfer process. A sentence to be translated is first parsed by the marker-normal-form grammar generated above. All leaf-nodes are replaced by their translations as defined by the context-sensitive dictionary representing their parent class. The system then proceeds to restructure the parse tree in strict bottom-up fashion. The children of a particular parent are reordered in keeping with the permutation function, and then the children's words are concatenated into a constituent phrase that replaces the (sub)tree of the parent.

The parent therefore is now a leaf and a child in its own right for another node, and its phrase will be incorporated into a larger phrase until the entire tree has been reordered and flattened into a translation of the entire source sentence. This sentence can either be presented to the user or compared against the target sentences in the example base for evaluation.

16.4 Experiments

The above formalism has been tested in a series of experiments designed to determine the strengths and limitations of the approach as well as the most efficient algorithms to use for error metrics and optimization techniques. We consider here the two most interesting from a linguistic or theoretical point of view. In the first experiment, artificial context-free grammars covering interesting and relatively complex subsets of French and English (including sentential complements, relative clauses, and gender distinctions) were created, and the system attempted to learn the appropriate transfer functions from English to French based on a 29-sentence artificial corpus developed and tested against the judgements of a native speaker of French. The system was then tested both against the training corpus and against novel sentences that had not been seen in the training phase.

The other experiment was designed as an attempt to model a "situated cognition" task, and to compare the performance of the system against a comparable task for humans, that of learning a second language (Urdu) by exposure to instructional documents. In particular, the system was given the vocabulary and grammar examples from a particular sample of instructional text (Lesson 2 from ur Rahman 1958) and told to learn appropriate transfer functions. As above, the resulting system was tested against both the training corpus and novel sentences (the exercises from the same lesson).

16.5 Evaluation

The problem of evaluating translations, whether human or machine, is difficult indeed. The following sections provide examples of two sorts of evaluations done on the system. The first, a black-box examination, is a simple comparison of the system's results with the correct translation on novel material. For most stochastic

MT systems, this is the only type of analysis that can be done, because the tables of probabilities are, to all practical purposes, opaque. This level of analysis will typically show the presence of errors, but not necessarily the source, the method of correction, or even what sorts of training data should be included to reduce them. However, because the system uses the symbolic information incorporated into the Marker Hypothesis (as well as a more linguistically plausible description in the form of a CFG), one can also do a glass-box examination of the details of the translation functions and use this additional information to identify the precise source (in many cases a single decision) of errors and correct them.

16.5.1 Black-box evaluation

In the English–Urdu experiment, the training data consisted of a vocabulary list for both languages and a set of seven sentences providing coverage for copula-locatives and imperative sentences. The training set was learned without errors, and the system was then tested on the exercises incorporated into Lesson 2 from ur Rahman (1958). Except in cases where an individual lexical item had not been included in the training data, the test set was also translated perfectly. Expansion of the training data to include the complete system vocabulary in context resulted in a perfect transfer function for the constructions studied.

As is to be expected, the higher syntactic complexity of the English–French data reduced system performance considerably. This experiment was performed six times, using different random seeds and annealing schedules. Over several trials, the system was usually able to reproduce between 30% and 70% of the sentences correctly. Typical error patterns were instructive, however. The system usually identified the verb correctly, and the most common errors were context-sensitive deletion errors, for instance of a pronominal direct object, a reflexive particle or a complementizer. Over the repeated experiments, only 5% of the sentences were translated as gibberish.

Trials on novel sentences seem to bear this out. The experiment with the longest amount of learning time was selected for further analysis, and presented with novel sentences developed by native English speakers from the system's vocabulary without knowledge of the experimental results. These sentences were post-edited to limit the sentences to syntactic forms present in the training data (for example, the system only saw *glass* as a noun, not an adjective) and presented to the system without further modification. The system correctly translated 46% of the novel sentences, and produced the minor deletion errors or simple lexical production errors on another 8%. (These numbers can be compared, respectively, with the 51% perfect and 44% minor errors that this particular trial achieved on the training data.) In particular, the system had the most difficulty with the areas where the French structure is the most different from English: in the preverbal (pronominal) direct and indirect objects, the non-optional sentence complementizers, and reflexive particles.

16.5.2 Glass-box evaluation

A major advantage of this approach is that it is possible to read a grammar directly and transfer functions from the output of the simulated annealing. This allows us to explain the behaviour of the system at a conceptual level appropriate to the task at hand. For example, by examining the set(s) of words used as grammatical markers, one can identify which words the system felt were used in similar contexts and identify mistakes in class identification. This allows us (or any user) to provide human guidance at any point in the learning cycle.

As an example of this approach, we examine a partial evaluation of the English–French transfer function discovered by the system. The fundamental unit for analysis should be a sentence, e.g. (2).

(2) The man washes the car.

The system attempts to translate this sentence by noting that words like *washes*, *falls*, *creates* comprise a class, and that everything before the appearance of the first word of such type should be translated as a unit. A similar process identifies the words *a*, *the*, *this* and *that* as another class that divides the third utterance of the sentence from the second, as in (3).

(3) (the man) (washes) (the car)

These utterances are themselves translated (4) and then permuted (via the identity permutation) and concatenated to form the French translation.

(4) (*le homme*)[1] (*lave*) (*la voiture*)

With this level of analysis, the reasons for certain types of errors are clearly shown. For example, the identity permutation learned above is applicable in some instances but not in others (pronominal objects, for instance), merely reflecting the most common rule in the training set. A more sophisticated system would have the capability of applying different permutations depending on the relevant utterances. It may be impractical on a large scale to list the verbs in a language explicitly, and some form of on-line tagging (e.g. Cutting et al. 1992) may be useful. The most serious flaw is that the classes learned are imperfect (for example, *woman* is misclassified as a verb, resulting in a serious mistranslation of (5)), but these are easily identifiable and correctable by more sophisticated search algorithms or by human intervention as necessary.

(5) * (the) (woman washes) (the car)

The error here is more sophisticated than merely garbage in the partition. Because the system is allowed to reuse the partition classes to allow for recursive productions, occasional local maxima are found where two classes are parsed and translated by the same function: in the case of this particular error, the set described above as "verbs" is also used to distinguish between masculine and feminine nouns so that articles can be correctly translated.

---

1. The process that converts *le homme* to *l'homme* is almost purely phonetic, and was ignored for the purposes of this experiment.

Some translations as performed by the METLA system are shown below. These illustrations show, for each language pair, sample source sentences (a), their initial division into components (b), their translated components (c), and the final sentence as translated (d). As can be seen, the Urdu sentences (6)–(9) are not only translated perfectly but also broken down into logical and linguistically cogent categories such as subjects, objects and prepositional phrases.

(6) a. the man is in the shop
b. ((the man) ((is) (in the shop)))
c. ((*admi*) ((*hai*) (*dukan men*)))
d. *admi dukan men hai*

(7) a. bring the letter from the shop
b. (bring) ((the letter) (from the shop))
c. (*lao*) ((*chitthi*) (*dukan se*))
d. *chitthi dukan se lao*

(8) a. wait in the office
b. (wait) (in the office)
c. (*thairo*) (*daftar men*)
d. *daftar men thairo*

(9) a. put the box on the table
b. (put) ((the box) (on the table))
c. (*rakho*) ((*sanduq*) (*mez par*))
d. *sanduq mez par rakho*

The results for the French (10)–(14) are not as uniformly positive, but for each of the incorrect sentences, it is possible to identify and explain the source of the errors.

(10) a. the glass touches a car
b. (the glass) (touches) (a car)
c. (*le verre*) (*touche*) (*une voiture*)
d. *le verre touche une voiture*

(11) a. she washes a cat
b. (she) (washes) (a cat)
c. (*elle*) (*lave*) (*un chat*)
d. *elle lave un chat*

(12) a. the man that touches a car touches a glass
b. (the man that) (touches) (a car touches a glass)
c. (*le homme qui*) (*touche*) (*une voiture touche un verre*)
d. *le homme qui touche une voiture touche un verre*

(13) a. that man washes a car that she creates
b. (that man) (washes) (a car that she creates)
c. (*ce homme*) (*lave*) *(*une voiture qui elle crée*)
d. * *ce homme lave une voiture qui elle crée*

(14) a. this cat washes
b. (this cat) (washes) ( )
c. (*ce chat*) (*lave*) ( )
d. * *ce chat lave*

For example, the division in (12) is incorrect: *the man that touches a car* is an entire component and the main verb of the sentence is the *second* token of *touches*. This is an artefact of the admittedly broken METLA-1 parsing algorithm, which divides at the first appearance of a given token. That this sentence is correctly translated at all is a tribute to the remarkable structural similarity between this sentence and its French translation. Sentence (14) is an example of a so-called "reflexive" verb: the proper translation should be (15),

(15) *ce chat se lave*

where *se* is a general pronoun meaning 'self'. In English, certain verbs can be intransitive when the subject and object of the verb are the same, for example (16).

(16) a. I shave (myself) every morning.
b. I wash.

Some of these verbs *must* be expressed with the reflexive particle in French but with an ordinary direct object otherwise. This leads, in turn, to another example of the multiple necessary permutation problem discussed above.

A similar analysis can be done for the early experiments in English–Urdu translation. In this case, errors not illustrated here can be tied directly to the fact that a certain noun, although learned as a single lexical item, was never presented *in context*, and the system had no way of identifying its grammatical class. When presented as part of the test data, the system determined (randomly) that it was a determiner, received no evidence to disprove this during training, and mistranslated accordingly. When the training data was extended to cover this case, the percentage correct rose to 100%.

It is important not to let the errors made by a prototype system overshadow the larger results. Despite having no *a priori* knowledge of semantic or syntactic categories, the system correctly identified the important grammatical constructs most of the time and built appropriate transfer functions. The errors were easily identifiable by examining the set of "marker words" used in parsing. Adding a new language to the system required only typing in the training data; no system modifications were required. If this approach scales well to larger corpora and vocabularies, this should cut the time necessary to develop and maintain large MT databases by a large fraction.

Some of these suggested improvements have been incorporated into the METLA-2 system (Juola 1995a,b). The METLA-1 parsing formalism has been replaced by a new, bottom-up formalism based on Categorial Grammar (Wood 1993). Syntactic ambiguity handling has been improved, and many minor improvements have been made to test and improve the scalability. Experiments have been performed, with similar levels of success, on children's literature from pre-computer corpora. These improvements lend credence to the basic soundness of the psycholinguistic approach, and specifically the Marker Hypothesis, as a valid method of learning to translate.

16.6 Conclusions

It may, at this point, be useful to revisit some of the differences between this work and some of the major projects in EBMT and statistical approaches. This work does not exclusively focus on grammatical induction. Although grammatical induction is an important part of the task, neither the problem (translation) nor the approach guarantees that the system will learn anything usable for grammaticality judgements. At the same time, the system would presumably be robust enough to translate malformed phone numbers without causing system errors. This is clearly an advantage in dealing with real-world input, where typographical errors and misphrasings are not uncommon. At the same time, this system includes grammatical structure that should result in more robust, understandable and linguistically plausible translation functions than the Markov chains developed by Brown et al. (1990).

Finally, although the system uses examples to develop its translation functions, there are several crucial differences between this work and the more mainstream EBMT paradigm. First, other than the notion of paired sentences, there is no pre-analysis of the translation database, which greatly reduces the load on the developers of the system. This system also produces a reduced database, explicitly extracting patterns rather than finding them as needed in on-line examples.

These results suggest that induction of transfer functions from untagged, unanalysed corpora is both theoretically and computationally viable as an approach for the development of MT systems. In particular, computer time can be substituted for human time if the appropriate bilingual corpus is available, as it is for most major languages in instructional text. The above formalism appears to work well and produces results that can be impressive in their own right as well as easily modified and improved.

References

Brown, P. F., J. Cocke, S. A. Della Pietra, V. J. Della Pietra, F. Jelinek, J. D. Lafferty, R. L. Mercer & P. S. Roossin 1990. A statistical approach to machine translation. *Computational Linguistics* **16**, 79–85.

Cutting, D., J. Kupiec, J. Pedersen & P. Sibun 1992. A practical part-of-speech tagger. In *Proceedings of the Third Conference on Applied Natural Lanugage Processing*, Trento, 133–40.

Green, T. R. G. 1979. The necessity of syntax markers: two experiments with artificial languages. *Journal of Verbal Learning and Verbal Behavior* **18**, 481–96.

Juola, P. 1994. *Self-organizing Machine Translation: example-driven induction of transfer functions*. Technical Report TR-722-94, Computer Science Department, University of Colorado.

Juola, P. 1995a. *Corpus-based acquisition of grammars and transfer functions for Machine Translation*. Technical Report TR-756-95, Computer Science Department, University of Colorado.

Juola, P. 1995b. *Learning to translate: a psycholinguistic approach to the induction of grammars and transfer functions*. PhD thesis, University of Colorado at Boulder.

Morgan, J. L., R. P. Meier & E. L. Newport 1989. Facilitating the acquisition of syntax with cross-sentential cues to phrase structure. *Journal of Memory and Language* **28**, 360–74.

Mori, K. & S. D. Moeser 1983. The role of syntax markers and semantic referents in learning an artificial language. *Journal of Verbal Learning and Verbal Behavior* **22**, 701–18.

Myers, E. W. 1986. An O(ND) difference algorithm and its variations. *Algorithmica* **1**, 251–6.

Nagao, M. 1984. A framework of a mechanical translation between Japanese and English by analogy principle. In *Artificial and Human Intelligence*, A. Elithorn & R. Barnerji (eds), 173–80. Amsterdam: North-Holland.

Sato, S. 1991. Example-based translation approach. In *International Workshop on Fundamental Research for the Future Generation of Natural Language Processing (FGNLP), Proceedings*, Kyoto, Japan, 1–16.

Smith, T. C. & I. H. Witten 1993. *Language inference from function words*. Technical Report 1993/3, University of Waikato, New Zealand.

Sumita, E., H. Iida & H. Kohyama 1990. Translating with examples: a new approach to Machine Translation. In *The Third International Conference on Theoretical and Methodological Issues in Machine Translation of Natural Language*, Austin, Tex., 203–12.

ur Rahman, A. 1958. *Teach yourself Urdu in two months*, 22nd ed. Karachi: Azizi's Oriental Book Depot.

Wood, M. M. 1993. *Categorial grammars*. London: Routledge.

17

A natural-language-translation neural network

NENAD KONCAR AND GREGORY GUTHRIE

17.1 Introduction

Machine Translation of natural languages (MT) has been tackled in many ways. This paper[1] discusses the usefulness of feed-forward neural networks to perform such tasks. Most conventional approaches to MT fail adequately to address the problem of allowing an MT system to learn from a human expert translator during its use. Most systems have hard-coded rules (with varying depth of meaning) that can be modified only by a knowledge engineer who is an expert in expressing such rules in the language of the computer. Neural networks, having the ability to learn from examples, are a possible solution to this problem. Research has already shown the usefulness of neural networks in various natural language processing tasks: Allen (1987), Jain (1991), Waibel (1988) and Waibel et al. (1991). If such a neural-network translation system wrongly translates a sentence it can be corrected and taught the proper translation by a user without any expert knowledge of how the computer stores and represents rules. This paper demonstrates the utility of neural networks in precisely this area on a small-scale translation problem.

1. We would like to thank all of those who have contributed ideas to this paper and have reviewed its manuscript giving many helpful comments.

17.2 Grammar used

The grammar used to generate the 24 750 English and corresponding Serbo-Croatian sentences was kept simple. Each English sentence consisted of up to eight words with two determiners, two nouns, a verb, an adverb, a preposition and an adjective. Each Serbo-Croatian sentence contained two nouns, a verb, an adverb, a preposition and an adjective for a total of six words (e.g. Fig. 17.1).

Det	Noun	Verb	Adverb	Prep	Det	Adjective	Noun
The	child	runs	quickly	to	the	large	house
	Dijete	*trći*	*brzo*	*do*		*velike*	*kuće*

Figure 17.1 *Example translation.* The first line shows the parts of speech in each of the sentences under it. The second line is the English sentence and the third line is the Serbo-Croatian sentence.

The training set was generated from a simple deterministic grammar by a program. The program can grade eight English components, with a total of $11 \times 5 \times 9 \times 2 \times 5 \times 5 = 24\ 750$ sentences (see Fig. 17.2). In addition to learning simple word-pair mappings, certain words change translation depending on context. The adjective and noun endings are different for different adjective and noun combinations in Serbo-Croatian, so this was a context rule that had to be learned by the neural network. The noun and adjective endings also changed when one of the two different prepositions was used, adding another context rule.

First noun (11 words): child man woman person actor driver doctor father mother brother sister
dijete čovjek žena osoba glumac vožak doktor otac majka brat sestra
Verb (5): runs walks strolls skips glides
trći hoda korača poskakuje klizi
Adverb (9) quickly slowly carefully hurriedly tiredly energetically instantaneously insecurely blissfully
brzo polako oprezno ubrzano pospano snažno trenutno nesigurno radosno
Preposition (2) to toward
do prema
Adjective (5) large big small nice beautiful
velik-e/-og/-om/-oj ogromn-e/-og/-om/-oj mal-e/-og/-om/-oj predivn-e/-og/-om/-oj lijep-e/-og/-om/-oj
Second noun (5) house car swimming-pool boat field
kuć-a/-e/-i aut-o/a/u bazen/-a/-u brod/-a/-u njiv-a/-e/-i

Figure 17.2 *Words used for each part of speech*

The positioning of the verb and the adverb in the English sentence was randomly chosen in order to add more variety to the training set. The training set was randomized after generation, because it was found that the neural network refused to learn after a certain time if the training set was not properly randomized. The translation was not a simple direct mapping because of the difference in the number of words and the context-sensitive change of the adjective and noun according to which preposition was used and which adjective and noun pair was used, and also the random change of verb and adverb positions in the English sentence.

17.3 Incremental search

Back-propagation (Rumelhart et al. 1986) seems to be the most widely used learning algorithm in feed-forward neural networks today. The back-propagation algorithm, being an algorithm that can only find a local minimum in weight space, has several limitations in terms of speed of training and modelling capability when one tries to address problems of growing complexity such as natural language translation. Initially we tried to use the back-propagation training algorithm to solve our MT problem, but results were not satisfactory, so we made a new heuristic algorithm with a back-propagation subroutine that searches for an optimal neural network topology and weights (Fig. 17.3). For a graphic representation of the neural network architecture used by the algorithm see Figure 17.4.

It has been shown (Lang & Witbrock 1988; Mirchandani & Cao 1989; Touretzky 1989) that the first layer of a back-propagation neural network serves as a feature detector and that successive layers try to combine these features in order to achieve the desired output. It has also been observed that if there are too many nodes in a layer then the ability to generalize is lost (Caudill 1990). This is the justification for the way layers are constructed one after the other in the "incremental search" algorithm. We need first to find out all the possible features from the data by using the first hidden layer. We will know when the first hidden layer is big enough when we observe no further improvement in generalization (i.e. when memorization starts to occur). Back-propagation learning generally slows down by an order of magnitude every time a layer is added to a network. This is because the error signal, generated at the output layer, is attenuated each time it flows through a hidden layer. Learning progress is therefore limited by the slow adaptation of units in the early layers of a multilayer network. To avoid this one can use short-cut connections to provide direct information pathways to all parts of the network (Lang & Witbrock 1988). This is why our algorithm connects each new added layer to all the previous layers. During the execution of the incremental search algorithm the architecture of the neural network is changed slightly by adding a new node or a new layer. The error surface (Tank & Hopfield 1989) will also change, allowing for an escape from a local minimum in the error surface that the learning algorithm might be in.

1. Create a feed-forward neural network (NN) that has only an input and an output layer with each having a number of nodes predefined by the training dataset. Initialize all the variables.
2. Create a new current hidden layer and place it just before the output layer.
3. Add one more node (or use "chunks" of *n* nodes as increments) to the current hidden layer and connect it with random weights to all nodes in all other layers.
4. **for** *num_randomizations* **do**
   (the purpose of this "for" loop is to try different random starting weights used by the back-propagation algorithm called in 4.1.1)
   - 4.1. **repeat**
     - 4.1.1. Train the NN using back-propagation over 1 presentation of the entire training set. During learning keep track of RMS (root mean squared) error on the training set (*RmsTrain*).
   - 4.2. **while** *RmsTrain* is decreasing (i.e. network is learning)
   - 4.3. Calculate RMS error (*RmsEval*) on the early test set (note: the early test set is different from the final test set).
   - 4.4. Update *RmsTrain_best* and *RmsEval_best* with the smallest values of *RmsTrain* and *RmsEval*. If an update was made then save the network architecture and the starting weights for that architecture.
   - 4.5. Re-randomize the newly added weights.
5. **if** *RmsEval_best<RmsEval_prev_layer* (RMS error on the early test set just before a new layer was added)
   then
   - 5.1. **if** *RmsEval_best>RmsEval_prev* (RMS error on the early test set just before a new node was added)
     then (memorization has occurred)
     - 5.1.1. Remove the node just added and restore the state (topology and weights) of the NN to the state just before the node was added.
     - 5.1.2. **goto** 2

     else
     - 5.1.3. **goto** 3

   else
   - 5.2. **if** *RmsEval_best≤RmsLimit*
     then (memorization has occurred)
     - 5.2.1. Inform the user that a network has been designed that can correctly generalize within the given error limit (*Rms_Limit*).

     else
     - 5.2.2. Inform the user that more training data is needed in order to achieve the desired error rate (*Rms_Limit*) on the early test set. (Also ask the user if the training data was properly randomized or not.)

Figure 17.3 *Pseudo-code for the "incremental search" algorithm.*

17.3.1 Optimal neural network

The incremental search algorithm does not guarantee an optimal neural network topology and weights (Judd 1987; Baum 1989) because it is a heuristic algorithm.

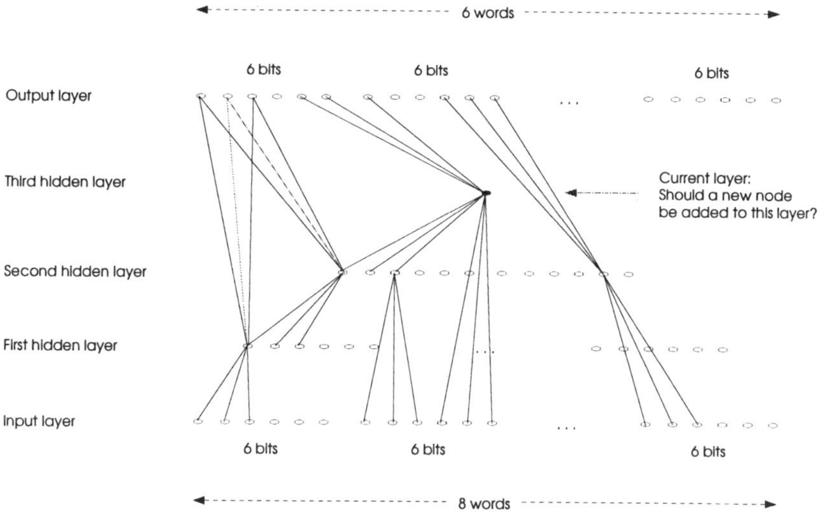

Figure 17.4 *Language-translation neural network.* Each circle represents one node in the neural network. The input layer consists of a total of 48 bits. Each group of 6 bits represents 1 word and thus there are 8 words in the input layer. These 8 words represent the English sentence. The output layer consists of a total of 36 bits which makes a total of 6 words in the output layer. These 6 words represent the Serbo-Croatian sentence. Each layer is fully connected to every previous layer.

However, our experiments show that it will produce a satisfactory network topology and weights for those problems where back-propagation fails.

17.3.2 Other growth/trimming algorithms

The Cascade–Correlation learning architecture (Fahlman & Lebiere 1990), the Tiling algorithm (Mezard & Nadal 1989), Optimal Brain Damage (Le Cun et al. 1990), and Burkitt's (1991) algorithm are some examples of existing growth and trimming algorithms for training neural networks and automatic neural network topology-formation. Our incremental search algorithm differs in very important details from all the above-listed algorithms. Our algorithm is capable of generalizing well when real-valued numbers are used as outputs whereas the Cascade–Correlation architecture does not do this well and the Tiling algorithm can deal with only binary-valued outputs. The Optimal Brain Damage algorithm and Burkitt's algorithm are both trimming algorithms that are fundamentally different from ours so that we cannot compare them.

17.4 Results

Each word in each language was assigned a unique binary code. Because the total number of words in one language did not exceed 64 it was possible to use 6 bits to encode all the words in one language. Figure 17.2 shows how this encoding scheme produced a total of 48 bits in the input layer and a total of 36 bits in the output layer of the neural network. The evaluation scheme used was very thorough. Word errors, sentence errors and part-of-speech errors were all evaluated and recorded. Any output greater than 0.5 was interpreted as a 1, any other as a 0.

The results that are shown in Tables 17.1 to 17.3 were achieved after training each neural network on a training set of 10 000 English sentences and their Serbo-Croatian translations. Each neural network was then evaluated on a set of 100 English and Serbo-Croatian sentences. It was shown that using the incremental search algorithm it was possible to achieve a high accuracy rate on the test set. The neural network architectures produced at different stages of the execution of the algorithm are listed in the tables. The left-most column of each table shows the network architecture that was evaluated. It was found that the results achieved were extremely sensitive to randomization of the input–output vector training pairs. If no randomization was present the neural network would learn certain words in the translation very quickly but would refuse to learn those words with a low frequency of change in the training set. It was also found that the random starting weights of each neural network architecture tested had a major influence on the accuracy of the resulting neural network solution.

All of the neural networks had the following parameters in common:

- Training file: 10 000 sentences
- Test file: 100 sentences
- Learning rule: Delta learning rate: 0.6
  Momentum: 0.9
- Number of presentations: 10 000

Note in Table 17.1 that as the size of the first hidden layer grows toward 70 nodes, the performance of the network improves, but then falls after further increasing the number of nodes. This is a clear indication that memorization of the training data is occurring. Thus a good approximation to the optimal number of nodes in the first hidden layer is 70 from the results observed. Because of the structure of the grammar used, it was easiest for the neural networks to learn how to translate the preposition (there were only two prepositions used). It was found that it was hardest to learn the grammar's context-sensitive rules between the adjective and the second noun. Furthermore, it was also slightly harder to learn the adverb because of the fact that the grammar randomly chose to interchange the positions of the verb and adverb in the training and test sets.

It can also be observed that a marked increase in network performance occurs each time a new layer is added. It must be noted that this performance increase is largely as a result of the fact that the weights of the previous layer are preserved and

Table 17.1 Performance measurement of three-layer neural networks. The second layer, i.e. the first hidden layer, was incrementally given more nodes and the resulting neural network performance was measured for each of these networks.

Network structure	Word error (%)	Sentence error (%)	Parts of speech errors (%)					
			Noun1	Verb	Adverb	Prep	Adj	Noun2
48-2-36	72.92	100	15.34	9.47	14.77	0.00	16.67	16.67
48-5-36	57.39	100	14.96	9.09	15.53	0.19	16.67	0.95
48-10-36	58.14	100	7.20	6.06	7.77	4.36	16.67	16.10
48-15-36	36.17	100	5.11	6.06	6.25	0.00	15.34	3.41
48-20-36	20.08	100	4.36	5.87	5.49	0.00	4.36	0.00
48-25-36	30.30	100	5.11	5.30	5.49	0.00	14.39	0.00
48-30-36	17.80	100	4.55	3.03	4.55	0.00	5.68	0.00
48-35-36	19.89	100	2.27	3.60	2.84	0.00	11.17	0.00
48-40-36	18.18	100	4.55	7.58	5.49	0.00	0.38	0.19
48-45-36	27.27	100	0.95	3.03	5.30	0.38	15.91	1.70
48-50-36	29.36	100	2.08	4.92	6.82	3.79	9.85	1.89
48-70-36	2.84	18	0.95	0.00	0.95	0.00	0.95	0.00
48-90-36	13.26	78	0.57	0.19	1.89	0.57	10.04	0.00
48-110-36	36.36	98	3.41	16.29	16.29	0.00	0.38	0.00
48-130-36	18.94	100	0.76	6.76	2.27	0.00	15.15	0.00

that the learning rate of the previous layer(s) is changed to zero (frozen) when the new layer is added to the neural network architecture.

17.5 Discussion

Allen (1987) has shown that neural networks have the capability to translate sentences from English to Spanish. Sentences used in Allen's research were generated using a very limited vocabulary and format. All sentences included a subject, verb, direct object and indirect object. The verb was either *give* or *offer* and three different verb tenses were used (present, past and past perfect). In the English sentences, the order of direct object and indirect object was randomly selected, while in the Spanish sentences the preferred sentence structure always placed the indirect object

Table 17.2 Performance measurement of four-layer neural networks. The third layer, i.e. the second hidden layer, was incrementally given more nodes and the resulting neural network performance was measured for each of these networks.

Network structure	Word error (%)	Sentence error (%)	Parts of speech errors (%)					
			Noun1	Verb	Adverb	Prep	Adj	Noun2
48-70-1-36	1.33	12.00	0.57	0.00	0.00	0.00	0.76	0.00
48-70-5-36	0.95	6.00	0.38	0.00	0.00	0.00	0.56	0.00
48-70-10-36	0.57	3.41	0.38	0.00	0.00	0.00	0.19	0.00
48-70-15-36	0.76	4.55	0.38	0.00	0.00	0.00	0.38	0.00
48-70-20-36	0.76	4.55	0.57	0.00	0.00	0.00	0.19	0.00

Table 17.3 Performance measurement of five-layer neural networks. The third layer, i.e. the second hidden layer, was incrementally given more nodes and the resulting neural network performance was measured for each of these networks.

Network structure	Word error (%)	Sentence error (%)	Parts of speech errors (%)					
			Noun1	Verb	Adverb	Prep	Adj	Noun2
48-70-10-1-36	0.00	0.00	0.00	0.00	0.00	0.00	0.00	0.00
48-70-10-5-36	0.19	1.14	0.00	0.00	0.00	0.00	0.19	0.00

after the direct object. Nouns referring to people (including two first names) and animals were used as subjects and indirect objects, while nouns referring to things were used for direct objects. Nouns were randomly modified by one of the two adjectives. A training set of 3 310 sentences and 33 test sentences were used to train and test a multi-hidden-layer 50–150–150–150–66 back-propagation network with learning rate of 0.01 and momentum 0.9. After two million presentations, training produced a root-mean-squared error rate of 0.027 over all the outputs. On the test set this trained network was incorrect on an average of 2.5 bits and 1.3 words.

17.5.1 The scalability problem

Sejnowski & Rosenberg (1987) used a context of seven characters (including the space) from a word as input to a neural network and the phoneme corresponding to the middle character as output. This same approach could be taken in using neural networks to perform real-world MT. The neural network would be given a sliding window of words from the source language and the neural network output would be a single word in the target-language text.

17.5.2 Words with multiple meanings

Context rules (i.e. for multiple-meaning words) of language translation would be captured by using Sejnowski & Rosenberg's (1987) method just as for the scalability problem. Requirements for the neural network size in terms of the number of neurons and hidden layers would also be reduced. If the sliding window of words from the source language is increased sufficiently to cover three or more sentences then inter-sentence information could be captured and used in translation.

17.5.3 Text attributes

There are some attributes that can be given to an entire text. If a text is written in old English then its attribute would be "old English". If the text is a legal document then its attribute would be that of a legal document, etc. Giving such attributes as input to the neural network during training and during its use by a skilled operator would greatly enhance the accuracy and versatility of translations that the neural network could perform.

References

Allen, R. B. 1987. Several studies on natural language and back-propagation: natural language translation. In *Proceedings of the First International Conference on Neural Networks*, San Diego, Calif., 338–9.

Baum, E. B. 1989. What size net gives valid generalization? *Neural Computation* **1**, 151–60.

Burkitt, A. N. 1991. Optimization of the architecture of feed-forward neural networks with hidden layers by unit elimination. *Complex Systems* **5**, 371–80.

Caudill, M. 1990. Using neural nets: diagnostic expert nets, pruning trained networks. *AI Expert* **5** (September), 45.

Fahlman, S. & C. Lebiere 1990. *The Cascade-Correlation learning architecture*. Technical Report, CMU-CS-90-100, Carnegie Mellon University, Pittsburgh, Pa.

Jain, J. S. 1991. Parsing complex sentences with structured connectionist networks. *Neural Computation* **3**, 110–20.

Judd, J. S. 1987. Learning in networks is hard. In *Proceedings of the First International Conference on Neural Networks*, San Diego, Calif., 685–92.

Lang, K. J. & M. J. Witbrock 1988. Learning to tell two spirals apart. In *Proceedings of the 1988 Connectionist Models Summer School*, Pittsburg, Pa., 52–9.

Le Cun, Y., J. Denker & S. Solla 1990. *Optimal brain damage. Advances in neural information processing systems 2*. San Mateo, Calif.: Morgan Kaufmann.

Mezard, M. & J. P. Nadal 1989. Learning in feedforward networks: the Tiling algorithm. *Journal of Physics A* **22**, 2191–2203.

Mirchandani, G. & W. Cao 1989. On hidden nodes for neural nets. *IEEE Transactions on Circuits and Systems* **36**, 661–4.

Rumelhart, D. E., G. E. Hinton & R. J. Williams 1986. Learning internal representations by error propagation. In *Parallel Distributed Processing: explorations in the microstructure of cognition. Vol. 1: Foundations*, D. E. Rumelhart, J. L. McClelland & the PDP Research Group (eds), 318–62. Cambridge, Mass.: MIT Press.

Sejnowski, T. J. & C. R. Rosenberg 1987. Parallel networks that learn to pronounce English text. *Complex Systems* **1**, 145–68.

Tank, D. W. & J. J. Hopfield 1989. Collective computation in neuronlike circuits. *Scientific American* **257**, 104–14.

Touretzky, D. S. 1989. What's hidden in the hidden layers? *Byte* **14** (August), 227–33.

Waibel, A. 1988. Connectionist glue: modular design of neural speech systems. In *Proceedings of the 1988 Connectionist Summer School*, Pittsburg, Pa., 417–25.

Waibel, A., A. N. Jain, A. E. McNair, H. Saito, A. G. Hauptmann & J. Tebelskis 1991. JANUS: a speech-to-speech translation system using connectionist and symbolic processing strategies. In *Proceedings of the 1991 IEEE International Conference on Acoustics, Speech, and Signal Processing*, Toronto, 793–6.

18

Direct parse-tree translation in co-operation with the transfer method

YOSHIHIRO MATSUO, SATOSHI SHIRAI, AKIO YOKOO AND SATORU IKEHARA[1]

18.1 Introduction

Up until now, most machine translation (MT) systems have been based on the transfer method, where translation is conducted in several phases such as morphological analysis, syntactic analysis, semantic analysis, transfer and generation. The semantic analysis and transfer phases mainly process words while the generation process combines the translations. Although phrase-transfer rules using syntactic information have also been used, such rules, which are described without strictly defined semantic attributes, sometimes cause unexpected side-effects. When the sentence is divided into the smaller units that are required by the semantic analyser, if there is excessive division the meaning of the input sentences can be changed.

1. The authors wish to thank the other members of the MT research group for several valuable discussions. They also wish to thank Miki Nakamura, Tomiko Hyoudou and Hiroko Inoue for their suggestions and valuable discussions.

Recently, example-based (Nagao 1992; Furuse & Iida 1992), knowledge-based (Tsujii & Ananiadou 1993; Nirenburg & Levin 1991) and pattern-based (Katoh & Uratani 1992; Maruyama 1993) translation systems have been proposed to replace the transfer method. Since these methods translate without excessive division, the meaning in the input sentence structure is conserved. However, there are problems with all these methods. The example-based method cannot readily calculate the similarity between input sentences and the examples, and also translation fails without sufficiently similar examples. It is not clear how to use and build a knowledge-base for knowledge-based translation. Pattern-based translation with morpheme patterns cannot be applied to free-word-order languages.

In order to conserve the meaning of an input sentence, translation units that cannot be divided prior to semantic analysis need to be appropriately defined. The Japanese–English translation system ALT–J/E, based on the multilevel translation method (Ikehara 1989), was developed to reduce unexpected division. This method employs three levels of abstraction for translating unit sentences,[2] and each level has its own transfer rules.[3] The least abstract rules are applied first. Other expressions such as noun phrases or adverbial phrases are translated based on a semantic analysis.

Since the three levels of rules for unit sentences require units that contain one verb and some case elements and the semantic analysers for noun or adverbial phrases require appropriate structures, the multilevel translation method must divide input sentences into several units. This makes it difficult to handle Japanese verbs with wide-ranging meanings such as *naru* or *suru* that are used frequently (similar to *do* or *make*), and special English expressions such as subjunctives, because the information needed for translation is often scattered between the units. In order to handle such scattered information, we have introduced direct parse-tree translation into ALT–J/E. The direct parse-tree translation uses pattern matching between the parse tree of an input sentence and parse trees in a dictionary. Since this is processed prior to the division process, information from the entire parse tree can be utilized.

It is possible to build a translation system using only this method, but such a system would have the following disadvantages:

- Since every kind of structure is treated as a simple tree, it is impossible to write suitable rules for structures such as noun phrases or unit sentences.
- It is not realistic to describe every phenomenon of a natural language, so it is difficult to ensure that the dictionary contains enough patterns.

Translation based on semantic analysis does not have these disadvantages. In order to integrate the two methods, direct parse-tree translation is mainly used to handle long-range dependency on the parse tree, which is difficult to treat with ordinary semantic analysis. This paper proposes a method of co-operative translation using both direct

2. A unit sentence is made up of a verb and "case elements".

3. The first-level rules translate idiomatic expressions (about 3 000 rules). The second-level rules are valence patterns (about 10 000 rules) which are described as relations between a verb and cases categorized by about 3000 semantic attributes. The third-level rules are the default translation rules for verbs.

parse-tree translation and the transfer method implemented in the Japanese–English MT system ALT–J/E.

18.2 Translation system overview

Direct parse-tree translation should capture the Japanese structure corresponding to an English expression. It is difficult to find a pattern of morpheme sequences because Japanese has almost no word-order dependency. Therefore, we introduce a pattern-matching function on the dependency structure of the input sentences.

Figure 18.1 shows an overview of the translation system. The whole system is made up of a pattern-matching part, some semantic-analysis-based translators and an English synthesizer.

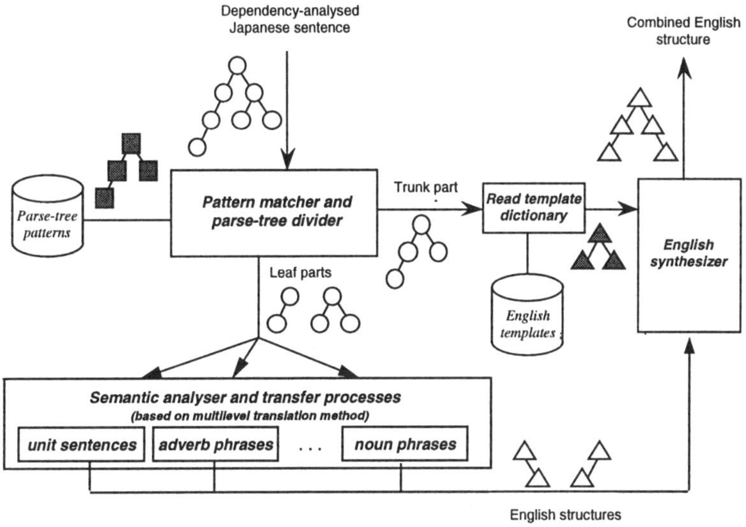

Figure 18.1 *Translation system overview.* A white circle represents a Japanese phrase and a tree of white circles represents a dependency-analysed Japanese sentence; a shaded square represents a rule that a Japanese phrase should satisfy; and a tree of shaded squares represents a parse-tree pattern. A white triangle represents an English word and a tree of white triangles represents the structure of the English sentence. A tree made up of shaded triangles represents an English template as described in the English template dictionary.

The pattern-matching part receives a dependency-analysed Japanese sentence and compares it with the Japanese parse-tree patterns described in the Japanese parse-tree dictionary. If the pattern matches the input tree, the tree is divided into a "trunk part" and some "leaf parts". The trunk part is the part that is translated as a whole, and the leaf parts are the rest of the input tree which will be translated by the semantic analysis-based translation. For the trunk part, since the scattered information has already been captured, no further deep analysis is required. The system merely uses the English template that corresponds to the pattern from the Japanese parse-tree dictionary. For each leaf part, the system invokes the relevant semantic analyser and transfer process needed to generate the English structures. The English synthesizer receives the English template read from the English template dictionary and the English structures generated by the transfer process, and combines them into a complete English sentence.

18.3 Matching and division process

The pattern-matching part compares the dependency-analysed Japanese sentence with parse-tree patterns. The dependency structures are represented as trees that contain words and phrases on their nodes. Therefore the parse-tree patterns are made of trees with attribute conditions on their nodes. The entire comparison examines all conditions on each node in the parse-tree pattern and the attributes of each node in the input sentence.

The result of the pattern matching is that each node of each parse-tree pattern has a part of an input tree as its value. The division process separates node values into leaf and trunk parts, but there may be more than one possible separation. Sentence (1) shows an example of a subjunctive expression, which cannot be represented by a more simple Japanese form.

(1) a. *Kare-wa marude nan-demo shitte-iru-ka-no-yōni hanasu.*
HE-subj ALMOST EVERYTHING KNOW-AS-IF TALK
b. 'He talks as if he knew everything.'

In this case, the key expressions that determine that this sentence is the subjunctive are the Japanese adverb *marude* and the compound made of an auxiliary verb *yōni* and particles *ka-no*. The Japanese sentence is parsed into the dependency structure shown in Figure 18.2a. To capture this structure, the parse-tree pattern of Figure 18.2b can be stored in the parse-tree dictionary.

The pattern-matching part supplies the result that X directly corresponds to *kare*, that Y directly corresponds to *shitte-iru* and that Z directly corresponds to *marude*. To generate the phrase *know everything*, Y should be *nan-demo shitte-iru*. Thus, the additional element *nan-demo* should be connected to variable Y. However, Z and W are parts of the trunk and are not translated using the transfer rules.

Another example, sentence (2), may be informative.

(2) a. *Kare-wa isu-no ashi-wo kumu.*
HE-subj CHAIR-gen LEG-obj COMBINE
b. 'He assembles chair legs.'
c. * 'He crosses chair legs.'

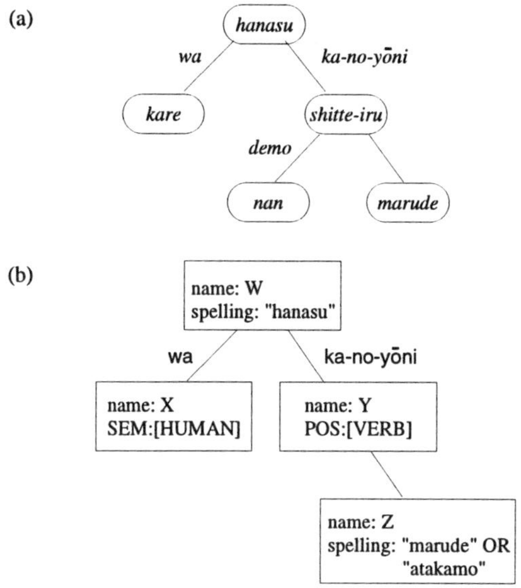

Figure 18.2 *Dependency structure of sentence (1) and example pattern.*

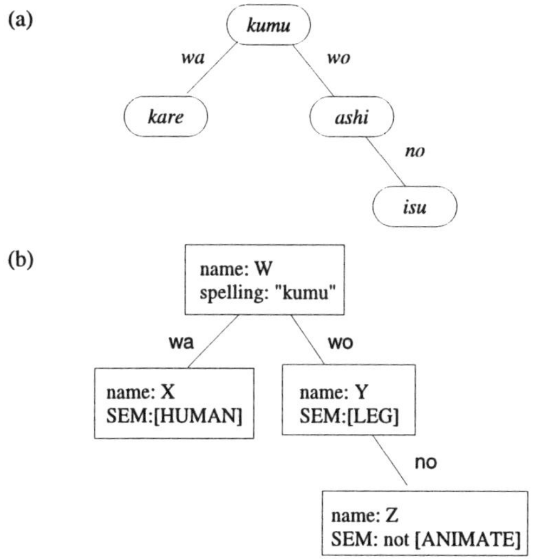

Figure 18.3 *Dependency structure of sentence (2) and example pattern.*

In this case, to translate *kumu* correctly as *assemble* requires that *ashi* does not refer to a part of an animal.[4] Thus the parse-tree pattern in Figure 18.3b should be stored in the parse-tree dictionary.

The result from the pattern-matching part is that X directly corresponds to *kare*, that Y directly corresponds to *ashi*, that Z directly corresponds to *isu* and that W directly corresponds to *kumu*. Since the input to generate the phrase *chair leg* in node Y is that Y is *isu-no ashi*, Z needs to be connected to variable Y.

These examples show that the Z in the pattern for sentence (2) should be treated differently from the Z in the pattern for sentence (1).

To do this, we introduce three types of node in the parse-tree pattern:

- *a-type*: This is the root of a leaf part. This node should be translated into English.
- *b-type*: This is a part of the trunk part. This node should not be translated into English, but is translated directly as a part of the template.
- *c-type*: This is a part of a leaf part, but not the root. This node should be connected to an upper node.

For a-type nodes, the system invokes the relevant semantic analyser as described in the parse-tree pattern (Figs 18.4 and 18.5). The b-type nodes are discarded. For all other elements in the input sentence (those that directly correspond to c-type nodes and any additional elements), the following sequence is performed:

1. Follow the parse tree toward the root until the root itself, an a-type node, or a b-type node is reached.
2. If an a-type node is reached, the element is a part of that node.
3. If a b-type node or the root is reached, the element is treated as a free element.

In the case of sentence (1), the nodes should be categorized as follows: X and Y are a-type and Z and W are b-type. X and Y are translated by the semantic analysis-based translator, and Z and W are discarded. The sequence shown above is performed for one additional node *nan* in the example sentence. Following the tree will stop at the node *shitte-iru*, which directly corresponds to a-type node Y. Therefore, the node *nan* is connected to *shitt-eiru* and the system determines that X consists of *kare* and Y consists of *nan-demo shitte-iru* (see Fig. 18.4).

In the case of sentence (2), the nodes should be categorized as follows: X and Y are a-type, Z is c-type and W is b-type. The node *isu* which corresponds to c-type node Z is treated by the above sequence and connected to *ashi*. The system determines that X consists of *kare* and Y consists of *isu-no ashi* (see Fig. 18.5).

---

4. For translating the verb *kumu*, ALT–J/E has several valence patterns. One of them is such that if the direct object has the semantic attribute [LEG] then the verb should be translated as *cross*, while another says that if the direct object has the semantic attribute [CONCRETE THING] then the verb should be translated as *assemble*. Since the semantic attribute of *ashi* is [LEG], the system without the direct parse-tree translation produces the incorrect translation (2c).

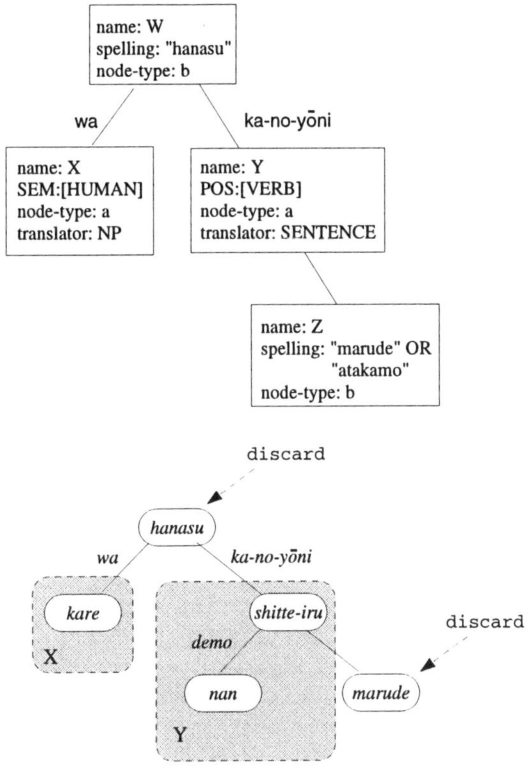

Figure 18.4 *Node-categorized pattern for sentence (1) and the result of identification of the node's value.*

18.4 Combining the "trunk" and the "leaves"

The English template dictionary contains the templates of English structures corresponding to the trunk parts. The template has one variable for each a-type node. The role of each variable such as SUBJ in SENTENCE or MODIFIER in NP is also described in the template. The part determined as the value of an a-type node is analysed semantically by the relevant analyser and is transferred by the relevant transfer process. Each result of the transfer process is connected to the template according to the role of the variable in order to build a complete English sentence. Figure 18.6 shows the English template used with the example pattern in Figure 18.5.

18.5 How to treat free elements

The pattern-matching part sometimes produces free elements. These need to be correctly translated into English using the semantic analyser and the transfer process,

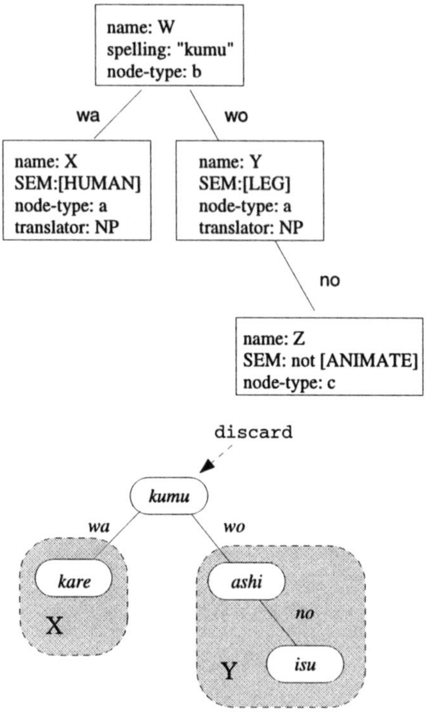

Figure 18.5 *Node-categorized pattern for sentence (2) and the result of identification of the node's value.*

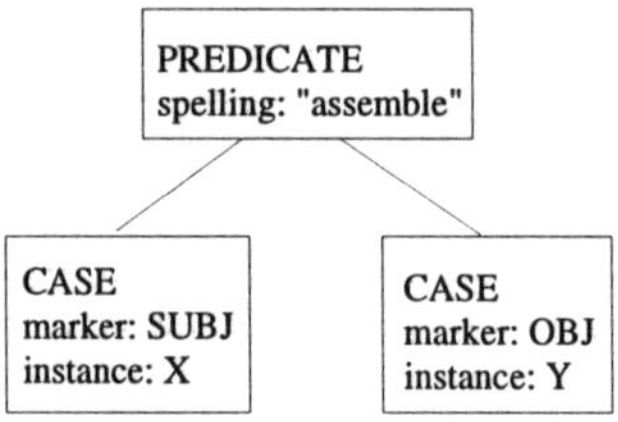

Figure 18.6 *Example of English template.*

and the result of the transfer process should be properly connected to the English structure. Our current system can treat free elements if the following two conditions apply:

- The resulting English structure has a predicate in its top level.
- The free element is an adverbial phrase or a case element.

When both these conditions are satisfied, the free element is translated as an adverbial phrase or a prepositional phrase connected to the predicate. Otherwise, the direct parse-tree translation fails and the whole sentence is translated normally using semantic analysis.

For example, sentence (3) has the free element *isoide*, 'in a hurry'. Because *isoide* is an adverbial phrase and there is a predicate in the sentence, the translation of *isoide* can be connected to the predicate. This gives sentence (3b).

(3) a. *Kare-wa isu-no ashi-wo isoide kunda.*
HE-subj CHAIR-gen LEG-obj IN-A-HURRY COMBINED
b. 'He assembled chair legs in a hurry.'

18.6 Applicability

We examined the translation of *naru* in a functional test set (Ikehara 1992) of about 3 700 sentences. Although ALT–J/E translates the verb *naru* with many valence patterns, it is difficult to translate. One of the reasons is that *naru* is sometimes translated into a phrase without a verb. The solution is to capture the structure around *naru* with an upper structure including another verb or to use a mechanism to convert a clause into a phrase. Both are impossible with simple valence patterns for unit sentences that cannot refer to external information. Another reason is that information distant from the verb is required to select the English structure. For example, to translate ... *suru jidai-ni naru* into *the age will come when ...* , the sequence ... *suru* should be treated together with *naru*.[5] But the division process in the transfer method would send ... *suru jidai* to the noun-phrase analyser on its own.

The test set has 146 sentences that include *naru*, of which about 60 sentences can be translated into acceptable English by ALT–J/E without direct parse-tree translation. We have obtained key expressions to capture the structure around *naru* for about 40 more sentences: rules using these are currently being refined and implemented.

References

Furuse, O. & H. Iida 1992. Transfer-driven machine translation. In *Proceedings of International Workshop on Fundamental Research for the Future Generation of Natural Language Processing (FGNLP)*, Manchester, 95–105.

Ikehara, S. 1989. Multi-level machine translation method. *Future Computing Systems*, **2**, 1269–79.

Ikehara, S. 1992. Criteria for evaluating the linguistic quality of Japanese to English MT system. In *Proceedings of MT Evaluation Workshop*, San Diego, Calif., 58–9.

5. With simple valence patterns, it will be translated as **It becomes the age that ...* .

Katoh, N. & N. Uratani 1992. Teikei-patān wo fukumu nyūsubun no chushutsu no sono einichi-kikai-honyaku [Extraction and machine translation of news sentences with fixed patterns]. In *Jōhō-shori-gakkai dai-44-kai taikai [Proceedings of 44th Annual Convention of the Information Processing Society of Japan],* Kanagawa, Japan, 3.133–4.

Maruyama, H. 1993. Pattern-based translation: context-free transducer and its applications to practical NLP. In *Proceedings of Natural Language Processing Pacific Rim Symposium*, Fukuoka, Japan, 232–7.

Nagao, M. 1992. Some rationales and methodologies for example-based approach. In *Proceedings of International Workshop on Fundamental Research for the Future Generation of Natural Language Processing (FGNLP)*, Manchester, 82–94.

Nirenburg, S. & L. Levin 1991. Syntax-driven and ontology-driven lexical semantics. In *Proceedings of the 1st SIGLEX Workshop*, Berkeley, Calif., 5–20.

Tsujii, J. & S. Ananiadou 1993. Knowledge-based processing in MT. In *Proceedings of Japan–US Workshop on Machine Aided Translation*, Washington, DC, 199–212.

Part V
Statistical approaches

19

Evaluating the information gain of probability-based PP-disambiguation methods

ROBERTO BASILI, MARIE-HÉLÈNE CANDITO, MARIA TERESA PAZIENZA AND PAOLA VELARDI

19.1 Introduction

Recently, several papers have been published on the automatic acquisition from corpora of PP-disambiguation methods (Basili et al. 1991, 1993a; Boggess et al. 1991; Grishman & Sterling 1992; Hindle & Rooth 1991, 1993; Jelinek et al. 1990; Resnik & Hearst 1993; Sekine et al. 1992). Though differences in the algorithms proposed may suggest arguments for a qualitative comparison, the definition of formal evaluation criteria is still a matter of discussion and criticism.

In the literature, the most popular evaluation parameters to compare the performance of "inductive systems" (from statistically based syntactic analysers to information retrieval systems, or pattern classifiers) are *accuracy* (also referred to as "efficiency" or "recall") and *precision*. "Accuracy" measures the number of correct decisions over the number of the expected decisions (or test cases). "Precision" is the number of correct decisions divided by the global number of automatic decisions. Almost all the aforementioned papers on PP-disambiguation use these measures to evaluate their methods.

When we focus on evaluation of a PP-disambiguation method it is useful to analyse it as a classification task. Syntactic disambiguation is the classification of a test case (i.e. an ambigous parse) in the class of correct and wrong parses, according to a set of suitable observations (i.e. training examples). In this view, accuracy and precision are particularly unsatisfactory for comparing different acquisition (i.e. observation) methods and disambiguation algorithms. As already observed by different authors, accuracy and precision do not provide a good measure of the quality of different inductive systems, since they are not sensitive to the *complexity of the decision task* at hand (Kononenko & Bratko 1991).

This criticism can be intuitively understood with the following example: say we wish to assign instances of some observed phenomenon to one of n classes. The "blind" probability of assigning the correct class in the absence of any decision strategy is $1/n$. Clearly, an inductive system that selects the correct class over n, with 80% precision, does in fact a much better job than one that exhibits a 90% precision at selecting from $n/2$ classes. What is missing here is an evaluation of the complexity of the learning task, i.e. of the induction of decision rules from the training set.

The absence of a notion of blind probability, called the *a priori*, or "prior", probability in Kononenko & Bratko (1991), renders the comparison of classification methods presented by different authors very difficult.

In this paper we show that modelling the PP-attachment problem as a classification task favours the definition of a more principled, and uniform, notion of performance. This evaluation framework provides a unified view of the different disambiguation methods, and allows a systematic study of performances in terms of *information gain*.

However, the linguistic nature of the classification problem at hand renders a formal definition of the prior (and posterior) probability rather more complex than for other "standard" classification tasks. For example, in the field of supervised learning systems, the prior probability of a given class is simply evaluated as the number of available training instances in the class (Kononenko & Bratko 1991). Furthermore, the test set is relatively small and well assessed. In the case of syntactic disambiguation, on the other hand, the acquisition of information is triggered by a noisy, unsupervised set of instances, i.e. the training corpus.

The focus of this paper will be to devise a formal definition of the information gain of the PP-disambiguation task. The definition will be applied to the evaluation of two disambiguation methods proposed in the literature, namely "lexical association" (Hindle & Rooth 1993) and "mutual conditioned plausibility" (Basili et al. 1993a, 1994). The purpose of the comparison will not be to argue in favour of one of the two methods, but rather to test and demonstrate the advantages of the proposed performance evaluation framework.

19.2 PP-disambiguation as a classification task

Let us considers a reference set of sentences Σ, each with one (or more) underlying parse tree $t(s)$. A given grammar Γ provides, for each sentence $s \in \Sigma$, a related forest $\gamma(s) = \{t\}$. In general, $t(s) \in \gamma(s)$.

The syntactic disambiguation of a sentence is equivalent to the task of partitioning the set of ambiguous parse trees $\gamma(s)$ into two distinct classes: G, the class of correct (or meaningful) trees, which express the expected structure assigned to s by any language user, and E, the class of wrong, or meaningless, parses.

More generally, for all the available sample sentences, we can consider the space of all trees (1) as partitioned into two distinct classes (2) and (3).

(1) $\Omega = \bigcup_{s \in \Sigma} \gamma(s)$

(2) $\mathrm{G} = \{t \in \Omega | \exists s : t(s) = t\}$

(3) $\mathrm{E} = \Omega - \mathrm{G}$

Given the sets E and G, the process of assigning the correct parse tree to a sentence s is thus equivalent to classifying members of $\gamma(s)$ into the sets E and G.

Please note that the above partition gives rise to two distinct sets of elementary syntactic structures embedded in the parses. In fact, trees are not the only structures involved in the disambiguation process. For example, in (4), the dominance of the verb *flies* over the prepositional modifier *by plane* in the correct parse tree (5) is a typical example of ambiguous structure V+P+N (verb + preposition + noun).

(4) John flies to London by plane.

(5) (John (flies (to London) (by plane))

An alternative reading in fact produces the structure N+P+N (6).

(6) (John (flies (to London (by plane))

Definition 1. Structure occurring in a tree: Given a sentence s, an elementary syntactic structure *ess* is said to "occur in a tree" $t \in \gamma(s)$ *iff* it denotes a syntactic relation also expressed by t.

According to Definition 1, the V+P+N structure (7) occurs in the correct tree, while the N+P+N structure (8) occurs in a wrong reading of the sentence s.

(7) (flies (by plane))

(8) (London (by plane))

The class of elementary structures can be partitioned into correct and wrong triples according to the correctness of the related parse tree. More formally:

Definition 2. ***ess*** **correctness:** Given a sentence $s \in \Sigma$, an elementary syntactic structure *ess* is correct *iff* it occurs in at least one correct parse tree $t(s) \in \gamma(s)$.

Definition 2 implies that (7) is a correct *ess* for the sentence *s* while (8) is a wrong one.

Definition 2 defines two sets of correct and wrong syntactic structures, which we will refer to as G_c and E_c, respectively. As Definition 2 is coherent with the definition of correct and wrong parse trees, whenever no ambiguity arises, we will use only G (and E) to denote both the set of correct (and wrong) syntactic structures and parse trees.

Evaluation can now proceed from full parses as well as from simpler syntactic structures. Let us now turn to the problem of evaluation. Whenever a known partition into wrong and correct parses is available then a systematic definition of the information gain is possible.

19.2.1 Information gain

The "information gain" of a classification task is defined in information theory as the average reduction in number of bits necessary to describe the correct classification or disambiguation. Information gain is based on the notion of "prior probability", i.e. the probability of a given classification antecedent to any inductive process (e.g. corpus processing in our case) and "posterior probability", i.e. the probability of a classification after the inductive process.

Whatever the inductive process is about, it is always possible to define a notion of prior and posterior probability and represent them by two distributions, respectively denoted by P(G) (or P(E)) and P′(G) (or P′(E)), that is, $P'(t \in G)$ (or $P'(t \in E)$): P(G) is the distribution of correct decisions (or positive examples) in the sample space, while P′(G) is the probability of being correct that the system assigns to the test cases. In our linguistic framework, P(G) (that is, $P(t \in G)$) expresses the distribution of correct parses *t* in the sample space, while P′(G) (that is, $P'(t \in G)$) expresses the lexical preference that the trained system assigns to parses. A decision (i.e. classification) is provided according to the increase of the posterior probability produced by the training process.

The definition of "information score" for our PP-disambiguation problem follows closely the general definition provided, for example, in Kononenko & Bratko (1991).

> **Definition 3. Useful, useless and misleading decisions**: Given a sentence *s*, a decision of the system for a correct parse $t = t(s)$ is "useful" *iff*
>
> $$P'(t(s) \in G) = P'(G) > P(G)$$
>
> For other wrong syntactic interpretations $t \in t(s)$ (which are ruled by P′(E)), the decision is "useful" *iff*
>
> $$P'(t) = P'(E) > P(E)$$
>
> A decision is "useless" when
>
> $$P(G) = P'(G) \text{ (i.e. } P(E) = P'(E),$$
>
> as no change in the related information about the phenomenon is implied. If a decision is neither useful nor useless, it is "misleading".

Definition 3 has been given in term of parse trees. It can be easily extended to elementary syntactic structures (*ess*'s) (e.g. SVO or V+P+N triples) just by substituting G and E by G_c and E_c. When no confusion arises, in the following we will refer to useful, useless and misleading decisions over syntactic structures, where E and G are meant as E_c and G_c.

For the sample sentence (4), the distribution P′ in (9) provides two useful decisions if (10) holds.

(9) a. P′((flies (by plane))) = 0.7
b. P′((London (by plane))) = 0.3

(10) P(flies (by plane))) = P((London (by plane))) = 0.5

Conversely, with the same prior probability P, the posterior probabilities in (11) imply two misleading decisions for the system.

(11) a. P′((flies (by plane))) = 0.35
b. P′((London (by plane))) = 0.65

A suitable definition for the information gain can now be given as follows.

Definition 4. Information score: Given any tree t from the sample space Ω, the information score (I) of a useful decision in the class G is

(12) $I = -\log P(G) + \log P'(G),\ t \in G$

or

(13) $I = -\log P(E) + \log P'(E),\ t \in E$

for the wrong cases, i.e. classification in E. If the corresponding decision is *misleading* then the information score (I) is a penalty, i.e.

(14) $I = -\log(1 - P(G)) + \log(1 - P'(G)),\ t \in G$

or

(15) $I = -\log(1 - P(E)) + \log(1 - P'(E)),\ t \in E.$

The overall performance index I_Σ over the test set Σ is the sum of the information scores of all the testing cases, i.e. the sum of the scores divided by their cardinality $|\Sigma|$.

The important aspect of Definition 4 is that I assigns to an inductive step a score as much positive as the classification is correct and the complexity of the task was high, and a penalty as strong as the classification is incorrect and the complexity of the task was low.

19.3 Modelling the prior probability

In this section we define the notion of "prior probability" under the specific perspective implied by the linguistic task at hand. In corpus linguistics, it is common to extrapolate the properties of a sublanguage $\mathcal{L}$ by analysing a reference corpus C. We can say that C embodies the model of use of $\mathcal{L}$. The majority of methods for automatic syntactic disambiguation, whose evaluation is the concern of this paper, rely on the following hypothesis:

> Hypothesis (H1): The more we observe a phenomenon in the corpus C, the more we can rely on the assertion that it is meaningful (= semantically plausible) for the related language $\mathcal{L}$. *Vice versa*: rare observations may be markers of inconsistency (or noise during the observation phase).

The observed phenomena, in the majority of methods proposed in the literature, are word collocations, augmented by syntactic markers. The type of syntactic structures observed may vary significantly, but in general they are rather simpler than a full parse tree. For example, they are productive triples like SVO or verb–prepositional modifier (V+P+N). We have called these structures "elementary syntactic structures" (*ess*'s).

In the following we propose a method of expressing the prior and posterior probabilities of correct and wrong parses according to the prior and posterior probabilities of elementary syntactic structures. The functional dependencies are shown in Figure 19.1.

	Prior probabilities	Posterior probabilities
Probabilities of *ess*'s	$P(ess \in G_c)$	$P'(ess \in G_c)$
	$\Downarrow$	$\Downarrow$
Probabilities of trees	$P(t \in G)$	$P'(t \in G)$

Figure 19.1 *Elementary structures vs parse trees.*

Once coefficients $P(ess \in G)$ are known for all *ess*'s occurring in a tree t, then $P(t \in G)$ can be consequently derived (operator $\Downarrow$) by composition of such coefficients.

Let us concentrate now on the definition of prior probability for elementary structures.

We can exploit (H1) as follows: given the set Ω_c of syntactic structures observed in a corpus C, $\Omega_c \in \Omega$, for each $ess \in \Omega$, we have (16),

$$
\begin{aligned}
(16)\ P(ess \in G) &= P(ess \in G|\Omega_c)P(\Omega_c|\Omega) + P(ess \in G|\overline{\Omega_c})P(\overline{\Omega_c}|\Omega) \\
&= P(ess \in G|\Omega_c)P(\Omega_c|\Omega) \\
\text{where } \overline{\Omega_c} &= \Omega - \Omega_c
\end{aligned}
$$

Equation (16) defines the blind probability, for an elementary syntactic structure, of being correct, i.e. belonging to G.

$P(ess \in G|\Omega_c)$ depends on the ambiguity of single sentences of the corpus: it is the probability of a syntactic structure being meaningful, given it has been observed. $P(\Omega_c|\Omega)$ models the "coverage" of the corpus: it quantifies the degree by which Ω_c approximates Ω.

When we focus on a given syntactic structure of type τ (e.g. SVO triples) we can focus on the subset Ω_T of Ω, including only structures of type τ. The probability of being meaningful for syntactic structures of type τ can be easily defined by (17),

$$(17)\ \mathrm{P}(\Omega_{c\tau}) = \frac{|\Omega_{cT}|}{|\Omega_\tau|}$$

(where | | denotes the cardinality of a set), and consequently by (18).

$$(18)\ \mathrm{P}(\Omega_c|\Omega) = \mathrm{P}(\Omega_c) = \mathrm{P}(\bigcup \Omega_{c\tau}) = \sum \mathrm{P}(\Omega_{c\tau})$$

To define the other component of the prior probability, $\mathrm{P}(ess \in \mathrm{G}|\Omega_c)$, it is necessary to rely on the notion of "collision set", or colliding tuples (for formal definitions, see Sekine et al. 1992 and Basili et al. 1994). Intuitively, every ambiguous segment of the corpus generates a non-empty set of collisions, i.e. mutually excluding syntactic structures. For example, in the sample sentence (4), wrong and correct *ess*'s (see Section 19.2) form the collision set (19).

(19) {N+P+N(*London,by,plane*),V+P+N(*fly,by,plane*)}

It seems reasonable to model the probability of a syntactic structure being correct as inversely proportional to the intrinsic ambiguity of the sentences in which it appears (20),

$$(20)\ \mathrm{P}(ess \in \mathrm{G}|X) = \frac{1}{|X|}$$

where $|X|$ is the cardinality of the collision set (see Basili et al. 1994) X for *ess*. Averaging over the whole corpus, we can approximate the notion of blind probability of being correct of an *ess*, given its observation, in at least one sentence, as (21),

$$(21)\ \mathrm{P}(ess \in \mathrm{G}|\Omega_c) = \frac{\sum_{X \in \Omega_c} \mathrm{P}(ess \in \mathrm{G}|X)}{C}$$

where C is the total number of collision sets X (ambiguous and non-ambiguous) observed in the corpus Ω_c.

Let us turn now to the definition of prior probability for parse trees *t*. The dependency operator $\Downarrow$ in Figure 19.1 should be expressed as a functional composition of the probabilites P(*ess* ∈ G). Is seems reasonable to define the prior probability of a given tree *t*, i.e. P(*t* ∈ G), as a composition of the corresponding probabilities of the *ess* ocurring in *t*. There is, however, a subtle problem with such a definition. Different trees generally give rise to a different number of syntactic structures. In other words, the cardinality of the sets of *ess*'s occurring in different parses of a given sentence is generally different. Composition of the members in such different sets is not well suited for direct comparison. The product operator, for example, will be penalizing for the larger set. A more careful definition for the prior probability of a tree follows.

Definition 5. Sentence support set of elementary syntactic structures: Given a sentence s, its support set, ESS(s) is the set of *ess*'s that occur in at least one tree of $\gamma(s)$, i.e.

(22) $\mathrm{ESS}(s) = \{ess|\exists t \in \gamma(s) \text{ such that } ess \text{ occurs in } t\}$

Definition 6. Score of a tree: Given a sentence s, and a tree $t \in \gamma(s)$, its evaluation $\mu(t)$ according to the probability of individual *ess*'s in ESS(s) is defined as

(23) $$\mu(t) = \prod_{ess \in \mathrm{ESS}(t)} \delta(ess, t)$$

where

(24) $$\delta(ess, t) = \begin{cases} \mathrm{P}(ess \in \mathrm{G}|X) \textit{ iff } ess \text{ occurs in } t \\ 1 - P(ess \in \mathrm{G}|X) \text{ otherwise} \end{cases}$$

Definition 7. Prior probability of a parse tree: The prior probability of a parse tree being correct is obtained by normalizing the score of trees in $\gamma(s)$. If M is the sum of $\mu(t)$ for $t \in \gamma(s)$, the prior probability of any parse tree $t \in \gamma(s)$ is:

(25) $$\mathrm{P}(t \in \mathrm{G}) = \frac{\mu(t)}{M}$$

Correspondingly we will have

(26) $$\mathrm{P}(t \in \mathrm{E}) = 1 - \frac{\mu(t)}{M}$$

Definition 7 expresses a probability that is uniform in the set $\gamma(s)$ of possible parses of a sentence s and is consistent with the syntactic relations expressed by each tree. If a syntactic relation ess_1 occurs in a tree t, an implicit piece of information in t is also the negation of the correctness of all the syntactic structures ess_i in the same collision set of ess_1. This is modelled by the operator δ in (23).

For the sentence (4), given

t_1: (John (flies (to London) (by plane)))

t_2: (John (flies (to (London (by plane)))))

and

ess_1: (John flies)

ess_2: (flies (to London))

ess_3: (flies (by plane))

ess_4: (London (by plane))

then (27) and (28) apply.

(27) $\mathrm{P}(t_1 \in \mathrm{G}) = \mathrm{P}(ess_1 \in \mathrm{G}) \times \mathrm{P}(ess_2 \in \mathrm{G}) \times \mathrm{P}(ess_3 \in \mathrm{G}) \times (1 - \mathrm{P}(ess_4 \in \mathrm{G}))$

(28) $\mathrm{P}(t_1 \in \mathrm{G}) = \mathrm{P}(ess_1 \in \mathrm{G}) \times \mathrm{P}(ess_2 \in \mathrm{G}) \times (1 - \mathrm{P}(ess_3 \in \mathrm{G})) \times \mathrm{P}(ess_4 \in \mathrm{G})$

19.4 Posterior probability of ambiguous parse trees

The posterior probability is the probability of being in a class (G or E), as it is assigned by the trained system to the instances of the test set (i.e. parse trees or *ess*'s). In order to express such a probability we need to model at first the corresponding probabilities for elementary syntactic structures, and then apply again a composition operator, as in (23). As such a compositon is not modified by the training process, i.e. the lexical acquisition or corpus-processing phase, it will be left unchanged in the expression of the posterior probability of trees. In order to derive the posterior probability of trees (i.e. $P'(t \in G)$ and $P'(t \in E)$) by (23) and (25), we just need to define the posterior probability of elementary syntactic structures (i.e. $P'(ess \in G)$ and $P'(ess \in E)$).

All the corpus-driven methods for automatic disambiguation assign some probabilistic score to extensive collections of data, i.e. syntactic patterns extracted from the raw texts. In order to use the information gain as a performance index of these methods we need to express the preference scores defined for each method as probability distributions P and P′. The problem is that each defined syntactic disambiguation operator has a probabilistic flavour *but is not a probability*.

Given any disambiguation score σ, if coll(s) denotes a collision set for the sentence s, the condition in (29) should hold for P′.

$$(29)\quad \sum_{ess \in \text{coll}(s)} P'_\sigma(ess \in G) = 1$$

where P'_σ denotes the posterior probability derived from the preference function σ. A possible definition of P′ from σ is the following:

Definition 8. Posterior probability of a syntactic pattern, given a disambiguation score σ: Given a disambiguation score σ, and a sentence s, we will say that the "posterior probability" of an $ess \in \text{ESS}(s)$ of being correct, given the preference function σ, is

$$\begin{aligned}(30)\quad P'_\sigma(ess \in G|\Omega_c) &= P'_\sigma(ess \in G)\\ &= P'_\sigma(ess \in G|\Omega_c)P(\Omega|\Omega_c)\\ &= \frac{\sigma(ess)}{M}P(\Omega|\Omega_c)\end{aligned}$$

where

$$(31)\quad M = \sum_{ess \in \text{coll}(s)} \sigma(ess)$$

Equation (30) is valid *for any disambiguation method*, given that an appropriate notion of collision set can be defined. In the following, we evaluate "lexical association" (Hindle & Rooth 1993) and "mutual conditioned plausibility" (Basili et al. 1993a, 1994) modelled in terms of probability distributions over sets of training instances. These two methods are chosen as a test-bed for studying the evaluation framework introduced in Sections 19.2 and 19.3, not to compare the methods against each other. Clearly, the applicability of this framework is not limited to such methods, since (30) can be easily extended to any corpus-based language-learning algorithm.

19.4.1 Posterior probability based on lexical association

Lexical association (LA) is a preference score introduced in Hindle & Rooth (1993) as an extension of the more classical *t*-score measure (Hindle & Rooth 1991). LA is used in ambiguous sentence frameworks like (32).

(32) verb + dirobj + prep + noun

If this score is (significantly) positive, preference is given to the verb attachment (verb + prep + noun); when negative, it suggests the opposite attachment (dirobj + prep + noun).

To summarize, we will recall the definition that models syntactic preference in sentences like (32). In this case the LA value is defined by (33).

$$(33)\quad \mathrm{LA}(verb; dirobj; prep) = \log_2 \frac{\mathrm{P}(prep|verb)\mathrm{P}(\varnothing|dirobj)}{\mathrm{P}(prep|bdirobj)}$$

where $\mathrm{P}(\varnothing|dirobj)$ is the probability of observing no prepositional modifier for *dirobj*. In this form, (33) is useful only within ambiguous-frame sentences such as (32). In order to extend its coverage to other ambiguous structures within the test set, we should also model sentence structures like (34) (i.e. chains of prepositional modifiers).

(34) word1 ... [prep1] word2 ... [prep2] word3 ... prep3 word4

Since in these cases alternative readings may give rise to more than two referents, we cannot use a single LA value. According to the definition (33), we will express a modified preference for a referent as follows. This preference score, which is slightly different from LA, fits our experimental purposes, and will be denoted σ_{LA}. When the referent of a postmodifier, e.g. (*prep3 word4*), is the closest word, i.e. *word3*, then the preference score follows the philosophy used for the denominator in (33):

$$(35)\quad \begin{aligned} \mathrm{P}'_{\mathrm{LA}}(ess \in \mathrm{G}) &= \mathrm{P}'_{\mathrm{LA}}(ess \in \mathrm{G}|\Omega_c)\mathrm{P}(\Omega_c|\Omega) \\ &= \frac{\sigma_{\mathrm{LA}}(w_1, p)}{M} P(\Omega_c|\Omega) \end{aligned}$$

where

$$(36)\quad M = \sum_{ess(w_1,p,w_2)\in \mathrm{coll}(s)} \sigma_{\mathrm{LA}}(w_1, p)$$

and coll(s) is the collision set of the sentence s to which *ess* belongs.

Otherwise, the score defined in (37) is preferable, as in the numerator in (33).

(37) $\sigma_{\mathrm{LA}}(w_1, p) = \mathrm{P}(p|w_i)\mathrm{P}(\varnothing|w_3),\ i \neq 3$

where w_i is the preferred referent in (34). This definition is a close approximation to the LA.

Definition 9. Posterior probability distributions based on lexical association: Given a sentence s, any syntactic structure $ess(w_1, p, w_2) \in \mathrm{ESS}(s)$ has a posterior probability based on LA, $\mathrm{P}'_{\mathrm{LA}}(ess(w_1; p; w_2) \in \mathrm{G})$ given by (35), (36).

19.4.2 Posterior probability based on mutual conditioned plausibility of syntactic patterns

In Basili et al. (1992a, 1993a,b) hybrid methods for deriving lexical and semantic information from a corpus have been defined. In particular, in Basili et al. (1993a), an algorithm to select between ambiguous referents of prepositional phrases is introduced. The method is hybrid since it relies on conditioned probabilities, but it is also knowledge-based because:

- sample data are derived by a (not so) shallow parser that collects syntactic triples (e.g. V+P+N, N+V+N, N+P+N, etc.) with a good approximation with respect to a full grammar (Basili et al. 1992b);
- collocation data are augmented with high-level conceptual tags τ for words, assigned manually or using on-line thesauri (e.g. "cognition", "instrumentality", "property", etc.). Conceptual tags allow the clustering of collocational data and improve the reliability of predictions.

The syntactic disambiguation method can be briefly summarized as follows. Given an elementary syntactic triple, $ess(w_1, w_2, w_3)$, and a given a conceptual tag τ for the word w_3, the "mutual conditioned probability" (MCP) is defined as (38),

$$(38)\quad \mathrm{MCP}(ess(w_1, w_2, w_3)) = \frac{freq(ess(w_1, w_2, \tau))}{freq(ess(\alpha, w_2, \tau))freq(ess(w_1, w_2, \alpha))}$$

where *freq* is the number of observations of a triple in the corpus, α is used to indicate a missing constraint on the corresponding argument, and clusters all the observations of words categorized by such class label. Hence, for example, in a sentence like (39), the *ess(fly,by,plane)* has the MCP(*ess(fly,by,plane)*) value (40) associated with it,

(39) John flies to Rome by plane.

$$(40)\quad \mathrm{MCP}(ess(fly, by, plane)) = \frac{freq(ess(fly, by, \mathrm{Ins}))}{freq(ess(fly, by, \alpha))freq(ess(\alpha, by, \mathrm{Ins}))}$$

where "Ins" ("Instrumentality" as in the WordNet on-line thesaurus (Miller 1990)) is the conceptual category assigned to the word *plane*. Alternative *ess*'s in a sentence are selected by comparing their MCP values. It is not the purpose of this paper to outline the advantages of this method over the others proposed in the literature, and in particular the LA. The interested reader may refer to the aforementioned papers.

In Basili et al. (1994) we introduced a more refined measure, called the "mutual conditioned plausibility" (MCPl). This score is a generalization of the MCP. It is evaluated from a model of graded syntactic significance assigned to syntactic structures during their extraction from (i.e. observation in) the corpus. The expression of the MCPl is obtained by replacing in (38) graded syntactic significance[1] (which is measured by a score named "syntactic plausibility") by frequency counts. More details can be found in Basili et al. (1994).

The "posterior probability based on MCPl" is the probability distribution obtained by the P'_{LA} (35) applied to MCPl over the support set.

Definition 10. Posterior probability distributions based on mutual conditioned plausibility: Given a sentence s, any syntactic structure $ess \in \mathrm{ESS}(s)$ has a posterior probability $P'_{\mathrm{MCPl}}(ess \in G)$, based on the mutual conditioned plausibility, given by

$$(41)\quad P'_{\mathrm{MCPl}}(ess \in G) = P'_{\mathrm{MCPl}}(ess \in G)P(\Omega_c|\Omega) = \frac{\mathrm{MCPl}(ess)}{M}P(\Omega_c|\Omega)$$

where

$$(42)\quad M = \sum_{ess \in \mathrm{coll}(s)} \mathrm{MCPl}(ess)$$

and coll(s) is the collision set of the sentence s to which ess belongs.

19.5 Discussion

The evaluation framework introduced in Sections 19.2 to 19.4 has been defined to compare disambiguation methods uniformly throughout different corpora and application domains. In order to study the impact of this experimental method we selected a common test set and performed the evaluation of precision, recall and the information score derived by using LA, and using MCPl in the disambiguation phase.

The test corpus Σ included 232 complex sentences from which 7871 parse trees were derived (an average of 33 parse trees per sentence). Sentences were taken from the legal domain in Italian and included about 500 000 words. The Italian grammar adopted in the test set was a DCG, including 103 rules. In the 7871 parse trees, 2782 elementary syntactic structures of interest were detected. The classes

1. In short, each observed *ess* has a weight inversely proportional to the cardinality of its collision set in the sentence in which it occurs.

of elementary syntactic structures of interest were the following: N+P+N, V+P+N, V+N, N+V, N+∅, V+∅. The test set was manually validated (i.e. class E and G were defined for the parse trees) by three human judges. The number of correct parses approximated the number of sentences (there was an average of 1.3 correct trees per sentence), while the number of correct elementary syntactic links was about 1540.

The experiment provided several interesting pieces of evidence on PP-disambiguation methods in general, and on the two analysed methods in particular. However, we will concentrate on the properties of the performance evaluation methods, rather than on those of the disambiguation methods, for the sake of space, and because the latter are not the focus of the paper (see Table 19.1).

Table 19.1 Experimental results: information score (I_Σ) vs accuracy

	MCPl	LA
I_Σ on all trees	−1.04	−0.93
I_Σ on correct trees	1.81	1.46
I_Σ averaged on sentences	0.32	0.20
I_Σ on all *ess*'s	0.26	0.18
I_Σ on correct *ess*'s	0.76	0.63
Accuracy over trees (%)	32.20	31.20
Accuracy over *ess*'s (%)	61.00	51.00

A first piece of evidence is the low-value information-score index (henceforth I_Σ), when calculated over all the trees (first row in the table). This is not surprising, since the *a priori* probability of the wrong trees is about 97%. It is very difficult for both systems to perform better than chance.

The third row shows a less penalizing measure that combines the average I_Σ for correct trees with the average I_Σ for wrong trees. Both methods perform rather well, as shown by the good information gain. To make a comparison, in Kononenko & Bratko (1991) the information gain of rather less complex classification tasks (e.g. with a prior probability of the most probable class not higher than 45%, and with supervised learning algorithms) is about 1.

Though this is not shown in the table, I_Σ values are not sensitive to the complexity of the test set. In fact, we did not observe significant changes in the I_Σ values for groups of sentences with a number of trees between 2 and 30, from 30 to 90, and over 90. Rather, I_Σ is sensitive to the complexity of the learning set, modelled by the denominators C and M in the formulae of the prior (21) and posterior (30) probabilities. I_Σ is also sensitive to the dimension of the learning set. We obtained improving performance for both methods when we increased the learning corpus from 200 000 to 500 000 words. This is intuitive, since all PP-disambiguation methods perform better as they gain evidence of linguistic patterns. It is our future objective to observe these dependencies more closely, by experimenting on different linguistic domains, and with fixed domains of increasing dimension (possibly, well over 1 million words).

The fourth row of Table 19.1 provides the same measure as in row 1, calculated over collision sets rather than over trees. This value is higher, as expected, since the the ratio between correct and wrong *ess*'s is lower than for trees.

Rows 6 and 7 provide the accuracy[2] of the two methods based on a simple maximum likelihood method. Again, the values in row 6 (accuracy at selecting the correct tree) are rather low compared with values in the subsequent line (accuracy at selecting the correct *ess* in a collision set). The average number of collision sets in each tree is 3.3. The composition operator used to assign a preference to a tree (see (23)) reduces the global confidence in each choice. Furthermore, neither of the tested preference scores provides a model of many ambiguity phenomena (e.g. anaphora, adjectival or adverbial PP referents). Suitable models of such phenomena should result in higher accuracy values.

As a final remark, we will briefly comment on the performances of the two methods. We have already stated that the performances of PP-disambiguation methods depend on the evidence they can gain of the observed linguistic patterns, i.e. the average frequency of the collected *ess*'s. This evidence, in turn, depends on the complexity and dimension of the learning corpus, which is accounted for in the I_{Σ} measure. However, it depends also on the type of *ess* observed by the specific method. Given a learning set, the LA collects word pairs while the MCPl collects word triples. Evidence of triples is obviously less than that of pairs. In all, 93 813 different triples and 22 404 different pairs have been derived from the corpus. This should penalize the MCPl. However, semantic tags allow triples to be clustered, thus increasing their evidence. Table 19.1 shows that adding semantics has a very positive effect on the performance of MCPl, despite the initial reduced linguistic evidence that was gained from the corpus.

References

Basili, R., M. T. Pazienza and P. Velardi 1991. Using word association for syntactic disambiguation. In *Trends in Artificial Intelligence*, E. Ardizzone, S. Gaglio and F. Sorbello (eds), 250–60. Berlin: Springer.

Basili, R., M. T. Pazienza & P. Velardi 1992a. Computational lexicons: the neat examples and the odd exemplars. *Proceedings of the Third Conference on Applied Natural Language Processing*, Trento, 96–103.

Basili, R., M. T. Pazienza & P. Velardi 1992b. A shallow syntactic analyzer to extract lexical information from corpora. *Literary and Linguistic Computing* **7**, 114–24

2. Since the methods are always forced to make a choice, accuracy and precision are here the same.

Basili, R., M. T. Pazienza & P. Velardi 1993a. Semi-automatic extraction of linguistic information for syntactic disambiguation. *Applied Artificial Intelligence* **7**, 339–64.

Basili, R., M. T. Pazienza & P. Velardi 1993b. Acquisition of selectional patterns in sublanguages. *Machine Translation* **8**, 175–201.

Basili R., A. Marziali & M. T. Pazienza 1994. Modelling syntactic ambiguity in lexical acquisition. *Journal of Quantitative Linguistics* **1**, 62–81.

Boggess, L., R. Agarwal and R. Davis 1991. Disambiguation of prepositional phrases in automatically labeled technical texts. In *Proceedings, 9th National Conference on Artificial Intelligence (AAAI)*, Anaheim, Calif., 155–9.

Grishman, R. & J. Sterling 1992. Acquisition of selectional patterns. *Proceedings of the fifteenth International Conference on Computational Linguistics: COLING–92*, Nantes, 658–64.

Hindle, D. & M. Rooth 1991. Structural ambiguity and lexical relations. *29th Annual Meeting of the Association for Computational Linguistics*, Berkeley, Calif., 229–36.

Hindle, D. & M. Rooth 1993. Structural ambiguity and lexical relations. *Computational Linguistics* **19**, 103–20.

Jelinek, F., J. D. Lafferty & R. L. Mecer 1990. *Basic methods of probabilistic context free grammars*. Research Report RC16374, IBM Yorktown Heights, NY.

Kononenko, I. & I. Bratko 1991. Information-based evaluation criterion for classifier's performance. *Machine Learning* **6**, 67–80.

Miller, G. 1990. Five papers on WordNet. Special Issue of *International Journal of Lexicography* **3**(4).

Resnik, P. & M. A. Hearst 1993. Structural ambiguity and conceptual relations. *Proceedings of the Workshop on Very Large Corpora: Academic and Industrial Perspectives*, Columbus, Ohio, 58–64.

Sekine, S., J. J. Carroll, S. Ananiadou & J. Tsujii 1992. Automatic learning for semantic collocation. *Proceedings of the Third Conference on Applied Natural Language Processing*, Trento, 104–10.

20
Automatic error detection in part-of-speech tagging

DAVID ELWORTHY

20.1 Introduction

Tagging by the Hidden Markov Model (HMM) is a successful technique for assigning grammatical information to words in a corpus. In outline, the tagger picks the most probable grammatical category, or "tag", for each word by combining the probability of possible tag sequences with the probability of each hypothesized tag for the words, considered in isolation from the context. There are two standard algorithms, known as forward–backwards (FB) and Viterbi. Viterbi achieves greater computational efficiency than FB by pruning out some hypotheses; FB has the advantage of assigning a score to every hypothesized tag. The model, in the form of the word–tag (lexical) and tag–tag (transition) probabilities may be estimated from a training corpus which has been tagged by some other means, for example by a human annotator. Alternatively, the model may be derived using a procedure called Baum–Welch re-estimation, which iteratively improves the quality of an approximate model using probabilities derived by the FB algorithm. The tagging algorithms are robust, in the sense that every word will receive a tag, even in ungrammatical text. For a more detailed description including the mathematical foundations of the technique, see Sharman (1990) and Cutting et al. (1992).

Tagging based on HMMs is capable of achieving a good success rate. Typically, about 90% of words that have more than one tag are assigned the correct part of speech (Cutting et al. 1992), equivalent to about 96% correctness over the whole corpus. While 96% sounds like a good success rate, it still represents one error in 25 words on average, and such accuracies are only achieved where the training and test corpora are of similar vocabulary and style. Furthermore, since the tagger always succeeds in assigning a tag to every word, there is no direct way of knowing where the errors are.

This paper[1] reports some experiments on the automatic detection of tagger errors. The basic idea is to use observable values from the tagging process to provide an indication of whether the chosen tag is likely to be correct. A similar approach can be applied to Baum–Welch re-estimation, in order to screen poor data out of the re-estimation process, and so hopefully improve the new model.

The suggestion that an appropriate threshold might enable errors to be detected is not a new one and some related work is discussed in a later section. The contribution of this paper is first to derive the data that suggests that an error detection technique can be made to work, and then to predict and verify the effects of various thresholds. As a consequence, it is possible to construct a tagger in which either the accuracy or the efficiency is supplied as a parameter.

20.2 The experiment

The proposed means of detecting and correcting tagger errors is to mark a tag as being unreliable if some observable value associated with it lies on the wrong side of a threshold. The most obvious observables to use are the probability of the tag and its entropy. Probability measures the likelihood compared to other hypotheses for the same word, and so a low probability may indicate that the tagger has not managed to make a clear disambiguation. Entropy (very roughly) gives a measure of the information content of the tag, which again is an indication of distinctness. To determine the suitability of these observables, the tagger was run on various corpora, and the distributions of the probability and entropy collected. We first introduce the tagger and corpora used in the experiment and then present the data that resulted.

20.2.1 The tagger and the corpora

The tagger is an implementation of the Viterbi, FB and Baum–Welch algorithms, written in C++. Three test corpora were constructed using parts of the *Wall Street Journal* corpus from the Penn Treebank (Marcus et al. 1993), referred to as WSJ1,

1. An earlier version of the techniques described here was tried out at Cambridge University Computer Laboratory, as part of ESPRIT BR Project 7315 "The Acquisition of Lexical Knowledge" (Acquilex-II). Ted Briscoe made a number of useful comments on those experiments. The work reported in the paper was carried out at Sharp Laboratories of Europe.

WSJ2 and WSJ3 below. WSJ1 was drawn from parts 4000 and 4100 of the WSJ in the treebank, WSJ2 from parts 0000 to 3900 inclusive and WSJ3 from 4200 and 4300. Each corpus was used separately to train the tagger. WSJ1 was then used as test data against the resulting models. The three tests represent the case where there is a very good match between the training and test data, where the match is less good but the training data is sufficiently large to provide reasonable quality, and where there is a poor match. Words that appeared in the test corpus but not in the training corpus were assigned all non-closed class tags.

The accuracy of the tagger on each test is given in Table 20.1, using the results from the FB algorithm. The "Proportion correct" column is the accuracy over the whole corpus, i.e. the proportion of words for which the tag chosen by the tagger was the correct one, and "Ambiguous correct" is the corresponding figure for words that have more than one hypothesized tag. The proportion of such word tokens is shown as "Amount of ambiguity". For most of the rest of this paper, accuracies are those of ambiguous words only. This is generally a more interesting figure than the overall accuracy, since it includes only those words where the tagger has to select between hypotheses. In passing, it is interesting to note that the tagger can achieve good performance even on the WSJ2 test, where 3 words out of 4 are ambiguous. Corpora WSJ1 and WSJ3 consisted of about 100 000 words, and WSJ2 of about 2 million words.

Table 20.1 Basic tagger accuracy on test corpus WSJ1.

Training corpus	Proportion correct (%)	Ambiguous correct (%)	Amount of ambiguity (%)
WSJ1	96.93	92.66	41.85
WSJ2	94.20	92.85	77.87
WSJ3	90.18	83.07	49.97

20.2.2 Empirical study

There are a number of observables that might prove to be useful in predicting when the tagger has made an incorrect choice. As already said, the most obvious is the probability p assigned to a tag by the FB algorithm. A second likely measure is the hypothesis entropy, defined as $-p \log_2(p)$, which gives an indication of how much information had to be contributed to make the choice compared with a purely random one. One further parameter to the study is whether to collect data for all hypotheses, or for just the one chosen by the tagger. The former is more useful for attempting to improve Baum–Welch re-estimation, and the latter for tagging itself. The results here are for the chosen tag only.

The results of the tests appear in Figures 20.1 and 20.2, which show the cumulative frequency distributions of hypotheses with the given measure, for ambiguous tokens. The scores assigned by the FB algorithm to the hypotheses

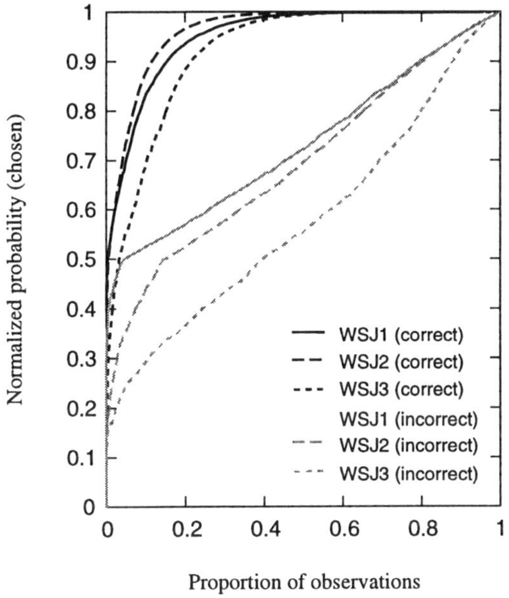

Figure 20.1 *Probability vs number of observations.*

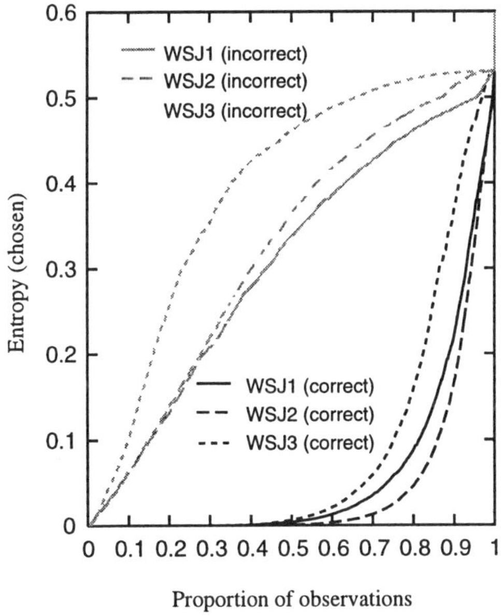

Figure 20.2 *Entropy vs number of observations.*

on a word do not sum up to 1, and in general are not comparable from one word to another. They were therefore normalized first.[2]

The important point is that the shapes of the graphs are broadly comparable across the three corpora. The WSJ3 test shows the greatest deviation from the others, since the test and training data correspond less well than in the other two tests. The distributions are generally quite "well behaved"; for example, they are monotonic and more or less smooth. These two facts give some reasonable confidence that a technique that is reliable, parameterizable and applicable across corpora can be developed.

20.3 Thresholding for error detection

The data of the previous section can be used to decide on suitable thresholds on the observable values, so that hypotheses that lie on the wrong side of the threshold are rejected. The ideal threshold is one that eliminates a large proportion of the incorrect hypotheses while retaining as many of the correct ones as possible. In the case of the probability, the threshold is used as a lower bound, i.e. hypotheses with lower probabilities are rejected. For entropy, it forms an upper bound, the inversion arising from the fact that the measured value is negated.

To evaluate the technique, we need a measure of *accuracy*. Two definitions are possible. If words with a rejected hypothesis are simply ignored, the accuracy is calculated by dividing the number of correctly tagged, non-rejected words by the total number of non-rejected words. Alternatively, if the existence of an "oracle" may be assumed, which will find the correct tag for any rejected words, the accuracy is found by summing the proportion of words that are correctly tagged and not rejected, and the proportion of words that are rejected and so handled by the oracle. Suppose s is the proportion of ambiguous words that are correctly tagged, c the proportion of correctly tagged ambiguous words that are (incorrectly) rejected, and i the proportion of incorrectly tagged ambiguous words that are (correctly) rejected, then the accuracy a on non-rejected ambiguous words, i.e. the first method of evaluation, is given in (1), and the second in (2).[3]

$$(1)\quad a = \frac{s(1-c)}{1 - sc - i(1-s)}$$

$$(2)\quad a = s + i(1-s)$$

2. This can be done without affecting the accuracy of the algorithm; in fact, it is sometimes used to ensure numerical stability (Cutting et al. 1992).

3. This can be seen as follows: c of the words in total are correct. Of these sc are rejected and $s(1-c)$ retained. $1-s$ are incorrect with $i(1-s)$ rejected and $(1-s)(1-i)$ retained. For the "ignore" measure the retained correct words are $s(1-c)$, and the retained words in total $s(1-c)+(1-s)(1-i)$. For the "oracle" measure, $s(1-c)$ correct words are retained and $sc+i(1-s)$ are supplied by the oracle.

A second figure for evaluating the process is the *efficiency* (also called "recall") of the tagger, defined as the proportion of ambiguous words actually labelled, whether correct or not. This gives a measure of how hard the oracle must work in the second case. The efficiency e is given by (3).

$$(3)\quad e = s(1-c) + (1-s)(1-i)$$

As a test to decide which of the proposed measures (probability, entropy) is best, the threshold that yields a specified accuracy was determined using Figures 20.1 and 20.2, and the corresponding efficiency found. The results are shown in Tables 20.2 and 20.3, for 95% and 99% (oracle) accuracy on ambiguous words.

Table 20.2 Efficiency for 95% accuracy on ambiguous words.

Training corpus	Measure	Threshold	Efficiency (%)
WSJ1	probability	0.629	94.8
	entropy	0.420	94.9
WSJ2	probability	0.577	96.2
	entropy	0.455	96.2
WSJ3	probability	0.710	79.2
	entropy	0.349	79.2

Table 20.3 Efficiency for 99% accuracy on ambiguous words.

Training corpus	Measure	Threshold	Efficiency (%)
WSJ1	probability	0.935	75.2
	entropy	0.888	75.2
WSJ2	probability	0.932	80.3
	entropy	0.094	80.4
WSJ3	probability	0.963	57.6
	entropy	0.516	57.9

With the proportions of ambiguous words as listed in Table 20.1, the success rates across the whole of each corpus would be as shown in Table 20.4.

Table 20.4 Success rates for the whole of each corpus.

Corpus	At 95%	At 99%
WSJ1	97.9	99.6
WSJ2	96.1	99.2
WSJ3	97.5	99.5

The tables show that the two measures give similar efficiencies, and that a lower efficiency results with low-quality training data (WSJ3). The WSJ1 and WSJ2 tests reject about 1 word in 20 to obtain 95% accuracy, or 1 word in 4 (WSJ1) or 5 (WSJ2) to obtain 99%.

Finally, the predictions were confirmed by running the tagger with the thresholds for 95% efficiency. The results are presented in Table 20.5.

Table 20.5 Measured accuracy and efficiency, WSJ1.

Training corpus	Measure	Threshold	Accuracy (%)	Efficiency (%)
WSJ1	probability	0.629	94.97	94.9
	entropy	0.420	95.01	94.8
WSJ2	probability	0.577	94.99	96.2
	entropy	0.455	95.01	96.1
WSJ3	probability	0.710	94.98	79.2
	entropy	0.349	95.04	79.1

The experimental results show close correspondence with the predicted ones. This confirms (for the test data, at least) that if we have evidence that allows a threshold to be chosen, then its effect can be predicted, allowing a controlled trade-off between efficiency and accuracy.

A follow-up experiment was conducted using the same thresholds and training corpora, but with WSJ3 as the test corpus rather than WSJ1. When training with WSJ2 the results were broadly comparable to the figures above, and with WSJ1 the results were similar to the values obtained with WSJ3 in the previous test, as would be expected. When WSJ3 was used as the training data, which could be expected to compare with the case of WSJ1 before, there was a poorer correspondence. This suggests that when we move to a significantly different corpus, then the frequency distributions must be collected afresh if the accuracy and efficiency are to be predicted accurately.

20.3.1 Related work

There are a number of references in the literature to the use of thresholds. Weischedel et al. (1993: 367) uses thresholds to eliminate tags from unknown words when their probability is less than $1/e^2$ that of the most likely tag. Garside et al. (1987: 51) apply thresholding to the output of the tagger CLAWS1, and retain tag ambiguities when the tag probabilities are judged too low to indicate a reliable result. Neither of these sources includes information about the distribution of probabilities or the accuracy–efficiency trade-off.

An examination of automatic error detection in more detail can be found in Macklovitch (1992) and the related work in Foster (1991). Macklovitch reports a comparison between two experiments on error detection and correction, one based on statistical information and the other employing linguistic knowledge. The statistical approach used an error detection technique developed by Foster, which assumes that "tagging errors correspond to situations in which the model assigns similar probabilities to competing alternatives" (Foster 1991: 75). He therefore compares the differences between scores on the best and second best hypotheses with a threshold. This can be seen to be roughly equivalent to the approach described above, as follows. Let p be the probability of the chosen tag. In the case where there are two hypothesized tags, the other tag has probability $1-p$. Then the difference between the probabilities is $p-(1-p) = 2p-1$, and hence comparing this against a threshold n is equivalent to comparing p against $(n+1)/2$. Similar remarks apply if the ratio is used rather than the difference. If there are more than two hypothesized tags, the equivalence between the two techniques is less exact, but in two common cases – where all hypotheses have similar probability, and where the third and remaining hypotheses all have very low probability – similar reasoning will apply. Macklovitch reports the statistical technique as having similar performance to the results quoted above: for example, it will detect all but 1% of the tagging errors while rejecting 15% of the tokens, i.e. there is 99% efficiency and 85% accuracy.

Macklovitch's linguistic, or knowledge-based, technique uses rules to flag potentially incorrect tagging of past and preterite verb forms – a common tagger error. The rules are based on linguistic principles; for example, a word tagged as "participle" is marked as being an error if it is the only verbal form in a sentence. Of the tags flagged by the rules, 68% were genuine errors, the remainder being spuriously flagged. Of the past–preterite errors made by the tagger, about 30% were detected by the rules. The statistical approach detected 49% of the tagger's errors when adjusted to give the same rate of errors in the detection.

The major argument in favour of using linguistic rules is that it is possible to specify how to correct the error as well as to detect it. However, there are some disadvantages to the knowledge-based approach. It is not parameterizable, in that one cannot choose a threshold to give a specified efficiency or accuracy. A second problem is that it introduces knowledge about the constructs of a specific language into the tagger, which is otherwise (barring the design of the tagset) language-independent. The knowledge is only applicable on the assumption of reasonably grammatical input. However, one of the strengths of HMM tagging is that such a requirement can largely be avoided in favour of an assumption that the training and test data are similar. Finally, it is likely that if a wide range of errors is to be detected, then many rules covering the different sources of error would be needed. The interactions between these rules might prove difficult to control.

20.3.2 Applications

Although the techniques described here have not yet been applied in anything other than an experimental system, a possible application area is as follows. In the Integrated Language Database project,[4] we are developing systems that will allow lexicographers and computational linguists to construct lexicons in which the lexical data is supported by evidence from analysed corpora. It is certainly reasonable to expect the corpora to have tens or hundreds of millions of words, providing instances of most lexical items in a variety of contexts. When using such data, it is more important to the lexicographer or computational linguist to know that the citations on which they are basing their decisions are reliable, even if this results in only a few examples. Consequently, the tagger can be run with a threshold that provides a certain degree of accuracy, accepting a reduced efficiency as a consequence, but still obtaining some citations of the word in question.

20.4 Thresholding to improve re-estimation

Thresholding can also be used to bring about a small improvement in Baum–Welch re-estimation, by excluding hypotheses on the other side of the threshold from the data used to re-estimate the model. Figures 20.3 and 20.4 present the probability distributions for all hypotheses, and not just the chosen ones as in Figures 20.1 and 20.2. The ideal threshold would be one that excludes as much of the incorrect data as possible while retaining most of the correct data. The graphs make it clear that entropy is not a useful measure, since the curves are too close together, but the probability is possible.

The technique was tested by setting a threshold that eliminates a given proportion of the incorrect hypotheses, using the data from Figure 20.3. The predicted effect of choosing various thresholds is shown in Table 20.6, for 90%, 95% and 98% of the incorrect hypotheses excluded.

The Baum–Welch experiments were then repeated with these thresholds, with the results shown in Table 20.7. In each case, the final tagging run with the re-estimated statistics did not make use of a threshold, that is, thresholding applies purely to the

4. The ILD project is a collaboration between Sharp Laboratories, Cambridge University Press, Cambridge University Computer Laboratory and Edinburgh University Language Technology Group, and part-funded under the UK Department of Trade and Industry's SALT programme.

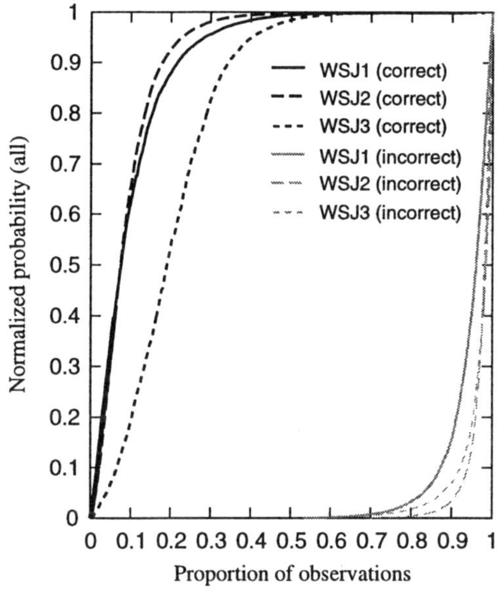

Figure 20.3 *Probability vs number of observations for all corpora.*

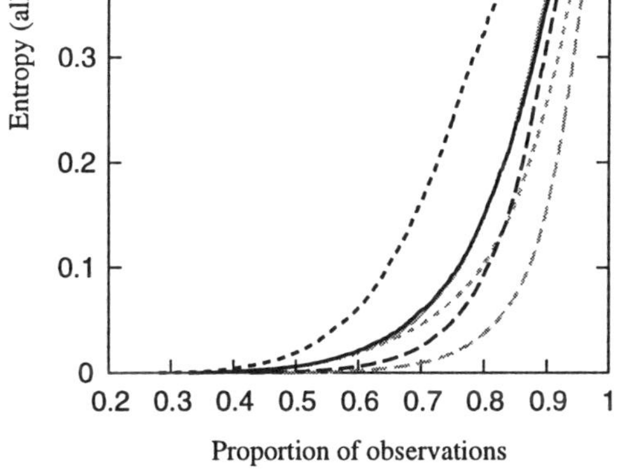

Figure 20.4 *Entropy vs number of observations for all corprora.*

Table 20.6 Probability thresholds for Baum–Welch re-estimation.

Training corpus	Threshold	Correct excluded (%)	Incorrect excluded (%)
WSJ1	0.155	2.5	90.0
WSJ2	0.035	1.1	90.0
WSJ3	0.070	5.2	90.0
WSJ1	0.408	6.1	95.0
WSJ2	0.139	2.8	95.0
WSJ3	0.185	9.9	95.0
WSJ1	0.735	12.1	98.0
WSJ2	0.460	7.0	98.0
WSJ3	0.443	17.2	98.0

Table 20.7 Effect of thresholds on Baum–Welch.

Training corpus	Threshold	Proportion correct (%)	Ambiguous correct (%)	Change
WSJ1	0.155	93.14	83.62	−3.86
WSJ2	0.035	88.45	85.47	−2.21
WSJ3	0.070	87.83	78.37	+0.46
WSJ1	0.408	95.33	88.86	+1.38
WSJ2	0.139	91.08	88.85	+1.17
WSJ3	0.185	88.21	79.12	+1.21
WSJ1	0.735	94.96	87.96	+0.48
WSJ2	0.460	92.08	90.14	+2.46
WSJ3	0.443	88.92	80.55	+2.64

re-estimation process and not to the tagging. When re-estimating a transition from hypothesis h to hypothesis i, the transition is included only if both h and i exceed the threshold. The final column of the table shows the improvement in the accuracy on ambiguous words compared with a test with no thresholding.

The conclusion from these results is that thresholding during re-estimation will bring about an improvement in the accuracy, but that careful choice of the threshold is needed. It is not clear why the first threshold reduced the accuracy with WSJ1 and WSJ2. As noted in Section 20.2.1, these are poor examples, since the training data is of sufficiently good quality that re-estimation lowers the accuracy.[5] The results with WSJ3 as training corpus are the more important ones, since they reflect a case where Baum–Welch might more reasonably be used. However, even in these cases, the improvement in accuracy that can be achieved is fairly small.

Raising the threshold too far will reduce the overall accuracy, since too much good-quality data is discarded. With a threshold on WSJ3 that excluded 98.5% of incorrect hypotheses, the accuracy rises by 1.66%; at the thresholds for excluding 99% and 99.5%, the accuracy falls by 0.72% and 5.26% respectively. This suggests that thresholding is, in general, less useful in re-estimation than it is in ordinary error correction.

20.5 Conclusions

We have seen the results of applying thresholds to hypothesis scores during tagging. Thresholding allows the accuracy of the tagger to be increased, at the cost of a reduction in efficiency. Depending on the quality of the training data, accuracies of 95% on ambiguous words can be achieved at efficiencies of 80–95%, or accuracies of 99% at efficiencies of 57–80%.

Two suggestions for extending this work are to collect data on probabilities for specific tags, as Garside et al. (1987) do for CLAWS1, and to examine the probability distribution on sequences of ambiguous words containing specific numbers of errors, with a view to selecting different thresholds in different circumstances. These techniques potentially allow better error detection, but at the cost of losing the simple relation between accuracy and efficiency and the corresponding tunability of the tagger.

References

Cutting, D., J. Kupiec, J. Pedersen & P. Sibun 1992. A practical part-of-speech tagger. In *Third Conference on Applied Natural Language Processing*. Trento, 133–40.

Elworthy, D. 1994. Does Baum–Welch re-estimation help taggers? In *Fourth Conference on Applied Natural Language Processing*. Stuttgart, 53–8.

Foster, G. F. 1991. *Statistical lexical disambiguation*. Master's thesis, School of Computer Science, McGill University, Montreal.

Garside, R., G. Leech & G. Sampson 1987. *The computational analysis of English: a corpus-based approach*. London: Longman.

Macklovitch, E. 1992. Where the tagger falters. In *Proceedings of the Fourth Conference on Theoretical and Methodological Issues in Machine Translation*. Montreal, 113–26.

5. For a more detailed examination of the relationship between the quality of the initial data and the effectiveness of re-estimation, see Elworthy (1994).

Marcus, M. P., B. Santorini & M. A. Marcinkiewicz 1993. Building a large annotated corpus of English: the Penn Treebank. *Computational Linguistics* **19**, 313–30.

Sharman, R. A. 1990. *Hidden Markov Model methods for word tagging*. Technical Report UKSC 214, IBM UK Scientific Centre, Winchester.

Weischedel, R., M. Meeter, R. Schwartz, L. Ramshaw & J. Palmucci 1993. Coping with ambiguity and unknown words through probabilistic models. *Computational Linguistics* **19**, 359–82.

21
A method of parsing English based on sentence form

JIM ENTWISLE AND MICHAEL GROVES

21.1 Introduction

A sentence is parsed by assigning syntax-tags to the words of the sentence and deducing the syntactic structures within the sentence. Most computer-parsing schemes begin by predesignating words of the sentence as "verb" and "noun" etc., but because of the fact that in English almost every inflectable word can operate as at least two of verb, noun and adjective, these particular classes cannot be used as a beginning classification scheme for a computer parser. These tags are frequently taken as a starting point in the higher-level parsing actions such as Categorial Grammar (Morrill et al. 1990) and the various generalizations of phrase-structure grammar (PSG) such as Gazdar et al.'s (1985) GPSG.

A pure syntax parser would work these tags out, not begin with them. The purpose of this paper is to demonstrate an acceptable starting point for parsing, one that is primitive enough to be a generally useful, highly extendible starting point.

Currently, amongst researchers who address parsing at this raw level, probability is the most usual method for deciding if a word has any particular tag. Such methods give an accuracy of 95–96% (Church & Hanks 1989) but it is not clear how this can be enhanced. We suggest that a thorough computer-analysis of the text can be done, carefully examining all possibilities without any recourse to semantics or probability in order to calculate all the possible tags exhaustively: essentially a computerized report of the raw text. Starting from the raw text, what can be observed with 100% certainty?

A further reason for such a thorough investigation is that syntax deduction is a rather straightforward exercise. Calculations that rely on semantics or probability as a source of syntax-tags are rather complex and never 100% safe. Algebraic precision is possible with pure syntactic arguments.

21.2 Word endings and tags in parsing

21.2.1 Inflections and English

In English, the inflection *narrows* the possible tags but does not make the word-tag unique, so parsing cannot be performed by examination of the words of the sentence in isolation. The inflection is clear just from inspection of the word and it does reflect, to a degree, the syntax-tag of the word: an *ing*-inflected word is never a verb, for example. This is not to say that English adheres only vaguely to its inflection rules. All inflection rules are followed precisely: an *ing*-inflected word is never a verb and an *s*-inflected word is never an adjective, etc.

The principal inflections of importance for parsing English are: *-s*, *-ed*, *-ing* and "null" (which means that the word has no inflection at all). There are other inflections: some words take an *-en* inflection instead of *-ed*: *take* has the two forms *taken* and *took* instead of **taked* but we classify both *taken* and *took* as *-ed* words for simplicity (we lose a small amount of information when we do this). A very few words do not permit full deduction of the inflection of the word: we will discuss this below.

Discussions of English are plagued by small numbers of exceptional cases but we have also found that sometimes the supposed "exception" is misnamed. Correct classification is important because an exception may be a special case whose premature handling can cloud and blur important issues, whereas a lack of handling on an important fundamental phenomenon (like the noun–verb question cited above) can lead to a poor solution that is essentially non-generalizable. Winston's third "criterion for success" applies:

> Is there a set of identifiable regularities or constraints from which the implemented procedure gets its power? If not, the procedure may be an ad hoc toy, capable perhaps of superficially impressive performance on carefully selected examples, but incapable of deeply impressive performance and incapable of helping you to solve any problem. Winston (1992: 13)

21.2.2 The Word Expert Parser

One natural language understanding (NLU) system that does not begin with a hard-wired lexicon is the Word Expert Parser (WEP) of Small & Reiger detailed in Small's (1980) thesis. The WEP divides each word separately into stem and inflection and then treats the inflection as the entity of importance: the inflections form the backbone of the parser and the uninflected word-base is placed on the periphery of the parser where it plays only a minor role.

The WEP permits words to contribute together in the deduction of the structure of the sentence. The parser, then, consists of a group of communicating entites that together form an analysis of the sentence. Specifically, these two qualities are of importance in the present paper:

> Individual words are active modular knowledge sources that coordinate the parsing process . . . Parsing knowledge is redundantly represented in word experts and inter-expert handshaking (lexical interaction). Small (1980: 12)

The inter-expert (read inter-word) handshaking is a powerful concept. The information that gives the tags of the words of a sentence is scattered throughout the sentence and needs to be collected. Inter-word handshaking allows it to be collected and formed into a tangible parse.

We note that the WEP performs a combination of both syntactic and semantic actions. In this paper we concern ourselves only with its syntactic actions.

In this approach to syntax parsing we also classify each punctuation mark as a separate closed-class word. Capitalization is used only to assist with the detection of proper nouns (but is only occasionally needed).

21.2.3 The classes of words

We divide the words of English into a number of classes (given in Table 21.1), just by inspection, and these classes satisfy exactly the starting point referred to in Section 21.1.

Each English word falls neatly into just one class, so these classes partition English (the fact that this happens so neatly is because of our particular choice of classes). Once classified, all words in any group will act in the same manner in a parser. So the class becomes representitive of the raw word.

The last entry is for the single-word classes: these last few words are so singular that each requires a category of its own. Note that the categories relate to slots in the sentence, not the (primary) character of the particular words.

21.2.4 Above the first line: the non-slashed classes

The non-slashed classes come directly from the WEP. We will discuss the inflection classes first. Each of the three inflections (*-ing*, *-ed*, *-s*) is a separate expert in the WEP and these are the only inflections that the creators of the WEP felt needed separate experts. We concur with this view: no other inflections are of such significance from the point of view of syntax.

Table 21.1 The classes.

Class	Examples
open-class-null	*run eat swim*
open-class-s	*walks flies*
open-class-ed	*stopped eaten*
open-class-ing	*singing eating*
preposition	*towards*
adverb	*quickly slowly*
subjunct	*purely*
determiner	*the a an my*
modal	*could would*
conjunction	*and but as-much-as because*
intensifier	*very*
open-class-ed/null	*set bit*
open-class-s/null	*sheep*
be-auxiliary/verb	*is are were*
do-auxiliary/verb	*do does did*
have-auxiliary/verb	*have has had*
preposition/particle	*in up on*
determiner/noun	*some these one*
interrogative/relative	*which who*
open-class/prep	*past behind*
intensifier/conjunction	*so*
intensifier/adverb	*fairly*
open-class/adverb	*fast last still*
modal/open-class-null	*can might will*
special-verb/open-class	*let make letting made*
single word	*what full-stop comma that to as*

For regularity we have added the null inflection as a separate inflection (though its symbol in English is vacuous it can still be viewed as just another inflection). This gave a huge step in the direction of generalizability. In the WEP, huge amounts of code needed to be repeated. The other non-slashed classes are either copies of other WEP experts or obvious generalizations (e.g. "preposition").

21.2.5 The slashed classes

The WEP's creators do not attempt to explain how one is to deal with words like *saw*. An examination of this word in isolation does not reveal whether it is null-inflected or *ed*-inflected. Thus we have special classes for the few words of this sort (but the majority of words will be handled by the classes above the line).

The one rather common below-the-line-class is "preposition/particle". Most of the prepositions fall into this rather unpleasant category. So, for our parser, the classification of (1a) by the WEP would be (1b) and this is *exactly* as much as needs to be extracted from this sentence: neither more nor less.

(1) a. The man eating peaches throws out a pit.
  b. fullstop the null ing s s particle/preposition a null fullstop

21.3 Constraints and parsing

One way of expressing this problem of trying to parse English using a word-by-word examination of the sentence is that the word in isolation lacks *constraint*. Parsing English, then, could be performed by attempting to increase the constraints on a word until its tag becomes unique (or, viewed another way, reducing the list of possible tags until the list has length 1).

The way to constrain a word, then, is to break the isolation. Again we refer to the WEP, this time Small's thesis:

> . . . instead of organizing the parsing system around rewrite rules, the system focusses on the individual word and on its idiosyncratic interaction with its context. The Word Expert Parser has done precisely that. Each word is represented as an active agent in its own right having the responsibility to fit itself into the overall meaning of the larger discourse structure in which it plays a part. Small (1980: 204)

21.3.1 Constraints from sentence form

We give a simple example to show some sources of constraints and the power of these. This example demonstrates a valid deduction of the syntax tag of the word *walk* in (2). The initial possible tags we will consider for *walk* are "noun", "verb", "adjective", "gerund", "past-participle".

(2) The walk is slippery.

- Constraint source: **inflection analysis**. When inflection analysis is applied, then *walk* cannot be a gerund, nor a past-participle.
- Constraint source: **word to the left: *the***. The word *walk* cannot possibly be a verb because *the* comes immediately before it.
- Constraint source: **word to the right: *is***. If the word to the right, *is*, is also taken into account, then the word cannot be an adjective.

So "noun" is the only possibility left. Longer sentences are correspondingly more difficult but it is not very difficult to diminish the tags quite markedly.

We give the sources of such constraints. We argue that together these constraints are sufficient to constrain the words of a sentence down to just one tag (in other words, to parse the sentence), or in the case of a syntactically ambiguous sentence, to a point where the correct parses can be listed off one by one. These constraints are far stronger than is generally believed and from the starting table given above, the following constraints will perform a complete parse. None of the constraints use probability: they are algebraic only.

21.3.2 Constraints from inflections

Inflections as a source of syntactic information are underrated. We give another example of their strength.

A word inflected with an *-s* may still be a noun, or it may yet be a verb. It cannot, however, be an adjective (a genuine constraint on open-class words). The *-s* inflection does provide a few constraints, which combined can parse a fragment of text. For example, for any fragment of seven *s*-inflected words in a row, there can only be one parse.[1] All seven words are required to force a strong enough constaint on the fragment. The fifth, sixth and seventh words have to be the verb, indirect object and object of a clause, and the first, second, third and fourth words have to be part of an embedded relative clause (object of a prepositional phrase, verb of the embedded clause and its indirect and direct objects respectively).

Sentence (3) is an example of this pattern of inflections. The very specific nature of this claim should be surprising. The inflections in English are not usually believed to have such a strong influence. This claim (i.e. the uniqueness of the parse), which we have yet to demonstrate, is evidence for our argument that the inflections provide a non-trivial source of syntax. That they have *some* significance is obvious, but their power (especially when augmented by other sources of constraint) has not been appreciated fully.

(3) . . . a person who at *times gives dogs bones gives cats bones* . . .

Getting useful constraints from inflections

The inflections do give genuine constraints but it is not really clear at first sight just what these are. The situation clarifies if two words in a row are examined (rather than seven). Table 21.2 gives all the possibilities of two *s*-words in a row, with an example sentence for each. (The validity of the remainder of our argument rests upon the completeness of this list.) The number on the end of the tag indicates the relative-clause level of the tag (0 is for words in the outermost sentence). Only two clause levels are discussed here (we will discuss deeper clause levels later).

1. Items such as commas could not be permitted to appear between the words, of course.

First word	Second word	Example sentence
indirect-object 0	object 0	He gives *students prizes.*
object-of-PP 0	verb 0	A man in evening *clothes stands* waiting.
subject 0	subject 1	The *cats dogs* chase get frightened.
verb 0	object 0	A man *eats chips.*
indirect-object 1	object 1	The man who gives *students prizes* waits.
object-of-PP 1	verb 0	A man who enjoys being in evening *clothes stands* waiting.
object-of-PP 1	verb 1	The man that the boy in *rags despises* is before him.
object 1	verb 0	The charity that gives *gifts sends* a representative.
verb 1	verb 0	A dog that *barks bites.*
verb 1	object 1	A man who *eats chips* will get fat.

Table 21.2 *Two successive s-inflected words.*

We term two words in a row being looked at in this manner a "junction" and for discussion purposes we use the join symbol "$\bowtie$" to designate these junctions. We would symbolize the previous junction as: $s \bowtie s$.

Across any such junction between two words there are certain constraints generated. The exact constraints vary from junction to junction. Each word will actually have a word on either side of it, so for any particular word there will be two sources of constraint. Next we examine a group of three *s*-inflected words together: $s \bowtie s \bowtie s$. In order to see what is constrained with three *s*-inflected words in a row, we join Table 21.2 with itself. By this we mean that we place a copy of the table beside the original and locate all tags shared by the two touching columns as in Figure 21.1.

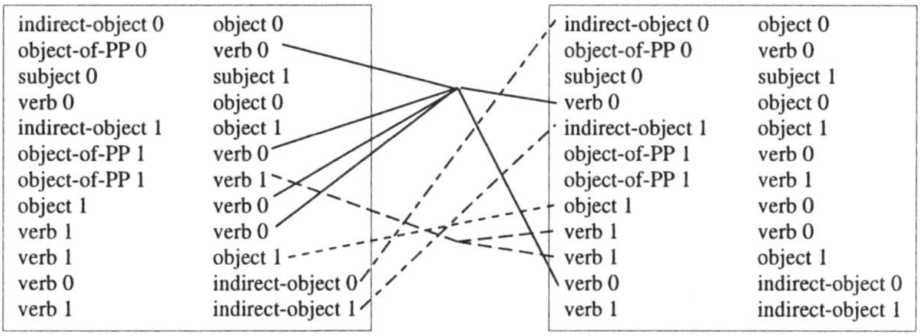

Figure 21.1 *The joining of two lists of constraints.*

The lines in Figure 21.1 indicate the shared tags. If the middle tag has no representative in both the touching columns then there is no connecting line between the tables. An examination of the possible tags available to each group shows that the list is decreasing as some tags did not get a match. For example, four patterns end in "object 0" and two begin with that tag, giving eight possible sequences of three *s*-words when the middle one is "object 0". This process is repeated with more and more *s*-inflected words in a row until, when seven *s*-words are in a row, there is only one parse left.

There are, of course, sets of constraints across all junctions of all of our classes listed above. Together these junction rules heavily constrain the words in an English sentence, frequently to just one tag each (i.e. they parse the sentence). Any two words (open or closed) that form a junction can have constraints put on either side.

We choose not to look further than one word either side of each word because the essential simplicity of the action would be lost. The dilemma is that unbounded dependencies *do* occur: words will at times have to interact with another word far along the sentence (Gazdar et al. 1985). The complexity of constraint parsing without this stricture is enormous (as in the "blackboard" of the WEP wherein the difficulty of working out what is really going on is very hard to calculate).

Our decision to keep this constraint is an important and fundamental decision. The question of a "window size" onto the sentence has, we feel, been rather arbitrarily answered in the past, at times: PARSIFAL (Marcus 1980) has a three-word window, for example, though the context-free grammars do a rather better job.

We show below a method by which *any* power that this stricture loses is fully recaptured.

21.3.3 Expressing tables as usable constraints

We do not store our constraint information in the tabular form given above. For each word we have lists of permitted tags given the words observed on either side. Thus if an *s*-inflected word found a "direct-object 0" to its right, we would consult the "$s \rightarrow$direct-object 0" constraint and constrain the *s*-inflected word accordingly. If Table 21.2 is consulted to calculate this constraint then the word itself can be seen to be constrainted to {verb 0, indirect-object 0}.

If the word-role to the right of the word under examination were not yet known, then only the weaker class-constraints could be applied, namely the $s \rightarrow s$ constraint which is {verb 0, indirect-object 0, object-of-PP 0, verb 1, indirect-object 1, object-of-PP 1, object 1, subject 1}.

Constraints occur on both sides of a word. In the junction $s \bowtie s$ the word on the right of the junction will apply the $s \leftarrow s$ constraint, which is {verb 0, indirect-object 0, object-of-PP 0, subject 0, verb 1, indirect-object 1, object-of-PP 1, object 1}.

21.4 Enhancing the power of the constraints

21.4.1 Case of the noun

If we add noun-case into the determiners, adjectives and nouns then the words both within and just beyond each noun phrase will have heavier constraints on them. If, in a sentence beginning as in (4), *the* is constrained to be a "the(subject)", then *cat* would be constrained to be {adjective(subject), noun(subject)} and then *cat* will put strong constraints on moves. The constraints are as in (5),

(4) "full-stop" The cat moves . . .

(5) ((adjective(subject)0$\leftarrow$*s*) $\cup$ (noun(subject)0$\leftarrow$*s*)) $\cap$ (null 0$\leftarrow$*s*)
= ({subject0} $\cup$ {verb 0, aux 0, linking-verb 0, subject 1})
$\cap$ {verb 0, aux 0, linking-verb 0, subject 0, object-of-PP 0, object 0, object-of-infinitive 0, subject 1}
= {subject 0, verb 0, auxiliary 0, linking-verb 0, subject 1}

whereas if the case of the noun were to be ignored then the constraint would only be as in

(6) (adjective 0$\leftarrow$*s*) $\cup$ (noun 0$\leftarrow$*s*) $\cap$ (null 0$\leftarrow$*s*)
= {verb 0, aux 0, linking-verb 0, subject 0, object-of-PP 0, object 0, object-of-infinitive 0, subject 1}

which is a much weaker constraint. The possibility that *cat* could also be the object of an embedded relative clause (via unbounded dependency) is ignored (see Section 21.5 for a note on "gap" and related matters).

We could be accused of solving a problem of our own making in that we do not permit a word to form junctions with words other than its neighbours. However, via the mechanism outlined, we can permit a *controlled* proliferation of constraints. The predictability of the constraints' actions is kept very high through this mechanism. We will show further mechanisms through which this controlled proliferation of constraints is enhanced (the impact of constraints as outlined so far is still too local).

In a simple sentence, there can only be one subject, one direct object and one verb. This makes an extra list of constraints that can be applied as desired. It can be applied whenever it is deduced that a word can only be the verb. At this point all other words can lose this option. These constraints must only be applied to full sentences and are meaningless on fragments. This action can be extended to include both compound and complex sentences.

21.4.2 Location of nonterminals

In the example of the seven *s*-inflected words, it was deduced that the first word was forced to be the object of a prepositional phrase. This means that the end of that prepositional phrase has been located. It is an achievement to be able to state unequivocally where a prepositional phrase ends (or to locate *any* nonterminal stably). Church & Hanks (1989) make a similar observation.

The ends of these nonterminal structures are often quite featureless, as in the example of seven *s*-inflected words above where the clause border is between the fourth and the fifth *s*-inflected words in a group of open-class words. The laws of English actually force these borders via the lists of constraints (in a totally non-obvious way: the combination of the constraints together forces this).

The vanishing nonterminals

When a prepositional phrase is located, then an extra junction is formed past it because the parse of the sentence has to remain the same both with and without the phrase (semantics may vary). When the phrase is joined over, the words on either side of it now form a junction and thus they can now create extra constraints with each other: a necessary action. This (eventually) allows words from far across the sentence to interact together in a tightly controlled manner. This action relates to constituent location in existing parsing systems such as GPSG. The location of such nonterminals is usually seen as the first step in parsing natural language. In the case of this constraint approach, it can never be done first, but the attempt to form such links is repeatedly tried throughout the whole constraint propagation process and the links appear and disappear as the word-roles change within the sentence, reflecting the changing state of the words at different points of the constraint calculations. The various branches of the constraint-tree of possible solutions have the links in different places.

If, for example, during the calculation of the parse of (7), the word *platform* is momentarily set to be the object of a prepositional phrase (for testing that possibility), then a link would immediately form between *child* and *sits*. If, however, the word *sits* is deduced to be the object of a prepositional phrase, then the link would appear between *child* and "fullstop" (which would cause a contradiction because the subject of a sentence would find a fullstop to its right so that that branch of the calculation would die out).

(7) The child on the platform sits "fullstop"

Adjectives, embedded clauses and nouns in apposition are also joined over, all with the aim of eventually getting the major verb of the simple sentence to form a junction with the subject of the sentence so that they constrain each other further. (Also, the article meets its head, the verb meets its object, etc.) The sentence gradually reduces until the bare framework of SVO (or whatever happens to be the underlying structure) is connected up. At this point the sentence is essentially parsed.

It is not always the case that a prepositional phrase should be joined over. If there is any doubt that the whole prepositional phrase has been located then it must stay. As always, the change has to be *proved* to be acceptable before it is allowed to happen. Any number of additional criteria can be added to ensure validity.

This demonstrates the versatility of the parsing actions of the vanishing nonterminals. Only when a nonterminal has been *unequivocally* located in its entirety is it correct to join over it. There is no necessity to join over any particular vanishing nonterminal at any particular time (not doing so only slows the parse). In (7), for example, once the relative clause has been located and joined, the stricture is off the prepositional phrase and it too can now be removed.

This joining action has a theoretical base in Deane's (1992) book *Grammar in mind and brain.* Its use there is initially to provide a more complete explanation for unbounded dependencies than the various existing theories of Kuno (1987), Erteshik-Sschir & Lappin (1979) and Takami (1989). We also extend its use here to include such phenomena. Further, the same linking structure can be implemented to handle that partial repetition of sentence that can be seen around the co-ordinating conjunctions: a very complete synthesis of Deane's approach to this one will be the subject of a forthcoming paper.

21.4.3 Combining sources of constraints

All the separate sources of constraint must be applied in turn or as needed to each major clause. They can be mixed freely: a very important observation. So if an optional constituent appears, then a junction is formed between the two words beyond the ends of the phrase and further constraints will now be generated.

If it is seen as desirable to apply any other source of constraint, then it, too, can be used to hasten (and even remove ambiguity from) the parse.

We have not specifically included semantics constraints as we find that the nature of these varies from application to application. Also, they flow over from sentence to sentence whereas each sentence is parsed as a stand-alone syntactic entity in this paper. Semantics constraints are classified as "informal constraints" for the purposes of this parser.

21.5 Implementation and performance

All aspects of the algorithm described above have been implemented in a computer program in Scheme. The constraint satisfaction is performed exactly by Waltz's (1975) local constraint propagation algorithm.

We have 600 test sentences all of which successfully parse, and we also use a few paragraphs from *War and peace* in order to test the work more fully. The parser currently reports accurately on its 600 test sentences. Furthermore, it accurately parses 12 contiguous lines of *War and peace*, the longest sentence being 75 words. It also parses the abstract of the original version of this paper (Entwisle & Groves 1994) correctly, neither reporting on extra parses nor removing the expected parse.

The conjunctions, and in particular *and*, have been carefully investigated and joined successfully into this parsing approach: a weakening of the rules is one aspect of this extension. The particle–preposition ambiguity resolution has also been investigated and worked out fully. The difficulties that the various different subcategories of verb and the corresponding "gap" phenomena are also handled. The handling of these three added features are the subject of a further paper.

This approach to parsing is, we argue, less arbitrary or *ad hoc* then many PSG-based approaches and should be extendible to other languages without difficulty, though, of course, an entirely new matrix will have to be derived, and so on. The location of closed-class words in a language, for example, is a fairly straightforward task and can be done by statistical and/or information-theoretic means (see Powers 1991 for an explanation of this process).

21.6 Conclusions

The observable phenomena of the English sentence are a useful starting point for the syntactic parsing of English. The power of the stable and straightforward argument that these offer should not be underrated. It can be applied repetitively in co-ordination with other natural language modules to refine further and further the interpretation of the sentence. In this fashion it bridges the gap between raw text and the PSGs and other grammars.

References

Church, K. W. & P. Hanks 1989. Word association norms, mutual information, and lexicography. In *Proceedings of the 27th Annual Conference of the Association of Computational Linguistics*, Vancouver, 76–83.

Deane, P. 1992. *Grammar in mind and brain.* Berlin: Mouton de Gruyter.

Entwisle, J. & M. Groves 1994. A method of parsing English based on sentence form. In *International Conference on New Methods in Language Processing (NeMLaP)*, Manchester, 116–22.

Erteshik-Sschir, N. & S. Lappin 1979. Dominance and the functional explanation of island phenomena. *Theoretical Linguistics* **6**, 41–86.

Gazdar, G., E. Klein, G. K. Pullum & I. A. Sag 1985. *Generalized Phrase Structure Grammar.* Oxford: Basil Blackwell.

Kuno, S. 1987. *Functional syntax.* Cambridge, Mass.: Harvard University Press.

Marcus, M. 1980. *A theory of syntactic recognition for natural language.* Cambridge, Mass.: MIT Press.

Morrill, G., N. Leslie, M. Hepple & G. Barry 1990. *Categorical deductions and structural operations.* Edinburgh Working Papers in Cognitive Science 5, Edinburgh University.

Powers, D. 1991. On the significances of closed classes and boundary conditions: experiments in lexical and syntactic learning. In *Proceedings of the Workshop on Natural Language Learning, IJCAI '91*, Sydney, 63–70.

Small, S. 1980. *Word expert parsing: a theory of distributed word-based natural language parsing*. PhD Thesis, Department of Computer Science, University of Maryland.

Takami, K-I. 1989. Preposition stranding: arguments against syntactic analyses and an alternative functional explanation. *Lingua* **76**, 299–335.

Waltz, D. 1975. Understanding line drawings of scenes with shadows. In *The psychology of computer vision*, P. H. Winston (ed.), 19–91. New York: McGraw-Hill.

Winston, P. 1992. *Artificial Intelligence*, 3rd edn., Reading, Mass.: Addison-Wesley.

22
A new approach to "center" tracking

RUSLAN MITKOV

22.1 The need for center determination in anaphora resolution

The notion of "center"[1] plays a crucial part in anaphora resolution. A decisive hypothesis used in the process of anaphora resolution is that the center (or alternatively "focus") of the sentence or clause is the prime candidate for pronominal reference.[2]

The syntactic and semantic criteria are not always sufficient to discriminate among a set of possible candidates for an antecedent. They should serve more as filters to eliminate unsuitable candidates than as proposers of the most likely candidates. In the case of antecedent ambiguity it is the center of a sentence (clause) that most frequently plays the decisive role.

As an illustration, consider the text (1).

1. The original use of this term (Grosz et al. 1983), and most of the subsequent related work has been in American English. We therefore retain the US spelling here, as most British work uses the term "focus".

2. The author expresses his gratitude to the Alexander von Humboldt Foundation for the financial support during his stay at IAI Saarbrücken as a Humboldt Fellow.

(1) Where previously the dataset to be transmitted was determined by the size, now the determining factor becomes the storage capacity of the network path, the so-called congestion window. It is expected always to be of smaller size.

The syntactic and semantic constraints are not sufficient to eliminate the ambiguity between *the determining factor*, *the storage capacity of the network path*, *the storage capacity*, *the network path* and *congestion window* as antecedents of the pronoun *It* in the last sentence. If discourse knowledge was applied, however, following one of the heuristics listed below, stating that a noun phrase (NP) after *so-called* tends to be the center of the subsequent discourse segment, the correct antecedent, *congestion window* would be easily distinguished. This example demonstrates that discourse knowledge, which also includes "know-how" to determine the center, is an integral part of any anaphora resolution system.

Certain ideas and algorithms for tracking the focus (Sidner 1983) or center (Brennan et al. 1987) have been proposed, although they require that one knows the focus or center of the first sentence in the segment. However, they do not try to identify this center. Our approach here determines the most probable center of the first sentence, and then tracks it all the way through the segment, correcting the proposed antecedent at each step.

Our new approach to determining the center of a discourse segment is part of a more extensive work on anaphora resolution described in Mitkov (1993, 1994) which concentrates on pronominal anaphora resolution in the sublanguage of computer science.

22.2 Empirical evidence

The present study considers a large computer-science corpus and the empirical observations allowed the development of efficient sublanguage-dependent heuristics (preferences) for center tracking in the sublanguage of computer science. The corpus contained 60 different documents in computer science and was hand-annotated. The independent opinions of five human experts provided estimations for the "true" centers. In the event of differing opinions, we considered the "true center" to be the NP with the majority of "votes". We summarize the most important conclusions as follows:

1. Consider the primary candidates for center from the priority list:subject, object, verb phrase.
2. Prefer the NP, representing a domain concept to the NPs, which are not domain concepts.
3. If the verb is a member of the "verbset" {*discuss*, *present*, *illustrate*, *summarize*, *examine*, *describe*, *define*, *show*, *check*, *develop*, *review*, *report*,

outline, *consider*, *investigate*, *explore*, *assess*, *analyse*, *synthesize*, *study*, *survey*, *deal*, *cover*}, then consider the object as a most probable center.

4. If a verbal adjective is a member of the "adjset" {*defined*, *called*, *so-called*}, then consider the NP it refers to as the probable center of the subsequent discourse segment.
5. If the subject is *chapter*, *section*, *table*, or a personal pronoun, *I*, *we*, *you*, then consider the object as the most likely center.
6. If an NP is repeated throughout the discourse section, then consider it as the most probable center.
7. If an NP occurs in the head of the section, part of which is the current discourse segment, then consider it as the probable center.
8. If an NP is topicalized, then consider it as a probable center.
9. Prefer definite NPs to indefinite ones.
10. Prefer the NPs in the main clause to NPs in the subordinate clauses.
11. Prefer an NP that is not a part of a PP to an NP that is part of a PP.

As far as rule 1 is concerned, the subject was found to be a primary candidate for center (in about 73% of the cases). The second most likely center would be the object (25%) and the third most likely one the verb phrase as a whole (2%).

There are certain "symptoms" that determine the subject or the object as a center with very high probability. Cases in point are 3 and 5. Other cases are not so certain, but are to some extent quite likely. For example, if a non-concept NP is in subject position and if a repeated concept NP, which is also in a head, is in object position, it is almost certain that the latter is the unambiguous center. Moreover, certain preferences or "considerations" are stronger than others. For example, an NP in subject position is preferred over an NP that is in a section head but not in subject position.

The empirical results (with approximating probability measures) and AI statistics-based techniques were used to develop a "proposer" module (within our anaphora resolution system) that identifies the most likely center. We must remember that even if we do not need one for immediate antecedent disambiguation, a center must still be proposed for each sentence, or else we will have to go all the way back to track it from the beginning of the segment when one is needed later on.

The rules stated above should be ordered according to their priority: this is a problem that is being currently investigated.

22.3 A new approach to calculating the probability that a noun (verb) phrase is the center

Based on the results described in the previous section, we propose a new approach to determining the probability that a noun (verb) phrase is the center of a sentence. Note that this approach allows us to calculate this probability in every discourse sentence, including the first one, and to propose the most probable center. This approach, combined with the algorithm for tracking the center (in Brennan et al. 1987), is expected to yield improved results.

Our model integrates an algorithm for calculating the probability of a noun (verb) phrase to be in the center of a discourse segment. The algorithm uses an inference engine based on Bayes's theorem (2),

$$\text{(2)}\ \mathrm{P}(H_k|A) = \frac{\mathrm{P}(H_k)\mathrm{P}(A|H_k)}{\sum \mathrm{P}(H_i)\mathrm{P}(A|H_i)}$$

for $k = 1, 2, \ldots$

Under the conditions of our model, Bayes's theorem allows the following interpretation. There are only two possible hypotheses for a certain noun (verb) phrase: that it is the center of the discourse sentence (clause) or that it is not. Let H_y be the positive hypothesis, H_n the negative hypothesis. If we call the presence of some of the pieces of evidence described in the previous section a "symptom", then A would signify the occurrence of that symptom with the examined phrase. $\mathrm{P}(A|H_y)$ would be the *a priori* probability of the symptom A being observed with a noun (verb) phrase that is the center (we will henceforth refer to this factor as P_Y). By analogy $\mathrm{P}(A|H_n)$ is the probability of the symptom being observed with a phrase that is not the center (henceforth referred to as P_N). The *a posteriori* probability $\mathrm{P}(H_k|A)$ is defined in the light of the new piece of evidence: the presence of an empirically obtained symptom, indicating the higher probability that the examined phrase is in the center of the discourse segment.

In other words, the inference engine based on Bayes's theorem draws an inference in the light of some new piece of evidence. This formula calculates the new probability, given the old probability plus some new piece of evidence.

Consider the following situation. According to our investigation so far, the probability of the subject being a center is 76%. Additional evidence (symptom), e.g. if the subject represents a domain concept, will increase the initial probability. If this NP is also the head of the section, the probability is increased further. If the NP occurs more than once in the discourse segment, the probability gets even higher.

An estimation of the probability that a subject, (direct or indirect) object or verb phrase (the only possible centers in our texts) is center, can be represented as a predicate with arguments: as in (3),

$$\text{(3) center}(X, \mathrm{P}_I, [s_1(wf_{1_1}, wf_{2_1}), \ldots, s_K(wf_{1_K}, wf_{2_K})])$$

where center(X, P_I, *list*) represents the estimated probability that X is the center of a sentence (clause), $X \in \{$subject, object_1, object_2, ... , verb phrase$\}$, P_I is the initial probability that X is the center of the sentence (clause), s is a symptom, and wf is a weight factor. Weight factor wf_1 is the probability of the symptom being observed with a noun (verb) phrase that is the center (we will henceforth refer to this factor as P_Y). Weight factor wf_2 is the probability of the symptom being observed with a noun (verb) phrase that is not the center (henceforth referred to as P_N).

Using our preliminary empirical results, we can write (4) and (5) for example in Prolog notation:

```
(4) center(object,25,[symptom(verbset,40,3),
      symptom(subjectset,40,2), symptom(domain_concept,95,80),
      symptom(repeated,10,5), symptom(headline,10,9),
      symptom(topicalized, 6,2), symptom(main_clause,85,30),
      symptom(definite_form,90,70)]).

(5) center(subject,73, [symptom (domain_concept,95,70),
      symptom(repeated,10,4), symptom(headline,10,8),
      symptom(topicalized,10,3), symptom(main_clause,85,30),
      symptom(definite_form,85,20)]).
```

The fact in (4) means that the object is the center in approximately 25% of the cases. In 40% of the cases where the center is the object the verb belongs to the set of verbs {*discuss*, *illustrate*, *summarize*, *examine*, *describe*, *define*, . . . } and it is possible with 3% probability for the verb to be a member of this set while the center of the sentence is not the object, and so on. The facts in (4) and (5) are part of a sublanguage knowledge base.

The process of estimating the probability of a given phrase being the center of a sentence (clause) is repetitive, beginning with an initial estimate and gradually working towards a more accurate answer. More systematically, the "diagnostic" process is as follows:

1. Start with the initial probability.
2. Consider the symptoms one at a time.
3. For each symptom, update the current probability, taking into account
   (a) whether the sentence has the symptom, and
   (b) the weight factors P_Y and P_N.

The probability that an NP is the center is calculated by the inference engine (using Bayes's theorem) which can be represented as a Prolog program as in (6).

```
(6) probability(center,Probability) :-
      center(center,P_current,Symptom_list),
      new_probability(P_current,Symptom_list,Probability).
    new_probability (P,[],P).
    new_probability (P_current,[Symptom|Tail],P_new) :-
      update(P_current,Symptom,P_updated),
      new_probability(P_updated,Tail,P_new).
    update(P_current,symptom(Symptom_name,Py,Pn),P_new) :-
      observed(Symptom_name),bayes(P_current,Py,Pn,P_new).
    update(P_current,symptom(Symptom_name,Py,Pn),P_new) :-
      not(observed(Symptom_name)), P1 is 100 - Py,
      p2 is 100 - Pn, bayes(P_current,Py,Pn,P_new).
    bayes(P,Py,Pn,Pdash) :- Top is 100 * Py * P,
      Bottom is (Py * P) + (Pn * (100 - P)), Pdash is Top/Bottom.
```

The inference engine operates on the basis of the sublanguage knowledge base and on the "local" knowledge base. The latter gives information on the current discourse segment. Initially, our program works with manual inputs. The local knowledge base has been represented as Prolog facts as in (7).

(7)
```
observed (headline).
observed (domain_concept).
observed (repeated).
% etc.
```

The inference engine's task is to match the expected symptoms of the possible syntactic function as center in the knowledge base of the sentence's actual symptoms, and produce a list of (reasonably) possible candidates.

The approach to center tracking presented here has been implemented as a program in the discourse module of an integrated architecture for anaphora resolution (Mitkov 1994) and preliminary experiments show that the decisions of the program on discourse segment centers coincide in almost 95% of the cases with the opinion of a human reader. As an evaluation corpus five tagged medium-length files were used taken from computer-science books. However, it should be pointed out that this figure should be regarded as approximate: because of the intuitive nature of the notion of center, human readers may differ in opinion as to which NP is to be made use of as the "true" center for comparison.

References

Brennan, S. E., M. W. Friedman & C. J. Pollard 1987. A centering approach to pronouns. In *Proceedings of the 25th Annual Meeting of the Association for Computational Linguistics*, Stanford, Calif., 155–62.

Grosz, B. J., A. Joshi & S. Weinstein 1983. Providing a unified account of definite noun phrases in discourse. In *Proceedings of the 21st Annual Meeting of the Association for Computational Linguistics*, Cambridge, Mass., 44–50.

Mitkov, R. 1993. *Anaphora resolution in natural language processing*. Internal Report, Universiti Sains Malaysia, Penang.

Mitkov, R. 1994. An integrated model for anaphora resolution. In *COLING 94: The 15th International Conference on Computational Linguistics*, Kyoto, Japan, 1170–6.

Sidner, C. 1983. Focusing in the comprehension of definite anaphora. In *Computational models of discourse*, M. Brady & R. Berwick (eds), 267–330. Cambridge, Mass.: MIT Press.

23 Structuring raw discourse

TADASHI NOMOTO AND YOSHIHIKO NITTA

23.1 Introduction

This paper describes a model for discovering coherent texts from unconstrained textual data.[1] The model is both linguistically and statistically motivated. It derives a linguistic motivation from the view that discourse consists of textual units called "discourse segments" (Nomoto & Nitta 1993), while, statistically, we are guided by ideas from the information retrieval literature (Salton 1988). As has been the case with research on information retrieval, previous quantitative approaches to text segmentation (Hearst 1993; Kozima 1993; Youmans 1991) have paid little attention to the linguistic structure of discourse and defined it away as a bag of words or sentences.[2] Part of our concern here is with explicating possible effects of a discourse segment on the quantitative structuring of discourse.

In what follows, we will describe some important features of discourse segments and see how they can be incorporated into a statistical analysis of discourse. Also, some comparison is made with other approaches such as Youmans (1991), followed by discussion of the results of the present method.

1. An unconstrained text here is meant to be a corpus with no grammatical or SGML-like annotations.
2. Lewis (1992) is an interesting exception.

23.2 Discourse segments

The theory of discourse segments is a theory of how written text is organized in Japanese (Nomoto & Nitta 1993). It claims that Japanese discourse is constructed from linguistic units called "discourse segments", which are two-part structures consisting of topic and comment. The topic corresponds to the subject matter and the comment to a discussion about it. It is also a fact that Japanese has a special way of marking the topic: by suffixing it with a postpositional particle *wa*. The comment part could become quite long, extending over quite a few sentences (Mikami 1960).[3] Furthermore, Japanese, although a free-word-order language, prefers the topic to precede the comment: thus normally topic and comment appear in that order. For the semantics of a discourse segment, Nomoto & Nitta (1993) observe an interesting tendency that cases of zero (elliptical) anaphora occurring within the segment do not refer across the segment boundary; that is, their references tend to be resolved internally.[4]

Now let us take a very simple view of how discourse is structured: syntactically, discourse is just a chronological juxtaposition of contiguous, disjoint blocks of sentences, each of which corresponds to a discourse segment, while, semantically, discourse is a set of anaphoric islands set side by side.[5] Furthermore, we do not intend the discourse structure to be anything close to what rhetorical theories of discourse (Grosz & Sidner 1986; Hobbs 1979; Hovy 1993; Mann & Thompson 1988) claim it to be; indeed we do not assume any functional relation, i.e. causation, elaboration, extension, etc., between the segments that constitute a discourse structure. The present theory is not so much about the rhetoric or the function of discourse as about the way anaphora is interpreted.

23.3 A quantitative structuring of discourse

23.3.1 The model

Let us suppose that a discourse looks something like Figure 23.1, where a discourse is made up of discourse segments G_i, which are in turn made up of terms $T_{i,j}$.

---

3. Japanese provides for a variety of ways to mark off a topic–comment structure; the *wa*-marking is one such, and a typographical device such as a line- or a page-break is another. For the present discussion, we take a discourse segment to be a block of sentences bounded by a text break and/or a *wa*-marked element.

4. For example:

   Tarō$_i$*-wa* 01_i *rojin*$_j$*-ni seki-wo yuzutte ageta node,* 01_i 02_j *orei-wo iwareta.*

   TARO-top OLD-MAN-dat SEAT-acc GIVE HELPED BECAUSE, THANK-acc SAY CAUSED

   'Because Taro did the old man the favour of giving him his seat, he thanked him.'

Here, 01 represents a subject (nominative) ellipsis, 02 an object (accusative) ellipsis. Note that all the instances of 01 and 02 have internal antecedents: *Taro* and *rojin*.

5. It is quite possible that a set of discourse segments is not aggregated into a single discourse but may have diverse discourse groupings (Nomoto & Nitta 1993). This happens when discourses are interleaved or embedded into each other. An interleaving or an embedding of discourse is often invoked by changes in the narrative mode such as direct or indirect speech, quoting, or interruption, which will cue the reader/hearer to suspend the current discourse flow, start another, or resume the interrupted discourse.

$$
\begin{array}{lllllll}
G_1 & T_{1,1} & T_{1,2} & T_{1,3} & T_{1,4} & \dots & T_{1,H} \\
G_2 & T_{2,1} & T_{2,2} & T_{2,3} & T_{2,4} & \dots & T_{2,K} \\
G_3 & T_{3,1} & T_{3,2} & T_{3,3} & T_{3,4} & \dots & T_{3,L} \\
G_4 & T_{4,1} & T_{4,2} & T_{4,3} & T_{4,4} & \dots & T_{4,M} \\
G_5 & T_{5,1} & T_{5,2} & T_{5,3} & T_{5,4} & \dots & T_{5,N} \\
\vdots & \dots & & & & &
\end{array}
$$

Figure 23.1 *Discourse structure.*

A discourse segment could then be represented as a "term vector" of the form (1),

$$(1)\quad G_i = (w(T_{i,1}), w(T_{i,2}), w(T_{i,3}), \dots, w(T_{i,t}))$$

where t represents a nominal occurrence in G_i and $w(t,i)$ the importance value, or weight of t_i.

In information retrieval terms, what happens here is that a discourse segment G_i is "indexed" with a set of terms $t_{i,1}$ to $t_{i,t}$; that is, we characterize G_i with a set of indices $t_{i,1}, \dots, t_{i,t}$. A term vector can either be "binary", where each term in the vector is 0 or 1, i.e. absence or presence, or is "weighted", where a term is assigned a certain importance value. In general, weighted indexing is preferable to binary indexing, as the latter is known to have problems with precision (Salton 1988).[6] The weighting policy that we will adopt is known as *tf•idf*. It is an indicator of the term's importance defined by (2),

$$(2)\quad w(T_{i,j}) = tf(T_{i,j}) \times idf(T_{i,j})$$

where *tf* (term frequency) is the number of occurrences of a term T_j in a document D_i; *df* (document frequency) is the number of documents in a collection of N documents in which T_j occurs; and the importance $w(T_{i,j})$ is given as the product of *tf* and the inverse of the *df* factor (*idf*), $\log N/df_j$. Note that

$$(3)\quad \log \frac{N}{df_j} = -\log \frac{df_j}{N}$$

and thus the *idf* is thought of as the self-information for the event that the term T_j is assigned to a randomly selected document D_i.

With the *tf•idf* policy, high-frequency terms that are scattered evenly over the entire document collection are considered to be less important than those that are frequent but whose occurrences are concentrated in particular documents.[7] Thus the

6. Precision measures the proportion of correct items retrieved against the total number of retrieved items. Problematically, binary indexing leads to too much retrieval.

7. Precision depends on the size of document collection: as the collection gets smaller in size, index terms become less extensive and more discriminatory. The *idf* factor could be dispensed with in such cases.

tf•idf indexing favours rare words, which distinguish the documents more effectively than common words.

With the indexing method in place, it is straightforward to define the coherence between two discourse segments. For discourse segments $X = x_1, x_2, \ldots, x_n$ and $Y = y_1, y_2, \ldots, y_m$, $n \leq m$, let the coherence be defined by (4),

$$(4)\ COH(X,Y) = \frac{2\sum_{i=1}^{m} w(x_i)w(y_i)}{\sum_{i=1}^{m} w(x_i)^2 + \sum_{i=1}^{m} w(y_i)^2}$$

where $w(x_i)$ represents a *tf•idf* weight assigned to the term $x_i \in X$, and similarly for $w(y_i)$. For any $n < k \leq m$, $w(x_k) = 0$. The measure is known as the "Dice coefficient".[8]

23.3.2 Experiments

In contrast to previous "bag-of-words" approaches to text partitioning (Youmans 1991; Hearst 1993; Kozima 1993), which work on an arbitrary block of words or sentences, we work on a block of discourse segments to determine the structure of discourse.

Let us now treat a discourse segment as a document unit by itself and then define the term frequency (*tf*), the document frequency (*df*), and the size of document collection (*N*) as usual. Coherence between a pair of segments will then be determined according to how many words the pair have in common and the weights the words carry. This means that one pair of segments will become more cohesive than another if the pair share more of the terms that are locally frequent.

The partitioning works as follows:

1. We collect all the nominal occurrences in a corpus,[9] and divide the collection into disjoint discourse segments.
2. We compare all pairs of adjacent blocks of discourse segments.
3. We assign a coherence/similarity value to each pair.
4. Finally, we examine the coherence curve for "hills" and "valleys" and partition it manually.

Valleys (i.e. low coherence values) are likely to signal a potential break in a discourse flow, whereas hills (i.e. high coherence values) would signal local coherency. Figure 23.2 shows how a coherence curve might appear.

8. Other measures standardly available in information retrieval include "inner product", "cosine coefficient" and "Jaccard coefficient". Our experiences with them suggest, however, that the choice of any particular measurement would not lead to a major difference in results.

9. This is done by JUMAN, a Japanese morphological analyser (available free from various `ftp` sites).

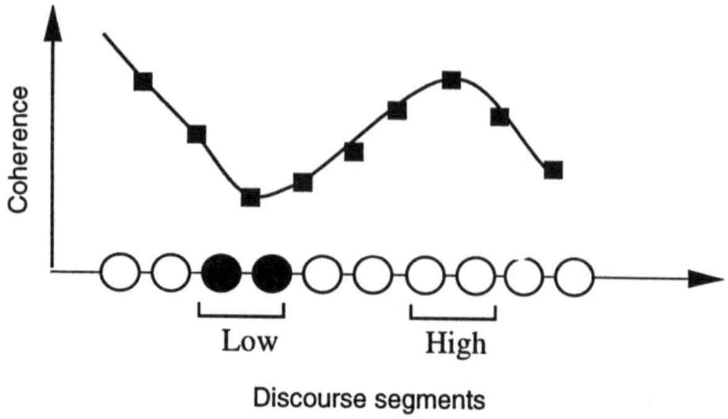

Figure 23.2 *A coherence curve.*

Coherence is measured at every segment break with a paired comparison window moving over segments. Or, more precisely, given a segment d_j and a block size n, what we do is compare a block spanning d_{j-n+1} to d_j and one spanning d_{j+1} to d_{j+n-1} (Fig. 23.3). The measurement is plotted at the jth position on the x-axis.

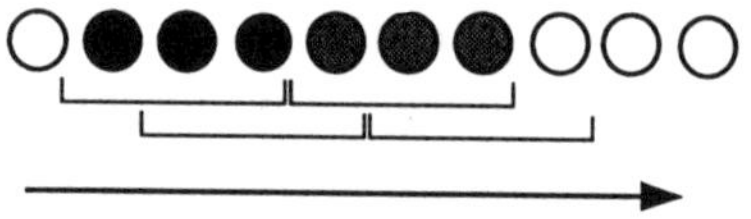

Figure 23.3 *A moving window pair.*

If either of the comparison windows is underfilled, then no measurement will be made. The graph that the procedure gives out is smoothed (with an appropriate width) to bring out its global trends. The length of a single segment, i.e. noun counts, varies from text to text, genre to genre, ranging from a few words (in a junior high-school science book) to somewhere around 60 words (in a newspaper editorial).

We performed experiments on a four-week collection of editorials from *Nihon Keizai Shinbun* (*Nikkei*, a Japanese financial newspaper) which contained a total of 1111 sentences with some 10 000 nouns, and 556 discourse segments. The corpus was divided into disjoint blocks of segments semi-automatically, and coherence was measured between pairs of adjacent blocks.[10] Coherence was measured for each adjacent pair of segments, using the Dice coefficient. It was found that a block size of 10 segments yields good results. Figure 23.4 shows a coherence graph covering about a week's worth of corpus material. The graph is smoothed with a width of 5. We see that article boundaries (vertical lines) coincide fairly well with major minima on the graph, with only one miss at 65, which falls on a paragraph boundary.

10. There is a problem in that some uses of the *wa* particle do not have the function of topic indicator and thus do not count as a boundary marker. These uses were removed from the corpus manually.

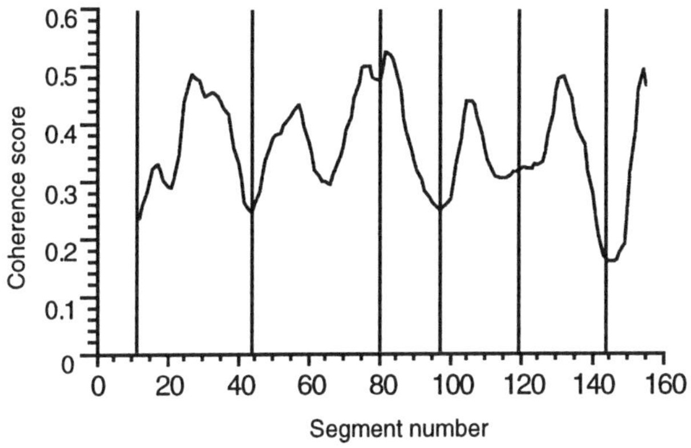

Figure 23.4 *A Dice analysis.*

Experiments with various block sizes suggest that the choice of block size relates in some way to the structure of discourse: an increasing block size would extract a more global or general structure of discourse.

Youmans (1991) has suggested an information measurement based on word frequency. It is intended to measure the ebb and flow of "new information" in discourse. The idea is simply to count the number of new words introduced over a moving interval and produce what he calls a "vocabulary management profile" (VMP), or measurements at intervals. Now, given a discourse $D = \{w_1, \ldots, w_n\}$, the *k*th interval of size Δ is defined by (5),

$$(5)\ I_k = \{w_k, \ldots, w_r\}$$

where

$$(6)\ r = \begin{cases} k + \Delta - 1 & \text{if } k \leq n - \Delta \\ n & \text{otherwise} \end{cases}$$

Measurements are made at intervals I_1 to I_{n-1}. What we want to see is how the scheme compares with ours. Figure 23.5 shows the results of a VMP analysis for the same nominal collection as above. The interval is set to 300 words, or the average length of a paired window in the previous analysis. The *y*-axis corresponds to the number of new words (types) and the *x*-axis to an interval position (tokens).

As it turns out, the VMP fails to detect any significant pattern in the corpus. One of the problems with the analysis has to do with its generality (Kozima 1993): a text with many repetitions or a limited vocabulary would yield a flattened VMP, which, of course, does not tell us much about its inner structure. We suspect that the VMP scheme fares better with short-term coherence than with long-term or global coherence.

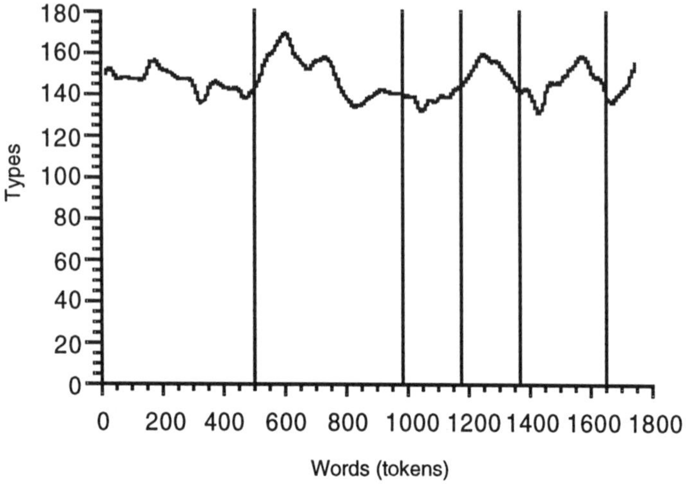

Figure 23.5 *A VMP analysis.*

23.3.3 Discussion

Figure 23.6 demonstrates the results of the Dice analysis on the *Nikkei* collection of editorial articles. What we see here is a close correspondence between the Dice curve and the global discourse structure. Evaluation here simply consists of finding major minima on the graph and locating them on the list of those discourse segments that comprise the corpus. The procedure is performed by hand.

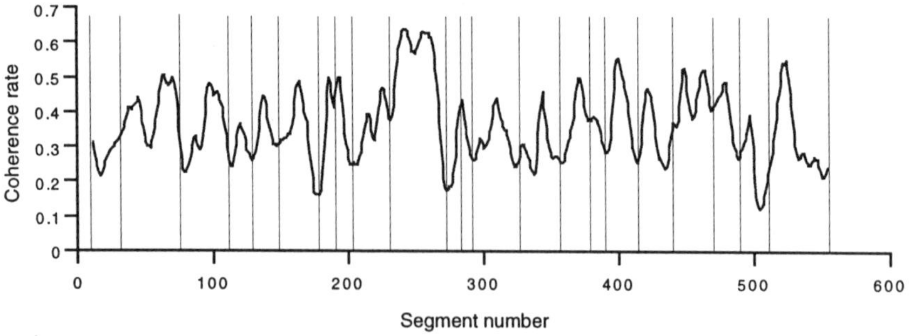

Figure 23.6 *The Dice analysis on the* Nikkei *corpus.*

Evaluation of correspondences has been problematical, since it requires human judgements on how discourse is structured, the reliability of which is yet to be demonstrated. It was decided here to use copious boundary indicators such as an article or a paragraph break for evaluating matches between the Dice analysis and the discourse. For us, discourse structure reduces to just an orthographic structure.[11]

In Figure 23.6, article boundaries are marked by dashes. Seven out of 27 local minima are found to be incorrect, which puts the error rate at around 25%. We obtained similar results for the Jaccard and cosine coefficients. A possible improvement would include adjusting the document frequency (*df*) factor for index terms; the average *df* factor we had for the *Nikkei* corpus was around 1.6, which is so low as to be negligible.[12] Another line to pursue would be to use an alternative weighting policy, for instance, the "weighted inverse document frequency" (Tokunaga & Iwayama 1994). The *widf* value of a term is its frequency within the document divided by its frequency throughout the entire document collection. Although the *widf* policy is reported to have a marked advantage over the *idf* for the text categorization task, the method fails to work for the text segmentation task (Fig. 23.7). The choice of weighting policy can have a crucial effect on the success of text segmentation.

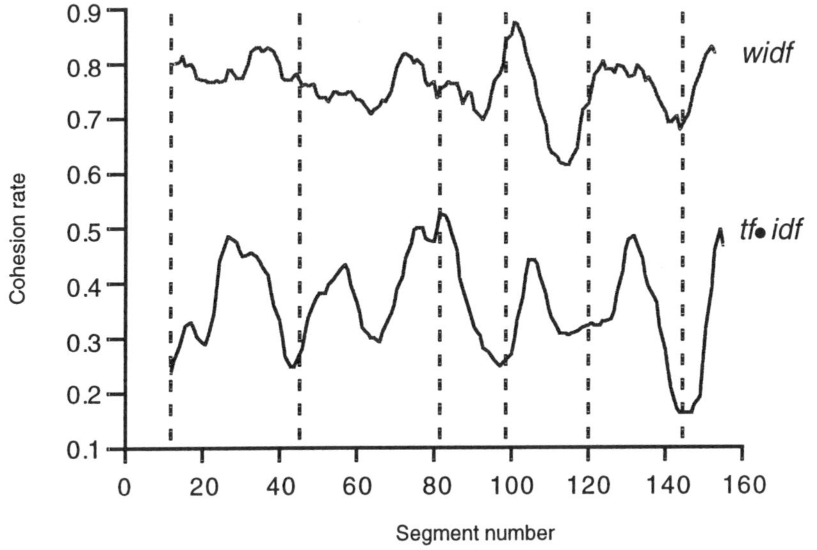

Figure 23.7 Widf *versus* tf•idf.

23.3.4 Recall and precision

As with the document analysis, the effectiveness of text segmentation appears to be dictated by recall–precision parameters where "recall" is the number of

11. However, there is some evidence that an orthographic structure is *linguistically* significant (Fujisawa et al. 1993; Nunberg 1990).

12. However, the average *df* factor would increase in proportion to the growth of corpus size. It is likely, therefore, that with a larger corpus we might get better results.

correct boundaries retrieved divided by the total number of correct boundaries, and "precision" is the number of correct boundaries retrieved divided by the total number of boundaries retrieved. A "boundary" here is meant to be a minimum on the coherence graph. Precision is greatly affected by the size of block or interval:[13] a large-block segmentation yields less boundaries than a small-block segmentation. Experiments were carried out with the *Nikkei* corpus to examine the effects of the block size parameter on text segmentation. The corpus was divided into equally sized blocks, ranging from 5 to 35 words in length. The window size was kept to ten blocks. The results are shown in Table 23.1.

Table 23.1 Block size (in words) and number of boundaries retrieved.

Block size	5	10	15	20	25	30	35
Boundaries	52	25	24	20	21	19	12

Shown in Figure 23.8 are the results given in terms of recall and precision. Also, a partitioning task with discourse segments, whose length varies widely, is measured for recall and precision, and the result is represented as *G*.

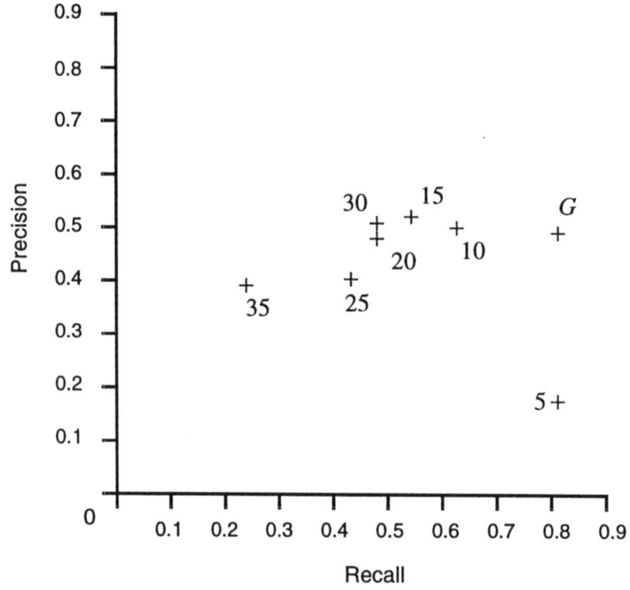

Figure 23.8 *Recall and precision.*

Averaging recall and precision values for each size gives an ordering as in (7).

(7) $35 < 25 < 20 < 5 < 30 < 15 < 10 < G$

13. "Block" here is intended to mean the minimal textual unit into which a discourse is divided and for which coherence is measured.

Highest ranked is *G*, and its average value, 0.66, is higher than any other. Second comes 10 (0.61).[14] (It is an interesting coincidence that the average length of discourse segments is 13.7 words.) One curious point about the result is that low recall does not mean high precision. Note that neither precision nor recall is high for the interval of 35 words.

23.4 Conclusion

In this paper, we have described a model for partitioning an unconstrained corpus into coherent textual units. We started out with the linguistic assumption that discourse is built up of disjoint units called "discourse segments" and tried to show how the notion is significant for the task of partitioning using a statistical measure. Results are evaluated based on how much coincidence there is between segmentations and actual boundaries, making possible an objective comparison of various segmentation models. Among problems that remain for future study is the question of how relevant the literary style of a particular domain is to text segmentation (a segmentation model for a financial newspaper may not work for corpora from other domains).

References

Fujisawa, S., Masuyama S. & Naito S 1993. Nihongo-bun no shōryaku-hokan ni kansuru danwateki-seiyaku no yukōsei no kenshō (An inspection on effect [*sic*] of discourse constraints pertaining to ellipsis supplement in Japanese sentences). In *Jōhō-Shori-Gakkai Kōen-Ronbun-Shū* [Proceedings of the Conference of the Information Processing Society of Japan], Kōgakuin University, Vol. 3, 199–200.

Grosz, B. & C. Sidner 1986. Attention, intentions and the structure of discourse. *Computational Linguistics* **12**, 175–204.

Hearst, M. A. 1993. TextTiling: a quantitative approach to discourse segmentation. *Sequoia 2000* 93/24, University of California, Berkeley.

Hobbs, J. R. 1979. Coherence and coreference. *Cognitive Science* **3**, 67–90.

Hovy, E. 1993. Automated discourse generation using discourse structure relations. *Artificial Intelligence* **63**, 341–85.

Kozima, H. 1993. Text segmentation based on similarity between words. In *Proceedings of the 31st Annual Meeting of the Association for Computational Linguistics*, Columbus, Ohio, 286–8.

14. In general, recall is inversely proportional to precision; high precision implies low recall and vice versa.

Lewis, D. D. 1992. An evaluation of phrasal and clustered representations on a text categorization task. In *Proceedings of the Annual International ACM SIGIR Conference on Research and Development in Information Retrieval*, Copenhagen, 37–50.

Mann, W. C. & S. A. Thompson 1988. Rhetorical Structure theory: toward a functional theory of text organization. *Text* **8**, 243–81.

Mikami, A. 1960. *Zō wa hana ga nagai.* Tokyo: Kuroshio Shuppan.

Nomoto, T. & Y. Nitta. 1993. Resolving zero anaphora in Japanese. In *Sixth Conference of the European Chapter of the Association for Computational Linguistics*, Utrecht, 315–21.

Nunberg, G. 1990. *The linguistics of punctuation.* Stanford, Calif.: Center for the Study of Language and Information.

Salton, G. 1988. *Automatic text processing: the transformation, analysis, and retrieval of information by computer.* Reading, Mass.: Addison-Wesley.

Tokunaga, T. and M. Iwayama 1994. Omomi-tsuki IDF wo mochiita bunsho no jidō-bunrui ni tsuite (Text categorization based on weighted inverse document frequency). In *Jōhō-Shori-Gakkai Kenkyū-Hōkoku* [Information Processing Society of Japan Research Report] 94–NL–100, 33–40.

Youmans, G. (1991). A new tool for discourse analysis: the vocabulary management profile. *Language* **67**, 763–89.

Part VI
Hybrid approaches

24

Coarse-grained parallelism in natural language understanding: parsing as message passing

NORBERT BRÖKER, MICHAEL STRUBE, SUSANNE SCHACHT AND UDO HAHN

24.1 Introduction

This paper[1] surveys ParseTalk, a grammar model for natural language analysis that combines lexical organization of grammatical knowledge with lexicalized control of the corresponding parser in an object-oriented specification framework. Our research takes into account recent developments in the field of linguistic grammar theory that have yielded a radical lexical decomposition of linguistic knowledge. We consider this rigid form of lexical modularization just as a starting point for the incorporation of lexicalized control at the grammar level. Such a local, distributed perspective on

1. The work reported in this paper was funded by grants from DFG (grant nos Ha 2097/1-1, 1-2, 1-3) and LGFG Baden-Württemberg (1.1.4-7631.0; M. Strube).

the behaviour of the grammar system contrasts with previous designs of lexicalized grammars (e.g. HPSG (Proudian & Pollard 1985), Lexicalized TAG (Schabes et al. 1988), Categorial Grammar (Hepple 1992)). In these approaches lexical items are considered as passive data containers whose contents are uniformly interpreted by globally defined operations (unification, tree adjunction, functional composition, etc.). Trying to exploit fully the potential of the object-oriented computation paradigm and thus pushing lexicalism to its limit, we assign complete procedural autonomy to lexical units. They are treated as active lexical processes, locally communicating with each other by message passing and dynamically establishing heterogeneous communication lines in order to determine each lexical item's functional role in the discourse. While the issue of lexicalized control has long been investigated in the paradigm of conceptual parsing (Riesbeck & Schank 1978), and in particular word expert parsing (Small & Rieger 1982), these approaches are limited in several ways. Systematic grammar development is hard as there is no common grammar theory available, generalizations over sets of lexical items cannot be expressed because of the lack of inheritance mechanisms, and lexical communication is based on entirely informal protocols that have no grounding in principles of distributed computing.

We intend to remedy these methodological shortcomings by designing a lexically distributed grammar on the basis of valency and dependency (these head-oriented notions already figure in various ways in many modern linguistic theories, e.g. as subcategorizations, case frames, theta roles; see Somers 1987), by introducing inheritance as a major organizational mechanism (for a survey of applying inheritance in modern grammar theory, see Daelemans et al. 1992), and by specifying a message-passing protocol for local and directed communication between lexical objects that is grounded in the actor computation model (Agha & Hewitt 1987). As this protocol allows for asynchronous message passing, concurrency enters as a theoretical notion at the level of grammar specification, not just as an implementational feature. Furthermore, the actor methodology allows for the balanced treatment of declarative and procedural specification items within a single formal framework, while still keeping both of these levels transparent. This is obviously in strong contrast to declarativist approaches which assign structural well-formedness conditions to the grammar level and leave their computation to (general-purpose) parsing algorithms.

After the introduction of the grammar and the computational model underlying the ParseTalk approach (Section 24.2), we will turn in Section 24.3 to three types of protocols in more depth: one for establishing sentence-level dependency relations, one for coping with structural ambiguities, and one for treating text-level anaphora. Their consideration should demonstrate how a message-passing-based model of natural language parsing can easily be adapted to more and more complex linguistic phenomena. In particular, we claim that any serious move from syntax-centred sentence parsing to discourse-level understanding must consider the interactions between multiple linguistic and non-linguistic knowledge sources involved. Accordingly, mechanisms must be supplied that account for these procedural aspects of natural language understanding as part of linguistic specifications proper, an issue that is not so pressing when monolithic grammar knowledge essentially boils down to sentence-level syntactic regularities.

24.2 Conceptual framework

In the exposition of the conceptual framework underlying the design of the ParseTalk model, we distinguish between the grammar model proper (various types of linguistic knowledge incorporated in composite valency and anaphora constraints, Section 2.1) and the computational model, building upon the formal foundations of the actor model and extending it according to the specific requirements imposed by natural language processing (Section 24.2.2).

24.2.1 The grammar model

The grammar model underlying the ParseTalk approach considers dependency as the fundamental notion of linguistic analysis at the sentence level (see Bröker et al. 1994 for an in-depth account). This choice is made for the following reasons:

- The declarative grammar specification is fully lexicalized, since only relations between lexical items are described; no rule component is necessary.
- The parsing procedure is fully distributed and inherently concurrent, since dependencies are established by independent local processes involving only two lexical items: the potential head and its associated modifier.
- Since dependencies are of a hierarchical nature, the flexibility required for the description of free-word-order languages (such as German) can be easily accounted for by additional specifications expressing linear ordering constraints, a design decision that results in a modular ID/LP-style grammar format.
- As we provide structured terminological concept representations for the domain knowledge, most language-specific dependency relations have close counterparts at the conceptual representation level; this suggests the simultaneous evaluation of linguistic and conceptual constraints and correspondingly leads to an incremental architecture without extra filtering.

Sentence-level relations

Co-occurrence restrictions between lexical items are specified as sets of valencies that express constraints on permitted grammatical relations within a sentence. Valencies are labelled by dependency relation names, $\mathcal{D} = \{$*specifier*, *attr*, . . . $\}$, and describe which types of modifiers a lexical head from a particular word class may govern. These specifications refer to:

- **Word classes**: (1) denotes the set of word classes, and (2) denotes the subclass relation which yields a hierarchical ordering among these classes.

(1) $\mathcal{C}$ = {*word, verbal, nominal, noun, adjective, . . .* }
(2) $isa_{\mathcal{C}}$ = {(*verbal,word*), (*nominal,word*), (*noun,nominal*), (*adjective,nominal*), . . . } $\subset \mathcal{C} \times \mathcal{C}$

Word classes represent the distributional properties of their instances (i.e. concrete words) and, thus, define the possible feature specifications for these words. In addition, word classes supply the behaviour of the word actors: they define the message repertoire that word actors can respond to (see Section 24.2.2 below).

- **Morphosyntax**: A common unification formalism is used in order to represent morphosyntactic regularities. It includes atomic terms from the set (3), complex terms associating labels from the set (4)[2] with embedded terms, value disjunction and coreferences.
  (3) $\mathcal{A}$ = {*nom, acc, . . . , sg, pl, . . .* }
  (4) $\mathcal{L}$ = {*agr, pers, num, gen, . . .* } $\cup \mathcal{D} \cup \{self\}$
  $\mathcal{U}$ denotes the set of allowed feature structures, ∇ the unification operation, and $\perp$ the inconsistent element. Two operations will be used subsequently: given $u \in \mathcal{U}$ and $l \in \mathcal{L}$, the "expansion" $[l : u]$ denotes the complex feature structure containing only one label, l, with value u. If $v \in \mathcal{U}$ is a complex feature containing l at top level, the "extraction" $v \setminus l$ is defined to be the value of l in v. Therefore, if $v = [l : u]$, then $v \setminus l = u$.
- **Concepts**: The concept hierarchy consists of the set of concepts (5) and the subclass relation (6).
  (5) $\mathcal{F}$ = {*Company, Hardware, Computer, Country, Japan, . . .* }
  (6) $isa_{\mathcal{F}}$ = {(*Computer,Hardware*), (*Japan,Country*), . . . } $\subset \mathcal{F} \times \mathcal{F}$
  Furthermore, the set of conceptual relation names (7) contains the labels of possible conceptual relations (a frame-style representation model is assumed).
  (7) $\mathcal{R}$ = {*hasPart, hasLoc, . . .* }
  The relation *permit* $\subset \mathcal{F} \times \mathcal{R} \times \mathcal{F}$ characterizes the range of actual slot fillers, e.g. (*Company,hasLoc,Country*) $\in$ *permit*.
- **Word order**: A (word-class-specific) subset of $(D \cup \{self\})^n$ contains n-tuples that express ordering constraints on the valencies of each word class. Legal orders of modifiers must correspond to an element of this subset. For established dependencies, a (word-specific) function maps valency names from $\mathcal{D} \cup \{self\}$ to the modifiers' text positions. These specifications appear at the lexical head only.

Figure 24.1 gives the conditions whose evaluation determines whether a concrete dependency relation can be established between a candidate head and a candidate modifier (the notation *object.attribute* denotes the value of the property *attribute* at *object*). Word actors are characterized by the attributes *features* $\in \mathcal{U}$, *concept* (corresponding conceptual instance), *order* $\subset (\mathcal{D} \cup \{self\})^n$ (legal orderings of modifiers), *occurs*: $\mathcal{D} \cup \{self\} \rightarrow N_0$ (mapping from dependencies to text positions),

2. The additional labels serve to partition the feature structures, with the features of the head embedded under the label *self*, and the modifiers' features embedded under the corresponding dependency label.

$$
\begin{array}{l}
\textit{DependencyTest}\ (\text{modifier, valency, head}) :\Leftrightarrow \\
\quad \text{modifier } isa_C{}^{*} \text{ valency.class} \\
\quad \wedge\ (([\text{valency.name} : (\text{modifier.features} \setminus \textit{self})] \\
\qquad \triangledown\ \text{valency.features})\ \triangledown\ \text{head.features}) \neq \bot \\
\quad \wedge \exists \text{ role} \in \text{valency.domain: (head.concept, role, modifier.concept)} \in \textit{permit} \\
\quad \wedge \exists\ \langle d_1, \ldots, d_n \rangle \in \text{head.}\textit{order}\text{: } \exists\ k \in \{1, \ldots, n\}\text{:} \\
\qquad (\text{valency.name} = d_k \\
\qquad \wedge \forall\ 1 \leq i < k\text{: (head.}\textit{occurs}(d_i) < \text{modifier.position)} \\
\qquad \wedge \forall\ k < i \leq n\text{: (head.}\textit{occurs}(d_i) = 0) \\
\qquad\qquad\qquad \vee\ (\text{head.}\textit{occurs}(d_i) > \text{modifier.position}))
\end{array}
$$

Figure 24.1 *Conditions for dependency.*

valencies (the set of valencies), *position* $\in N_0$, and *head* (the grammatical head, another word actor). Valencies, on the other hand, have the attributes *name* $\in \mathcal{D}$, *class* $\in \mathcal{C}$, *features* $\in \mathcal{U}$, and *domain* $\subset \mathcal{R}$. If *DependencyTest* is satisfied, a dependency relation *valency.name* is established between the head and the modifier. Thus, valencies represent co-occurrence constraints to be fulfilled at the word-class (grammar) level, while dependencies characterize actual relations between concrete lexical items (parser). If a dependency is established, a predicate holds that is written as *modifier valency.name head.*

Text-level relations

Complementary to dependency relations at the sentence level, anaphoric relations between discourse elements can be determined by the evaluation of predicates at the text level of analysis. These predicates also incorporate notions from the grammar model, namely, word classes, morphosyntax and concepts. *PronAnaphorTest* covers pronominal anaphora (Fig. 24.2), while *NomAnaphorTest* accounts for nominal anaphora (Fig. 24.3).

$$
\begin{array}{l}
\textit{PronAnaphorTest}\ (\text{pro, ante}) :\Leftrightarrow \\
\quad \text{ante } isa_C{}^{*}\ \textit{Noun} \\
\quad \wedge\ ((\text{pro.features} \setminus \textit{self} \setminus \textit{agr} \setminus \textit{gen})\ \triangledown\ (\text{ante.features} \setminus \textit{self} \setminus \textit{agr} \setminus \textit{gen}) \neq \bot) \\
\quad \wedge\ ((\text{pro.features} \setminus \textit{self} \setminus \textit{agr} \setminus \textit{num})\ \triangledown\ (\text{ante.features} \setminus \textit{self} \setminus \textit{agr} \setminus \textit{num}) \neq \bot) \\
\quad \wedge\ ((\text{pro.features} \setminus \textit{self} \setminus \textit{agr} \setminus \textit{pers})\ \triangledown\ (\text{ante.features} \setminus \textit{self} \setminus \textit{agr} \setminus \textit{pers}) \neq \bot) \\
\quad \wedge \exists\ v \in \text{pro.head.valencies} : \exists\ r \in v\text{.domain} : \\
\qquad \text{pro } v\text{.name pro.head} \wedge (\text{pro.head.concept}, r, \text{ante.concept}) \in \textit{permit}
\end{array}
$$

Figure 24.2 *Conditions for pronominal anaphora.*

$$\begin{array}{l} \textit{NomAnaphorTest}\ (\text{defNP, ante}) :\Leftrightarrow \\ \ \text{ante}\ \textit{isa}_C{}^*\ \textit{Noun} \\ \ \wedge\ ((\text{defNP.features} \setminus \textit{self} \setminus \textit{agr} \setminus \textit{num})\ \nabla\ (\text{ante.features} \setminus \textit{self} \setminus \textit{agr} \setminus \textit{num}) \neq \bot) \\ \ \wedge\ \text{ante.concept}\ \textit{isa}_F{}^*\ \text{defNP.concept} \end{array}$$

Figure 24.3 *Conditions for nominal anaphora.*

In the case of pronominal anaphora, the pronoun and its antecedent (a noun) must agree in gender, number and person. Furthermore, the selected antecedent must be permitted in those conceptual roles connecting the pronominal anaphor and its grammatical head. In the case of nominal anaphora, the concept to which the antecedent refers must be subsumed by the concept to which the anaphoric noun phrase refers. Additionally, a test must determine whether the definite NP agrees with the antecedent (a noun) in number.

24.2.2 The computational model

The actor model of computation (Agha & Hewitt 1987) aims at the methodologically clean combination of object-oriented features with concurrency and distribution. It assumes a collection of independent objects, "actors", communicating via asynchronous, point-to-point "message passing". Each actor has an identity (its mail address), a state (i.e. its local variables, called "acquaintances") and a behaviour (i.e. its repertoire of possible reactions to incoming messages). The arrival of a message at an actor is called an "event": it triggers an action described by the corresponding method definition, a composition of the following atomic actions:

- creating a new actor;
- sending a message to an acquainted or a newly created actor;
- specifying new acquaintances for itself.

An actor system is dynamic, since new actors can be created at run time and the communication topology is reconfigurable in the course of actor computations. The actor model does not contain synchronization primitives, but we assume one-at-a-time serialized actors for our specification, i.e. actors that cannot process more than one message at a time and that process each message step by step (see Hewitt & Atkinson (1979) for the expression of this policy in terms of patterns of simple actors). The distribution of computations among the collection of actors is thus the only source of parallelism. Furthermore, in order to compute complex, but well understood and locally determined conditions and functions, such as unification of feature structures and querying a (conceptual) knowledge base, we establish a synchronous request–reply protocol (see Lieberman 1987).

The ParseTalk model extends the basic actor model according to the requirements set up by the natural language processing application (see Schacht et al. (1994) for an in-depth account). The extensions are expressed in terms of the primitives supplied by the basic model. We distinguish between word actors, relations between word actors and a special set of messages that word actors may exchange.

Word actors

The grammatical knowledge associated with each lexical item is represented in a word-actor definition. Upon instantiation of a specific word actor (caused by stepwise scanning of lexical items from the text input), the acquaintances specified in the definition will be initialized with actors that stand for the lexical item's morphosyntactic features, its conceptual representation, valency constraints and, after instantiation and subsequent parsing events, governed lexical items and further grammatical, e.g. anaphoric relations.

Word-actor relations

Acquaintances of word actors are tagged according to linguistic criteria in order to serve as navigation aids in linguistic structures (cf. the message distribution mechanism described below). For instance, anaphoric relations (Section 24.3.3) are distinguished from linear adjacency and hierarchical dependency relations. Tagging imposes a kind of "typing" mechanism onto acquaintances that was missing from previous actor systems.

Word-actor messages

In contrast to simple messages which trigger the execution of the corresponding method at the receiving actor in an unconditioned way, we define complex word-actor messages as fully fledged actors with independent computational capabilities. Departure and arrival of complex messages are actions that are performed by the message itself, taking the sender and the target actors as parameters. Upon arrival, a complex message determines whether a copy of itself is forwarded to selected acquaintances of its receiver and whether the receiver may process the message on its own. Hence, we redefine an arrival event to be an uninterruptable sequence of a "computation event" and "distribution events".

The computation event corresponds to an arrival of a simple message at the receiving word actor, i.e. an event in the basic model: it consists of the execution of an actor's method that may change the actor's state and trigger additional messages. The distribution events provide for the forwarding of the message by creating new complex messages. The events refer to the (unchanged) state of the receiving actor or to the result of the computation event and take place before and after the computation event respectively. This extension accounts for the complexity of interactions typical of the language understanding task. In order to structure the message repertoire, message definitions are organized in an inheritance hierarchy, too. Inner nodes in this hierarchy encode distribution strategies. As an example, consider the *SearchAntecedent* message (Section 24.3.3) which expresses structural restrictions on both types of anaphoric antecedents to be considered below.

24.3 Parsing as message passing

We will now introduce in turn various types of protocols, each adapted to particular linguistic phenomena with increasing complexity. We start with the basic protocol for establishing dependency relations at the sentence level (Section 24.3.1), then turn to an extension that accounts for structural (syntactic) ambiguities (Section 24.3.2), and, finally, consider anaphoric relations at the text level of analysis (Section 24.3.3). Note that we abstract from some complexities of the grammar specifications (in particular, the syntax–semantics interface) and concentrate instead on the message passing mode of executing control in the lexicalized parser.

24.3.1 Establishing dependency relations

The following protocol (messages and associated actions) for establishing dependencies at the sentence level ensures incremental generation of dependency trees, encodes structural restrictions of the dependency structure (which guarantee projectivity) and yields a domesticated form of concurrency.

Consider a newly instantiated word actor w_n searching bottom-up for its head by sending a *SearchHead* message to its immediate left neighbour, w_{n-1} (Fig. 24.4). *SearchHead* is recursively moved forward by a sequence of distribution events to the head of each receiving actor (i.e. w_{n-1}, w_k, w_j); messages only pass the outer fringe of the already established dependency tree. Hence, only projective trees are generated.

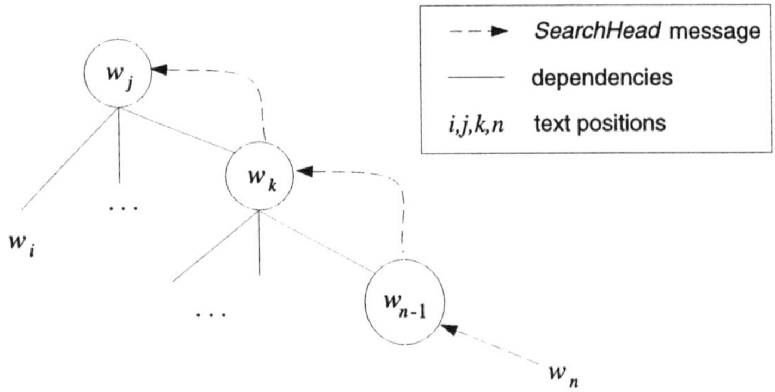

Figure 24.4 *Forwarding a* SearchHead *message.*

Each word actor w_k receiving the *SearchHead* message evaluates the predicate *DependencyTest* (Fig. 24.1) to determine whether it may govern w_n or not. If the restrictions of some valency are fulfilled, w_k replies by sending a *HeadFound* message to w_n. If this is the first *HeadFound* message w_n receives, it will reply to w_k by sending a *HeadAccepted* message, thereby establishing the dependency relation (any subsequent *HeadFound* message signals a case of structural ambiguity, see Section 24.3.2).

Because of a special receipt protocol, the termination of all processes triggered by the initial *SearchHead* message is guaranteed (Schacht 1995) before the next word actor w_{n+1} is instantiated, thereby ensuring incrementality. Concurrency is here restricted to the parallel processing of *SearchHead* messages at different actors. Alternative attachments result in structural ambiguities which are also processed in parallel.

24.3.2 Coping with structural ambiguities

A structural ambiguity arises if there are two possible heads for a word actor *w*. This is detected by *w* when it receives more than one *HeadFound* message. At this point, one attachment has already been established (or is under construction and cannot be blocked). For the second (and any further) attachment(s) to be established, first, all actors that will represent this reading must be created. w therefore copies itself (giving $\overline{w}$), requests that all its modifiers copy themselves, and asks the prospective head to copy itself, too. The copies of the modifiers accept $\overline{w}$ as their new head using the familiar *HeadAccepted* message, while the new copy of the head retries to govern $\overline{w}$ by sending *HeadFound.* Thus, there are only two new message classes to consider (Hahn et al. (1994) contains a more detailed description of the protocol for handling ambiguities):

- *CopyStructure* messages are sent to word actors that consequently duplicate themselves and their modifiers and are further required to reply with a *HeadAccepted* message, if completed. The duplication of all (transitive) modifiers is achieved by recursively sending *CopyStructure* messages to each of them.
- *DuplicateStructure* messages are sent to word actors that consequently duplicate themselves, their modifiers, and their heads. A *HeadFound* message is expected from the copy of each receiving actor. The duplication of the modifiers is achieved by *CopyStructure* messages, while the duplication of all (transitive) heads results from recursively sending *DuplicateStructure* messages to the head until an ungoverned actor is addressed.

Usually, a packed representation of ambiguous structures is preferred in the parsing literature (Tamura et al. 1991). This is feasible when syntactic analysis is the only factor determining the occurrence of partial structures. If conceptual restrictions are incorporated (as in our model), however, different syntactic attachments result in different conceptual descriptions possibly influencing further syntactic attachments. Consequently, no common structure is accessible that can be shared (Akasaka (1991) raises a similar argument). We represent ambiguities unpacked, with the expectation that the parallel evaluation of conceptual restrictions considerably reduces the amount of (syntactic) ambiguities.

24.3.3 Establishing anaphoric relations

The protocol described in this section accounts for the anaphoric relationship between pronouns or definite noun phrases and their associated antecedents at the text level of analysis.[3] Besides adjacency and dependency, an additional type of relation needs to be considered, namely, one which explicitly links the antecedent and its corresponding anaphor via an intersentential textual relation. In order properly to account for that relation our exposition will be based on the well-known focus mechanism (Sidner 1983; Grosz & Sidner 1986). Accordingly, we distinguish:

- each sentence's unique "focus", with the group of sentences continuously referring to the same focus constituting a so-called discourse segment (the hierarchical focus structure of a text is reflected in the corresponding stack of discourse segments);
- a complementary list of alternative "potential foci" composed of discourse elements of that particular sentence immediately preceding the currently considered one;
- a "history list" composed of discourse elements not in the list of potential foci but occurring in previous sentences of the current discourse segment.

Within ParseTalk, the focus structures are realized as acquaintances of sentence delimiters, e.g. the full stop. Each has the acquaintances *Focus*, *PotFoci* and *HistList* in order to restrict the search space beyond the sentence to the relevant word actors. Once an anaphor is resolved, the word actor representing the full stop sends a *SetFocus* message to the next sentence delimiter in order to update its associated acquaintances *Focus*, *PotFoci* and *HistList*. In the following discussion, emphasis is laid on the accessibility of the information contained in these acquaintances on the basis of message passing mechanisms, while the issue of stacking and unstacking discourse segments is not further dealt with.

The discussion of the protocol for establishing relations based on text-level anaphora refers to example (8) (see Fig. 24.5).

(8) *Das neue Powerbook ist mit leistungsfähigen Akkus ausgerüstet.*
Technoland vertreibt es / den Rechner *in Bayern.*
'The new Powerbook is equipped with powerful rechargeables. *It / This computer* is distributed in Bavaria by Technoland.'

Note that in the subsequent discussion "[ ]" stands for the word actor associated with a particular lexical item. Now, n the case of pronominal anaphora the search for the antecedent is triggered by the occurrence of the personal pronoun *es*. As this word actor is instantiated, a *SearchPronAntecedent* message will be sent. In the case of nominal anaphora the search for the antecedent is triggered by the attachment of the definite article *den* to the noun *Rechner*: upon receipt of a *HeadAccepted* message (sent by the definite article) at the noun, a *SearchNomAntecedent* message will be sent. Since the structural criteria for the position of both anaphors are the same, the distribution of the *SearchPronAntecedent* message and the *SearchNomAntecedent* message will be described by their common superclass, namely, *SearchAntecedent*.

3. Here, we will not consider the grammar specifications for intrasentential anaphora, the resolution of which takes additional criteria into account. The most relevant ones require anaphor and antecedent not to be modifiers of the same head. The anaphor must not occupy the position of the reflexive pronoun. See Strube & Hahn (1995a) for a description of constraints on intrasentential anaphora (including the analysis of reflexive pronouns) in terms of the ParseTalk dependency grammar.

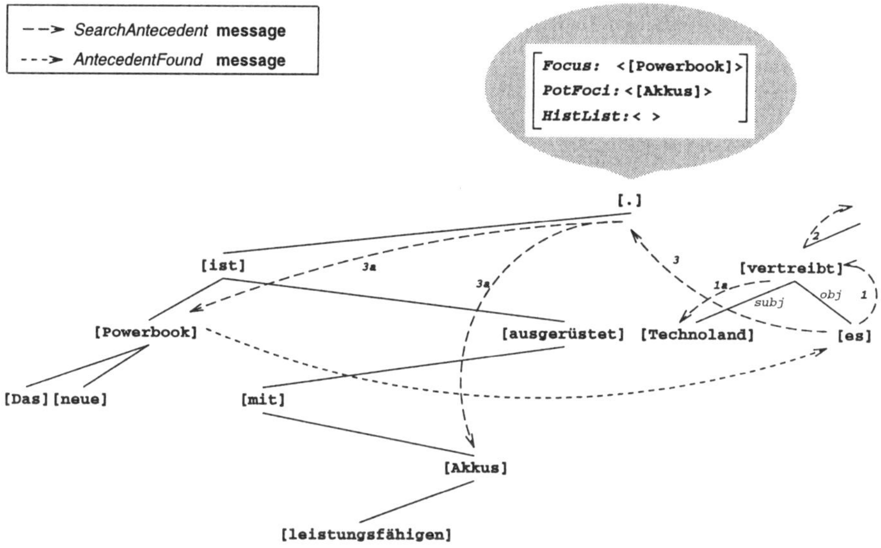

Figure 24.5 *Sample communication protocol.*

The distribution strategy represents the syntactic restrictions on the appearance of the anaphor and the antecedent, respectively.

A *SearchAntecedent* message (and therefore any instance of its specific subclasses) controls the distribution in its own responsibility. The message takes on some states ("phases") that reflect the structural restrictions. Figure 24.5 shows a corresponding sample parse that has proceeded up to the instantiation of the word actor [*es*].

In Phase 1, the message is forwarded from its initiator [*es*] to the finite verb [*vertreibt*] which is the head of the innermost verbal phrase. When the message reaches [*vertreibt*], two further messages with Phases 1a and 2 are sent simultaneously, and the message in Phase 1 terminates. In Phase 1a the left modifiers of the initiator's head [*vertreibt*] are tested in order to determine if any of these modifiers have modifiers themselves. In the given example, the test fails, and the message in Phase 1a terminates. If the test succeeds, the message will be forwarded to these modifiers, where the anaphor predicate *PronAnaphorTest* has to be evaluated in parallel.

In Phase 2, the path of the message leads from the verb [*vertreibt*] to the word actor that represents the sentence delimiter of the *current* sentence. Since on that path the message does not encounter a finite verb that governs [*vertreibt*], it terminates. If the message, however, reaches another finite verb, a new message with Phase 2a will be created. In Phase 2a, it is checked whether there are modifiers of this verb that might be antecedents of the pronoun [*es*].

Independently from Phases 1 and 2, Phase 3 is triggered. Its path leads directly from the initiator [*es*] to the sentence delimiter of the *previous* sentence, where its state is set to Phase 3a. In this phase are checked possible antecedents that have been stored as the acquaintances *Focus* and *PotFoci* of the sentence delimiter. We do not yet exploit the distinction between *Focus* (usually prioritized) and *PotFoci* (usually considered only if the focus element does not apply), but preserve it for later use by preference models. Thus, in our case [*Powerbook*] and [*Akkus*] are equally likely candidate antecedents for which *PronAnaphorTest* will be evaluated in parallel. [*Powerbook*] is then determined as the only valid antecedent of [*es*], because *PronAnaphorTest* succeeds only in this case: [*Powerbook*] agrees in gender, number and person with the anaphor [*es*], and fulfils the conceptual constraints as indicated by the variable assignments shown in (9) (see Fig. 24.2).

(9) pro = [*es*], *v*.name = *obj*, pro.head = [*vertreibt*],
pro.head.concept = *DistributeEvent*, *r* = *isDistributor*,
ante.concept = *Powerbook* isa_F* *Product*

SearchAntecedent is an obvious example of a complex word-actor message (see Section 24.2.2). During Phases 1, 2 and 3 the message is distributed without triggering computation events. In Phases 1a, 2a and 3a computation events of the receivers take place, depending on which message has been sent: *SearchPronAntecedent* evaluates *PronAnaphorTest*, while *SearchNomAntecedent* evaluates *NomAnaphorTest* (see p. 305). Only nouns or personal pronouns respond to these messages and test whether they fulfil the required criteria for an anaphoric relation.

If the test succeeds, the antecedent sends a direct *AntecedentFound* message to the initiator of the *SearchAntecedent* message. This message carries the concept identifier of the antecedent. The initiator of the *SearchAntecedent* message, namely the anaphor, changes its concept identifier accordingly upon receipt of the *AntecedentFound* message. The update of the concept identifier is the final result of the anaphora resolution and accounts for the coreference between concepts denoted by different lexical items at the text level among which an anaphoric relation holds.

The proposal above is an improvement over previous approaches in two ways. First, we are able to integrate the focusing mechanism homogeneously into our distributed grammar specification framework and do not consider it an add-on to some monolithic sentence grammar, a view prevailing hitherto. As should be obvious from the considerations above, phrasal, sentence and text-level analyses are highly interactive and proceed incrementally, a view that is also evidenced by various psycholinguistic studies (e.g. Thibadeau et al. 1982). Second, through the parallel search for antecedents we prevent possible errors in terms of lacking recognition of referential ambiguities that may arise in the original serial model when only one antecedent is searched for and only one solution for anaphora resolution actually needs to be determined.

24.4 Comparison with related work

In contrast to constituency-based models of lexicalized grammars, the ParseTalk approach considers dependency as the primary notion for grammatical specifications. Unlike other dependency parsers (Hellwig 1986; Starosta & Nomura 1986; Jäppinen et al. 1988; McCord 1990; Fraser & Hudson 1992), ParseTalk provides a specification platform for the integration of syntactic and non-syntactic (conceptual and domain) knowledge into the grammar and assigns equal opportunity to access different knowledge sources. The co-ordination of these accesses requires explicit communication primitives, a major issue already dealt with by conceptual parsers (Riesbeck & Schank 1978), and, in particular, word expert parsing (Small & Rieger 1982). The ParseTalk model, however, offers both a linguistically sound specification framework and facilities to balance the interaction of linguistic and extralinguistic knowledge properly. Message passing as an explicit control mechanism is inherent in various object-oriented implementations of standard rule- or principle-based parsers (cf. Phillips (1984) for augmented PSG, Lin (1993) for GB, or Yonezawa & Ohsawa (1994) for context-free PSG). Actor-based parsers have also been provided for LFG (Uehara et al. 1985), GB (Abney & Cole 1986) and word expert systems (Hahn 1994). Furthermore, a parallel implementation of a rule-based, syntax-oriented dependency parser has been described by Akasaka (1991), but these proposals offer concurrency at the implementational, i.e. programming-language level only. The consideration of concurrency at the grammar-specification level has also been investigated by Milward (1992) who properly relates notions from categorial and dependency grammar with a state logic approach, a formal alternative to the event-algebraic formalization underlying the ParseTalk model (cf. Schacht et al. 1994). For a general survey of parallel computation models for natural language processing, see Hahn & Adriaens (1994).

The object-oriented ParseTalk approach constitutes a coarse-grained parallel model of natural language understanding which is in contrast to the fine-grained (or massive) parallelism underlying connectionist models. Connectionist methodology (see the survey by Selman (1989) of some now classical connectionist natural language parsing systems and a later compilation of connectionist natural language processing studies by Reilly & Sharkey (1992)) is restricted in two ways compared with object-oriented computing. First, its communication patterns – after the learning cycle – are determined by the hard-wired topology of connectionist networks, whereas in object-oriented systems, and actor systems in particular, the topology is flexible and reconfigurable each time the system is started. Second, the type and amount of data that can be exchanged in a connectionist network is restricted to marker and value passing, together with severely limited computational logic (*and*-ing and *or*-ing of Boolean bit markers, determining maximum or minimum values, etc.), while none of these restrictions apply to message passing models. These considerations equally extend to spreading-activation models of natural language parsing (Charniak 1986; Hirst 1987) which are not as constrained as connectionist models but less expressive than the general message-passing models underlying the object-oriented and actor paradigms.

24.5 Conclusions

The ParseTalk model of natural language understanding emphasizes dependency and full lexicalization as fundamental notions of grammar design and considers an object-oriented computation model and concurrency essential for a corresponding parser design. Based on these methodological premisses parsing is viewed as communication between and within different knowledge sources (grammar, domain and discourse knowledge). The main specification elements of the grammar model are categorial, morphosyntactic, conceptual and word-order constraints attached to single lexical items to which the computation of concrete dependency and anaphoric relations refers. The associated concurrent computation model is based on the actor paradigm of object-oriented programming, with several extensions relating to special requirements of natural language processing.

The ParseTalk model has been experimentally validated by a prototype system, a text parser for German. The current full-form lexicon contains a hierarchy of 100 word-class specifications and nearly 3000 lexical entries. The parser's coverage incorporates the analysis of complex assertional sentences and the treatment of anaphora and ellipses (Strube & Hahn 1995a,b). It is implemented in Smalltalk-80 with extensions that allow for coarse-grained parallelism through physical distribution in a workstation cluster (Xu 1993) and asynchronous message passing. The ParseTalk system is coupled with the LOOM knowledge representation system (MacGregor & Bates 1987) via a set of request and update primitives. We currently supply two knowledge bases with approximately 900 and 500 complex concepts and relations covering the domains of information technology and medicine, respectively.

References

Abney, S. & J. Cole 1986. A government-binding parser. In *Proceedings of North-Eastern Linguistic Society 16*, University of Massachusetts at Amherst.

Adriaens, G. & U. Hahn (eds) 1994. *Parallel natural language processing*. Norwood, NJ: Ablex.

Agha, G. & C. Hewitt 1987. Concurrent programming using actors. In Yonezawa & Tokoro (1987), 37–53.

Akasaka, K. 1991. Parallel parsing system based on dependency grammar. In Brown & Koch (1991), 147–57.

Bröker, N., U. Hahn & S. Schacht 1994. Concurrent lexicalized dependency parsing: the *ParseTalk* model. In *COLING 94: The 15th International Conference on Computational Linguistics*, Kyoto, Japan, 379–85.

Brown, C. G. & G. Koch (eds) 1991. *Natural language understanding and logic programming III*. Amsterdam: North-Holland.

Charniak, E. 1986. A neat theory of marker passing. In *AAAI-86: Proceedings of the Fifth National Conference on Artificial Intelligence, Volume 1: Science*, Philadelphia, Pa., 584–8.

Daelemans, W., K. De Smedt & G. Gazdar 1992. Inheritance in natural language processing. *Computational Linguistics* **18**, 205–18.

Fraser, N. & R. Hudson 1992. Inheritance in Word Grammar. *Computational Linguistics* **18**, 133–58.

Grosz, B. & C. L. Sidner 1986. Attention, intentions, and the structure of discourse. *Computational Linguistics* **12**, 175–204.

Hahn, U. 1994. An actor model of distributed natural language parsing. In Adriaens & Hahn (1994), 307–49.

Hahn, U. & G. Adriaens 1994. Parallel natural language processing: background and overview. In Adriaens & Hahn (1994), 1–134.

Hahn, U., S. Schacht & N. Bröker 1994. Concurrent, object-oriented dependency parsing: the *ParseTalk* model. *International Journal of Human–Computer Studies* **41**, 179–222.

Hellwig, P. 1986. Dependency unification grammar. In *11th International Conference on Computational Linguistics: Proceedings of Coling '86*, Bonn, 195–8.

Hepple, M. 1992. Chart parsing Lambek grammars: modal extensions and incrementality. In *Proceedings of the fifteenth International Conference on Computational Linguistics: COLING-92*, Nantes, 134–40.

Hewitt, C. & R. Atkinson 1979. Specification and proof techniques for serializers. *IEEE Transactions on Software Engineering* **SE-5**, 10–23.

Hirst, G. 1987. *Semantic interpretation and the resolution of ambiguity*. Cambridge: Cambridge University Press.

Jäppinen, H., E. Lassila & A. Lehtola. 1988. Locally governed trees and dependency parsing. In *COLING BUDAPEST: Proceedings of the 12th International Conference on Computational Linguistics*, Budapest, 275–7.

Lieberman, H. 1987. Concurrent object-oriented programming in Act 1. In Yonezawa & Tokoro (1987), 9–36.

Lin, D. 1993. Principle-based parsing without overgeneration. In *31st Annual Meeting of the Association for Computational Linguistics*, Columbus, Ohio, 112–20.

MacGregor, R. & R. Bates 1987. *The LOOM knowledge representation language*. Technical Report ISI/RS-87-18, Information Sciences Institute, University of Southern California, Marina del Rey, Calif.

McCord, M. C. 1990. Slot grammars: a system for simpler construction of practical natural language grammars. In *Natural language and logic*, R. Studer (ed.), 118–45. Berlin: Springer.

Milward, D. 1992. Dynamics, dependency grammar and incremental interpretation. In *Proceedings of the fifteenth International Conference on Computational Linguistics: COLING-92*, Nantes, 1095–9.

Phillips, B. 1984. An object-oriented parser. In *Computational models of natural language processing*, B. G. Bara & G. Guida (eds), 297–321. Amsterdam: North-Holland.

Proudian, D. & C. Pollard 1985. Parsing head-driven phrase structure grammar. In *23rd Annual Meeting of the Association for Computational Linguistics*, Chicago, 167–71.

Reilly, R. & N. E. Sharkey (eds) 1992. *Connectionist approaches to natural language processing*. Hove, England: Lawrence Erlbaum.

Riesbeck, C. & R. Schank 1978. Comprehension by computer: expectation-based analysis of sentences in context. In *Studies in the perception of language*, W. J. M. Levelt & G. B. Flores d'Arcais (eds), 247–93. Chichester, England: John Wiley.

Schabes, Y., A. Abeillé & A. K. Joshi 1988. Parsing strategies with 'lexicalized' grammars: application to tree adjoining grammars. In *COLING BUDAPEST: Proceedings of the 12th International Conference on Computational Linguistics*, Budapest, 578–83.

Schacht, S. 1995. Proving properties of actor programs using temporal logic. In *16th International Conference on Application and Theory of Petri Nets, Workshop on "Object-Oriented Programming and Models of Concurrency"*, Turin.

Schacht, S., U. Hahn & N. Bröker 1994. Concurrent lexicalized dependency parsing: a behavioral view on *ParseTalk* events. In *COLING 94: The 15th International Conference on Computational Linguistics*, Kyoto, Japan, 489–93.

Selman, B. 1989. Connectionist systems for natural language understanding. *Artificial Intelligence Review* **3**, 23–31.

Sidner, C. L. 1983. Focusing in the comprehension of definite anaphora. In *Computational models of discourse*, M. Brady & R. C. Berwick (eds), 267–330. Cambridge, Mass.: MIT Press.

Small, S. & C. Rieger 1982. Parsing and comprehending with word experts (a theory and its realization). In *Strategies for natural language processing*, W. Lehnert & M. H. Ringle (eds.), 89–147. Hillsdale, NJ: Erlbaum.

Somers, H. L. 1987. *Valency and case in computational linguistics*. Edinburgh: Edinburgh University Press.

Starosta, S. & H. Nomura 1986. Lexicase parsing: a lexicon-driven approach to syntactic analysis. In *11th International Conference on Computational Linguistics: Proceedings of Coling '86*, Bonn, 127–32.

Strube, M. & U. Hahn 1995a. ParseTalk about sentence- and text-level anaphora. In *Seventh Conference of the European Chapter of the Association for Computational Linguistics*, Dublin, 237–44.

Strube, M. & U. Hahn 1995b. ParseTalk about textual ellipsis. In *International Conference: Recent Advances in Natural Language Processing*, Tzigov Chark, Bulgaria, 62–72.

Tamura, N., M. Bos, H. Murakami, O. Nishida, T. Yoshimi & J. Jelinek 1991. Lazy evaluation of preference on a packed shared forest without unpacking. In Brown & Koch (1991), 13–26.

Thibadeau, R., M. A. Just & P. A. Carpenter 1982. A model of the time course and content of reading. *Cognitive Science* **6**, 157–203.

Uehara, K., R. Ochitani, O. Mikami & J. Toyoda 1985. An integrated parser for text understanding. In *Natural language understanding and logic programming*, V. Dahl & P. Saint-Dizier (eds), 79–95. Amsterdam: North-Holland.

Xu, W. 1993. *Distributed, shared and persistent objects*. PhD thesis, Department of Computer Science, Queen Mary and Westfield College, University of London.

Yonezawa, A. & I. Ohsawa 1994. Object-oriented parallel parsing for context-free grammars. In Adriaens & Hahn (1994), 188–210.

Yonezawa, A. & M. Tokoro (eds) 1987. *Object-oriented concurrent programming*. Cambridge, Mass.: MIT Press.

25
A stochastic Government–Binding parser

ANDREW FORDHAM AND MATTHEW CROCKER

25.1 Introduction

Both principle-based parsing and probabilistic methods for the analysis of natural language have become popular in the last decade. The former borrows from advanced linguistic specifications of syntax, and constructs its theories on the basis of native-speaker intuition rather than samples of actually occurring language use. This is partly as a result of the competence–performance distinction (Chomsky 1986) which states that the language that humans produce is not a pure manifestation of the knowledge of the grammatical rules being put to use.

Probabilistic approaches, however, have been more concerned with extracting distributional regularities from language, often without reference to the human knowledge that linguists assume is behind the production of this language. These approaches are practical rather than theoretical in nature, and have been used to aid the implementation of NLP systems and the analysis of corpora. Techniques used range from simple bi-gram models of word tagging (Marshall 1987) to the selection of the best syntactic parse for a structurally ambiguous phrase (Briscoe & Carroll 1991).

These symbolic and statistical approaches are beginning to draw together as it becomes clear that one cannot exist entirely without the other: the knowledge of language posited over the years by theoretical linguists has been useful in constraining and guiding statistical approaches, and the corpora now available to linguists have resurrected the desire to account for real language data in a more principled way than has previously been attempted.

This paper falls directly between these approaches, using statistical information derived from corpus analysis to weight syntactic analyses produced by a "principles and parameters" parser. The use of probabilistic information in principle-based grammars and parsers is considered, including discussion on some theoretical and computational problems that arise. Finally a partial implementation of these ideas is presented, along with some preliminary results from testing on a small set of sentences.

25.2 Government–Binding theory

The principles and parameters paradigm in linguistics is most fully realized in the Government–Binding theory (GB) of Chomsky (1981, 1986) and others. Unlike phrase-structure grammars, the knowledge of language is heterogeneous, with the grammar divided into modules, each concerned with a specific aspect of the grammaticality of a sentence. These modules, and the principles that they contain, interact during parsing to license grammatical structures and filter out ungrammatical structures at various levels of representation; standard GB posits four representational levels – phonetic form (PF), logical form (LF), D-structure and S-structure – which are related by general transformations. PF is the "input" level, LF the interface with semantics, and D- and S-structures the deep and surface syntactic forms. A sketch of the organization of GB (the "T-model") is shown in Figure 25.1.

Little work has been done on the complexity of algorithms used to parse with a principle-based grammar, since such grammars do not exist as accepted, mathematically well-defined constructs. It has been estimated that, in general, principle-based parsing can only be accomplished in exponential time, i.e. $\mathcal{O}(2^n)$ (Berwick & Weinberg 1984; Weinberg 1988). Although this could be viewed as an efficiency problem, a GB grammar is very small when compared to a context-free grammar for a language such as English (Grover et al. 1989). Grammar size is a variable that is often overlooked in calculations of efficiency, but is one that will undoubtedly affect the speed of a parser if the difference in size is great.

Another feature of GB theory is its language-independence. The grammar principles are designed to be universal and much research has gone into the way in which these principles work in different languages. The language learner is assumed

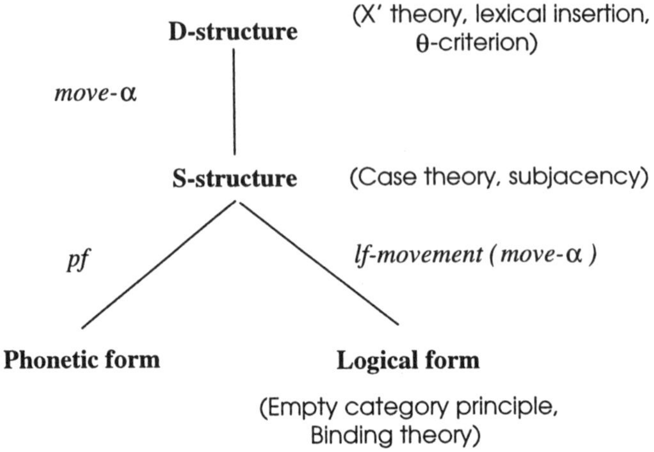

Figure 25.1 *The T-model of grammar.*

to be equipped with a set of switches or parameters, and the learning of the grammar of a language is merely the setting of these switches in a particular configuration. The size of a GB grammar will therefore stay reasonably constant between languages, whereas a new context-free rewrite grammar will be needed for each language, with those for non-configurational (free-word-order) languages being significantly larger than, for example, one for English.

A feature of principle-based grammars is their potential to assign some meaningful representation to a string that is strictly ungrammatical. It is an inherent feature of phrase-structure (PS) grammars that they classify the strings of words from a language into two (infinite) sets, one containing the grammatical strings and the other the *un*grammatical strings. Although attempts have been made to modify PS grammars/parsers to cope with extragrammatical input, e.g. Carbonell & Hayes (1983), Douglas & Dale (1992), this is a feature that has to be "added on" and tends to affect the statement of the grammar. Dealing with ungrammaticality in a GB parser, however, will be a matter for the parser, effectively relaxing the constraint that all modules must license a parse, and should therefore not affect the grammar.

25.2.1 Proper branches

Because of the lack of an accepted formalism for the specification of principle-based grammars, Crocker & Lewin (1992) define the declarative "proper branch" formalism, which can be used with a number of different parsing methods.

A proper branch is a set of three nodes – a mother and two daughters – that are constructed by a structure-proposing engine in the parser, e.g. a simple mechanism such as a shift–reduce interpreter. This proper branch is then "licensed" by the principles of grammar. A complete phrase marker of the input string can then be constructed by following the manner in which the mother node from one proper branch is used as a daughter node in a dominating proper branch.

Each proper branch is a binary branching structure, and so all grammatical constraints will need to be encoded locally. Crocker & Lewin develop

> . . . a 'representational' reformulation of the transformational model which decomposes syntactic analysis into several representation types – including phrase structure, chains, and coindexation – allowing one to maintain the strictly local characterisation of principles with respect to their relevant representation types. (Crocker & Lewin 1992: 511)

This local encoding of structure obviates the need for the parser to specifically construct a parse tree of the input except for output purposes. The inspection of the various levels of representation is also not required, since all the information encoded at the different levels can be made available locally.

By using the proper branch method of axiomatizing the grammar, the structure-building section of the parser is only constrained in that it must produce proper branches; it is therefore possible to experiment with different interpreters (i.e. structure-proposing engines) while keeping the grammar constant.

25.3 The grammar and the parser

A small principle-based parser was built, following the proper-branch formalism developed in Crocker & Lewin (1992). Although the grammar is very limited, the use of probabilities in ranking the parser's output can be seen as a first step towards implementing a principle-based parser using a more fully specified collection of grammar modules.

The grammar is loosely based on three modules taken from GB theory: X-bar theory, Theta theory and Case theory. Although these embody the spirit of the constraints found in Chomsky (1981) they are not intended to be entirely faithful to this specification of syntactic theory. There is also only a single level of representation (which is explicitly constructed for output purposes but not consulted by the parser). This representation is interpreted as S-structure.

Explanations of the knowledge contained within each grammar principle is given in the following sections.

25.3.1 X-bar theory

The version of X-bar theory used here employs a set of schemata to license local subtrees. These schemata resemble rewrite rules in context-free grammars but are used in our parser to rule out illegal proper branches that have already been generated by the structure-proposing engine, rather than generating the structures themselves. We use a parameterized version of the X-bar schemata, using unification to match each node in a proper branch with a feature bundle in a schema. There are five schemata, corresponding roughly to (1) specifier attachment, (2) and (3) complement attachment (depending on whether the head-word's θ-grid is about to be saturated), and (4) right- and (5) left-adjunction:

(1) $X^{-}_{-} \rightarrow Y^{-}_{-}\ X^{+}_{-}$

(2) $X^{S}_{+} \rightarrow X^{S}_{+}\ Y^{-}_{-}$

(3) $X^{S}_{-} \rightarrow X^{S}_{+}\ Y^{-}_{-}$

(4) $X^{S}_{-} \rightarrow X^{S}_{-}\ Y^{-}_{-}$

(5) $X^{S}_{-} \rightarrow Y^{-}_{-}\ X^{S}_{-}$

Each node is a feature bundle containing the following features:

- category: the standard category names are employed;
- specifier (SPEC): specifies whether the head of the phrase requires a specifier;
- complement (COMP): specifies whether the head of the phrase requires any complements;[1]
- the head (i.e. lexical item);
- the head's θ-grid, and a "government list" containing a list of the items on the grid that have already been discharged.

The probabilities for occurrences of the X-bar schemata were obtained from sentences from the preliminary Penn Treebank corpus of the *Wall Street Journal*, chosen because of their length and the head of their verb phrase (i.e. the main verbs were all from the set for which θ-role data was obtained); the examples were manually parsed by the authors.

The probabilities were calculated using (6),

$$(6)\quad P\left(X^{S_i}_{C_i} \rightarrow Y^{S_j}_{C_j}\ Z^{S_k}_{C_k} \mid \overline{X}\right) = \frac{C\left(X^{S_i}_{C_i} \rightarrow Y^{S_j}_{C_j}\ Z^{S_k}_{C_k}\right)}{C(A \rightarrow B\ C)}$$

where $P(X \mid Y)$ denotes the probability of X occurring, given Y; $C(X)$ is a count of the number of occurrences of X in the data; $X^{S_i}_{C_i} \rightarrow Y^{S_j}_{C_j}\ Z^{S_k}_{C_k}$ is a specific schema; $\overline{X}$ is the set of X-bar schemata; and A, B and C are variables over category, SPEC and COMP feature bundles.

This is different to the manner in which probabilities are collected for stochastic context-free grammars (SCFGs), where the identity of the mother node is taken into account, as in (7).

$$(7)\quad P\left(X^{S_i}_{C_i} \rightarrow Y^{S_j}_{C_j}\ Z^{S_k}_{C_k} \mid \overline{X}\right) = \frac{C\left(X^{S_i}_{C_i} \rightarrow Y^{S_j}_{C_j}\ Z^{S_k}_{C_k}\right)}{C\left(X^{S_i}_{C_i} \rightarrow B\ C\right)}$$

1. This feature is strictly redundant since this information is handled by Theta theory. The COMP feature is used merely to limit the number of superfluous proper branches to be considered by the other modules. This is obviously only of use if X-bar theory is the first constraint to be checked.

This would result in misleading probabilities for the X-bar schemata since the use of schemata (3), (4) and (5) would immediately bring down the probability of a parse compared to a parse of the same string that happened to use only (1) and (2).[2]

The overall (X-bar) likelihood of a parse can then be computed by multiplying together all the probabilities obtained from each application of the schemata, in a manner analogous to that used to obtain the probability of a phrase marker generated by an SCFG. Using the schemata in this way suggests that the building of structure is category-independent, i.e. it is just as likely that a verb will have a (filled) specifier position as a noun.

The work on SCFGs suggests a different set of results, in that the specific categories involved in expansions are all important. While SCFGs will tend to deny that all categories expand in certain ways with the same probabilities, they make this claim while using a homogeneous grammar formalism. When a more modular theory is employed, the source of the supposedly category-specific information is not so obvious. The use of lexical probabilities, to represent the likelihood of specific heads (i.e. lexical items) occurring as specifiers and complements to a word, could exhibit properties that appear to be category-specific, but are in fact caused by common properties that are shared by lexical items of the same category.[3] Since it can be argued that the probabilistic information on lexical items will be needed independently, there is no need to use category-specific information in assigning probabilities to syntactic configurations.

25.3.2 Theta theory

Theta theory is concerned with the assignment of an argument structure to a sentence. A verb has a number of the thematic roles (or "θ-roles") which must be assigned to its arguments. These roles are either external (subject position) or internal (complement position): e.g. a transitive verb has two θ-roles to "discharge" which must each be assigned to an NP. In the grammar used here, we only concerned ourselves with probabilities for internal θ-roles, as this information was much more easily obtainable than that for external θ-roles.

With the binary branching formalism employed, or indeed any such formalism where the arguments of an item and the item itself are not necessarily all sisters, the problem of when to access the probability of a θ-application is presented. The easiest method of obtaining and applying θ-probabilities will be with reference to whole θ-grids. Each θ-grid for a word will be assigned a probability that is not dependent on any particular items in the grid, but rather on the occurrence of the θ-grid as a whole.

A preliminary version of the Penn Treebank bracketed corpus was analysed to extract information on the sisters of particular verbs. Although the Penn Treebank data is unreliable since it does not always distinguish complements from adjuncts, it was the only suitable parsed corpus to which the authors had access. Although

2. The probabilities for schemata (1) and (2) would be 1 as they have unique mothers.

3. It is of course possible to store these cross-item similarities as lexical rules, but this alone does not entail that the properties be specific to a category, cf. the θ-grids of verbs and their "related" nouns.

the distinction between complements and adjuncts is a theoretically interesting one, the process of determining which constructions fill which functional roles in the analysis of real text often creates a number of problems (see Hindle & Rooth 1993 for discussion on this issue regarding output of the Fidditch parser).

The probabilities for each verb's θ-grid were calculated using (8),

$$(8)\ \ P(s_i \mid v) = \frac{C(v, s_i)}{C(v, S)}$$

where $P(s_i \mid v)$ is the probability of the θ-grid s_i occurring with the verb v, (v, s_i) is an occurrence of the items in s_i being licensed by v, and S ranges over all θ-grids for v. Some example statistics for θ-grids can be found in Table 25.1 (only five or more occurrences of a particular grid are recorded).

Table 25.1 Sample θ-grid statistics.

	appear	*believe*	*come*	*find*	*go*	*keep*
0					21	
AdjP	12				9	7
AdvP			7		11	
NP		10	6	38	10	18
NP AdjP				6		
NP PP				11	7	21
NP VP						8
PP	8	6	116		84	7
PP PP			16		10	
S	29		6		88	
$\bar{\text{S}}$		73	13			
VP			12			7
Total	60	91	213	86	283	89

25.3.3 Case theory

In its simplest form, Case theory invokes the Case filter to ensure that all noun phrases (NPs) in a parse are assigned (abstract) case. Case theory differs from both X-bar and Theta theory in that it is category-specific: only NPs require, or indeed can be assigned, abstract case. If we are to implement a probabilistic version of a modular grammar theory incorporating a Case component, a relevant question is: "Are there multiple ways of assigning Case to noun phrases in a sentence?", i.e. "Can ambiguity arise through the presence of two candidate Case assigners?".

Case theory suggests that the answer to this is negative, since Case assignment is linked to Theta theory via visibility, and it is not possible for an NP to receive more than one θ-role. As a result, the use of Case probabilities in a parser would be at best unimportant, since some form of ambiguity is needed in the module (i.e. it must be possible to satisfy the Case filter in more than one way) for probabilities associated with the module to be of any use. While having a provision for using probabilities deduced from Case information, the implemented parser does not in fact use Case in its parse ranking operations.

25.3.4 Local calculation

The use of a heterogeneous grammar formalism and multiple probabilities invokes the problem of their combination. There are at least two ways in which each mother's probabilities can be calculated; first, the probability information of the same type can be used: the daughters' X-bar probabilities alone could be used in calculating the mother's X-bar probability. Alternatively, a combination of some or all of the daughters' probability features could be employed, thus making, e.g. the X-bar probability of the mother dependent upon *all* the stochastic information from the daughters, including θ- and Case probabilities, etc.

The need for a method of combining the daughter probabilities into a useful figure for the calculation of the mother probabilities is likely to involve trial and error, since theory thus far has had nothing to say on the subject. The former method, using only the relevant daughter probabilities, therefore seems to be the most fruitful path to follow at the outset, since it does not require a way of integrating probabilities from different modules while the parse is in progress, nor is it as computationally expensive.

25.3.5 Global calculation

The manner in which the global probability is calculated will be partly dependent upon the information contained in the local probability calculations.

If the probabilities for partial analyses have been calculated using only probabilities of the same types from the subanalyses – e.g. X-bar, θ – the probabilities at the top level will have been calculated using informationally distinct figures. This has the advantage of making "pure" probabilities available, in that the X-bar probability will reflect the likelihood of the structure alone, and will be "uncontaminated" by any other information. It should then be possible to experiment with different methods of combining these probabilities, other than the obvious multiplication techniques, and this could result in one type of probability emerging as the most important.

On the other hand, if probabilities calculated during the parse take all the different types of probabilities into account at each calculation – i.e. the X-bar, θ-, etc. probabilities on daughters are all taken into account when calculating the mother's X-bar probability – the probabilities at the top level will not be pure, and a lot of the information contained in them will be redundant since they will share a large subset of the probabilities used in their separate calculations. It will not therefore be easy to gain theoretical insight using these statistics, and their most profitable method of combination is likely to be a more haphazard affair than when more pure probabilities are used.

The parser used in testing employed the first method and therefore produced separate module probabilities for each node. For lack of a better, theoretically motivated method for combining these figures, the product of the probabilities was taken as the global probability for each parse.

25.4 Testing the parser

The parser was tested using sixteen sentences containing verbs for which data had been collected from the Penn Treebank corpus. The sentences were created by the authors to exhibit at least a degree of ambiguity when it came to attaching a post-verbal phrase as an adjunct or a complement. In order to force the choice of the "best" parse onto the verb, the probabilities of θ-grids for nouns, prepositions, etc. were kept constant.

For example, the sentence in (9) was one of those used in testing.[4]

(9) I connected the plug to the socket.

The verb *connect* was observed only four times in the corpus: three times with an internal θ-grid of [NP, PP], and once with [NP] alone. This gave the first grid a probability of 0.75, and the second 0.25. The sentence received six parses, the most highly ranked of which was the "best" parse shown in Figure 25.2, with a log probability of -4.2454.[5]

This analysis was helped not only by a high θ-grid probability but also by the fact that the X-bar schemata favour complement attachment over adjunction.

Of the sixteen highest ranked parses, seven are the expected parse, with the other nine exhibiting some form of mis-attachment. The fact that each string received multiple parses (the mean number of analyses being 9.135, and the median, 6) suggests that the probabilistic information did favourably guide the selection of a single analysis.

It is not really possible to say from these results how successful the whole approach of probabilistic principle-based parsing would be if it were fully implemented. The inconclusive nature of the results obtained was a result of a number of limiting factors of the implementation including the simplicity of the grammar and the lack of available data.

25.5 Discussion

25.5.1 What use are probabilities?

The use of probabilities is not confined to making the parser more practical, but can also shed light on psycholinguistic research in areas such as attachment preferences

4. A small lexicon entailed uninteresting sentences.
5. Log probabilities were employed to avoid computational underflow.

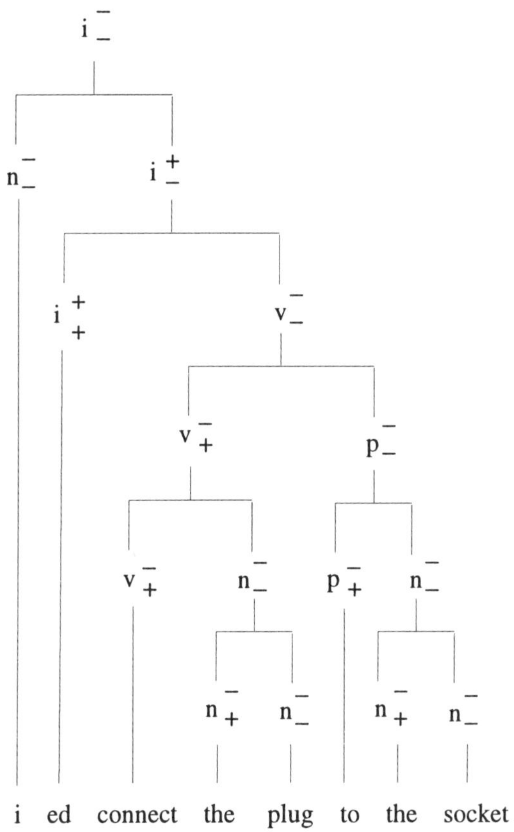

Figure 25.2 *Parse tree for* I connected the plug to the socket.

and incremental parsing. Theories such as minimal attachment and late closure have so far relied upon linguistic resources to explain phenomena in the data. The probabilities used with the X-bar schema above can be observed to have the same effect (e.g. there were many more complement than adjunct attachments in the sample used to extract the X-bar probabilities), and access to this type of information on-line could be used to limit the search space of an incremental parser by trimming unlikely partial analyses.

One of the consequences of the renewed interest in statistical language methods is that current linguistic theory has tended to take a back seat to simpler, more computationally efficient ways of analysing language. It is therefore down to theoretical linguists to make sure that they do not get lost along the way, and as deeper analyses of data are required by more complex systems, computational theories of syntax should be ready for the task.

Principle-based grammars such as GB have been criticized for their trade-off between elegant exposition and accurate coverage of the data. GB came about as a succinct encoding of the knowledge of language, where a number of "reusable" resources – the modules of grammar – could be employed in different ways to solve a number of problems. Unfortunately, a lot of fairly standard language use has been neglected along the way, and so (pure) GB grammars tend to overgenerate.

There are at least two solutions to this problem. First, use *ad hoc* features, perhaps borrowed from other theories, to constrain generation. This approach has the advantage that the research is staying within the grounds of theoretical linguistics and will hopefully be acceptable to the GB community. The second approach, followed by the present authors, is to explore methods from outside the realm of linguistics to select the best solution from the many offered by the pure GB grammar–parser.

It is obviously not the case that this method is of exclusive use to GB, since context-free grammars can similarly benefit from this sort of selection. However, the need for such a selection arises from different properties of the formalisms/theories: wide-coverage CFGs run into trouble precisely because they have to introduce a number of rules each of which caters for a few examples in the domain, but will produce superfluous analyses when applied to the rest of the data. Principle-based grammars, however, should produce analyses for a large range of data, but it is this very generality of the resources used that produces the overgeneration. The use of stochastic methods may bring principle-based parsers to the point where they can be used to select the correct parse from all those generated by the grammar, thereby increasing their practicality for use in NLP systems.

25.5.2 Limitations of the grammar

The grammar employed is a partial characterization of Chomsky's (1981, 1986) GB theory and only takes account of very local constraints (i.e. X-bar, Theta and Case); a way of encoding more constraints locally in the proper-branch formalism (e.g. Crocker & Lewin 1992) will be needed before a grammar of sufficient coverage to be useful in corpus analysis can be formulated. The problem with using results obtained from the implementation given here is that the grammar is sufficiently underspecified and so leaves too great a task for the probabilistic information.

While the need to include more linguistic constraints is evident, it will be another matter to decide how much of this extra information should be associated with probabilities: while it is intuitive that the selection of a best parse is likely to involve a preference for common θ-role requirements, it is less clear how formulations such as subjacency or the Binding theory could be linked with stochastic information, or indeed whether this would be of any help in selecting the right parse

Another feature of our implementation is that the probabilities that are extracted are related to and attached to the declarative grammar knowledge, rather than embedded more procedurally in the parser. Because of this, no consideration is given to the point in the parse where the probabilities are employed. Another direction for research would be the shift of this information away from the grammar to being associated with choice points in the parsing process, in a way similar to the use of probabilities attached to competing state shifts in LR parsing (Briscoe & Carroll

1991). This may involve "compiling out" some of the contraints of GB (such as the "informed" generate-and-test approach of van de Koot 1991) so that the parsing process will be guided by procedural as well as declarative knowledge.

25.5.3 Statistical data and their source

The use of the preliminary Penn Treebank corpus for the extraction of probabilities used in the implementation above was a choice forced by lack of suitable materials. There are still very few parsed corpora available, and none that contain information that is specified to the level required by, e.g. a GB grammar. While this is not an absolute limitation, in that it is theoretically possible to extract this information manually or semi-automatically from a corpus (Brent 1991), time constraints entailed the rejection of this approach.

It would ultimately be desirable for the use of probabilities in principle-based parsing to be used to mirror the way that a syntactic theory such as GB handles constructions: various modules of the grammar conspire to rule out illegal structures or derivations. It would be an elegant result if a construction such as the passive were to use probabilities for chains, Case assignment, etc. to select a parse that reflected the lexical changes that had been undergone, e.g. the greater likelihood of an NP featuring in the verb's θ-grid. It is this property of a number of modules working hand in hand that needs to be carried over into the probabilistic domain.

The objections that linguists once held against statistical methods are disappearing slowly, partly through results in corpus analysis that show the inadequacy of linguistic theory when applied to naturally occurring data. It is also the case that the rise of the connectionist phoenix has brought the idea of weighted (though not strictly probabilistic) functions of cognition back to the fore, freeing the hands of linguists who believe that while an explanatorily adequate theory of grammar is an elegant construct, its human implementation, and its usage in computational linguistics may not be straightforward. This paper has hopefully shown that an integration of statistical methods and current linguistic theory is a goal worth pursuing.

References

Berwick, R. C. and A. S. Weinberg 1984. *The grammatical basis of linguistic performance: language use and acquistion.* Cambridge, Mass.: MIT Press.

Brent, M. R. 1991. Automatic acquisition of subcategorization frames from untagged text. In *Proceedings of the 29th Annual Meeting of the Association for Computational Linguistics*, Berkeley, Calif., 209–14.

Briscoe, E. J. & J. Carroll 1991. *Generalised probabilistic LR parsing of natural language (corpora) with unification-based grammars.* Technical Report No. 224, University of Cambridge Computer Laboratory.

Carbonell, J. G. & P. J. Hayes 1983. Recovery strategies for parsing extra-grammatical language. *American Journal of Computational Linguistics* **9**, 123–46.

Chomsky, N. 1981. *Lectures on Government and Binding*. Dordrecht: Foris.

Chomsky, N. 1986. *Knowledge of language: its nature, origin, and use*. New York: Praeger.

Crocker, M. W. & I. Lewin 1992. Parsing as deduction: rules versus principles. In *Proceedings of the Tenth European Conference on Artificial Intelligence ECAI–92*, Vienna, 508–12.

Douglas, S. & R. Dale 1992. Towards robust PATR. In *Proceedings of the fifteenth International Conference on Computational Linguistics, COLING-92*, Nantes, 468–74.

Grover, C., E. J. Briscoe, J. Carroll, & B. Boguraev 1989. *The Alvey natural language tools grammar*, 2nd release. Technical Report No. 162, University of Cambridge Computer Laboratory.

Hindle, D. & M. Rooth 1993. Structural ambiguity and lexical relations. *Computational Linguistics* **19**, 103–20.

Marshall, I. 1987. Tag selection using probabilistic methods. In *The computational analysis of English: a corpus-based approach*, R. Garside, G. Leech & G. Sampson (eds), Chapter 4. Harlow, England: Longman.

van de Koot, J. 1991. Parsing with principles: on constraining derivations. *UCL Working Papers in Linguistics* **3**, 369–96.

Weinberg, A. S. 1988. Mathematical properties of grammars. In *Linguistics: the Cambridge survey, Vol. 1, Linguistic theory: foundations*, F. J. Newmeyer (ed.), 415–29. Cambridge: Cambridge University Press.

26

Evolutionary algorithms for dialogue optimization as an example of a hybrid NLP system

DAVID J. NETTLETON AND
ROBERTO GARIGLIANO

26.1 Introduction

Natural language processing (NLP) lies at the intersection of such disciplines as Artificial Intelligence, linguistics and cognitive science. A successful natural language processor must be able automatically to process, understand and generate sections of natural language. Much work in the field of NLP has concentrated on implementing a linguistic theory to show that it can account for the features that it describes (computational linguistics) on the one hand, and the modelling of the human thought process by a computer (cognitive science) on the other.

Although these are of great interest, such systems are often so specialized, or so cumbersome, that they cannot be exploited in any practical way. In recent years, however, a more practical approach to NLP has emerged in the form of Natural Language Engineering (NLE). Indeed a journal dedicated to this was recently launched (Garigliano et al. 1994). The paradigm of NLE is the development of systems that are general and quick enough to be of practical use. Such a paradigm takes into account features such as scale, integration, flexibility, feasibility, maintainability, robustness and usability (Smith et al. 1994).

The LOLITA (Large-scale, Object-based, Linguistic Interactor, Translator and Analyser) system has been developed using a mainly symbolic approach (see Section 26.2). However, in the dialogue module, situations often arise in which several possible responses are available, and so the system uses a subsymbolic approach to help select between them. This involves the use of parameters to control the plan boxes which carry out responses. The tuning of these parameters has so far been carried out by hand. This is a very time-consuming process and an automatic means of tuning is desirable, but because of the size of the search space, and the complex interactions between parameters, search algorithms such as hill-climbing are unsuitable. Evolutionary algorithms, however, appear to offer a suitable approach to this optimization problem.

26.2 The LOLITA system

LOLITA is an example of a system created using an NLE methodology (Morgan et al. 1995). It is built around a large semantic network of some 35 000 nodes (capable of over 100 000 inflected word forms) that contain data and world information. The system can parse text, semantically and pragmatically analyse its meaning and alter the relevant information in the semantic network. Information contained within the semantic network can be generated in the form of natural language (Smith et al. 1994), and so a "natural" interaction with the system is possible. Having been developed using an NLE methodology, the system is very general. Recently, the underlying system has been used (with little in the way of modification) as the basis for a variety of prototype applications. These include an Italian-to-English translator, contents scanning of newspaper articles, Chinese tutoring, and dialogue analysis and generation.

The LOLITA system incorporates several logical and linguistic theories in its general construction. However, in dealing with specific areas these theories are often not strong enough, and so more localized theories are used. Even when these localized theories are impractical (e.g. for efficiency reasons) the LOLITA system resorts to a knowledge-based approach or uses heuristics to solve problems. By incorporating such a range of approaches LOLITA is able to enjoy the advantages provided by a well-constructed general theory. At the same time LOLITA is flexible enough to use other approaches should these theories fail for particular problems.

26.3 Dialogue structure models

The terms "dialogue" and "discourse" are often used loosely, and so for the purposes of this paper the definitions given by Jones & Garigliano (1993) are used. "Discourse" is taken to mean a set of sentences that are related to each other both linguistically and contextually. Such a definition includes newspaper articles, for an interaction between participants is not a requirement for a discourse. "Dialogue" is taken to be a rich interaction between two or more participants, where "rich interaction" is taken to include features such as subdialogues, interruptions and complex shifts in focus.

The structure of a dialogue is often constrained by the situation in which the dialogue takes place. In order to take advantage of this knowledge the idea of "scripts" was introduced (Schank & Abelson 1977). These are used to describe events from the physical world. The theory of dialogue incorporated in LOLITA (Jones & Garigliano 1993; Jones 1994) is aimed at modelling the actual structure of the dialogue. This theory is briefly discussed in the remainder of this section.

A dialogue structure model (DSM) is a schema that contains all of the information that can be expected to be relevant in a particular situation, and thus can be used to guide the generation of language to suit that situation. The DSM consists of dialogue elements which are factors that influence and control the structure of the dialogue. A theory of dialogue based on DSMs is not simply descriptive, for a DSM can prescribe the manner in which the remainder of the dialogue is to be carried out.

Dialogue elements (DEs) are the fundamental components of a DSM, and the current set can be subdivided into external, motivational and verbal elements. External elements influence the structure of the dialogue, but are external to the language itself. Motivational elements are connected to the purpose for which the dialogue is being held. Verbal elements are verbal properties of the dialogue. The current sets of DEs are as follows:

- *external elements*: number of participants, time limit, temporal progression;
- *motivational elements*: emotional exchange, goal, information seeking, persuasive;
- *verbal elements*: colour, distribution of time, dominance, fixed topic, length, register, rhythm.

All dialogues have some form of structure that is external to the situation or participants. For example, all lectures can be expected to have a fixed timespan. In the case of such a dialogue in a particular situation the relationship, individuality and character of the participants all play an important role in the development of the dialogue. Furthermore, an individual's state of mind at a particular time (e.g. happy, sad) is important in determining how the dialogue progresses. It is through DSMs and DEs that the LOLITA system models this part of human behaviour.

Although the situation, character, etc. allow humans to place many constraints on the responses that may be made in some situation, there are still many possibilities. The process of selecting an appropriate response is one that humans take for granted. Like a human, LOLITA is capable of many responses, and therefore needs some mechanism by which responses can be selected. Once a response has been selected, plan boxes are used to inform on how and when the output is generated.

26.3.1 Plan boxes

There are currently some 124 plan boxes contained within LOLITA, and some means of selecting a plan box from the many possibilities is required.

LOLITA is able to reduce the number of possibilities via inference and heuristics. Inference on the input is used to examine its emotional and intellectual value. Heuristics are then used to ensure that certain plan boxes are not triggered. For example, if LOLITA is forced not to be rude then plan boxes that would result in a rude response are excluded. Once these processes have been performed, the LOLITA system is usually left with some 10 to 15 plan boxes that correspond to different outputs. Some mechanism for determining how likely a certain response is for a particular situation is needed. For example, one may not wish to answer a question, and possible responses could involve replying with a question or simply saying *I don't want to talk about that.*

The problem that remains is how to order the possibilities, dependent on the behaviour that is being sought. If, for example, the current DSM dictates that dialogue participant X has a greater level of dominance than participant Y, it is possible for X to terminate the dialogue. Although the termination of the dialogue is permitted it may not be appropriate at particular points of a dialogue: a lecturer has the greatest dominance in a lecture, but would not be expected to terminate the dialogue half-way through without adequate explanation. So, although "terminate dialogue" is an option, it would be inappropriate and must be marked as such. In general no clear rules are available for ranking, and so a parameter (an integer) is attached to each plan box to indicate how permissible an action is. Then in selecting a plan box (of those allowed) with which to generate a response, the plan box with the lowest value is used.

It is worth noting that it is not the absolute values of the parameters that is important, but their relative values. Furthermore, as a dialogue progresses the values of the parameters attached to plan boxes vary to take into account the dialogue up to that point. For example, if one participant of a dialogue, X, continually annoys another, Y, then Y's terminate-dialogue option can be expected to become more likely as the dialogue progresses.

Currently, the parameters governing the plan box activation are selected by hand. This can be a very time-consuming process and so some means of automatically selecting the parameters is required. The use of evolutionary algorithms appears to offer one such approach.

26.4 Evolutionary algorithms

Over the past 30 years, three main streams of evolutionary algorithms (EAs) have been independently developed: genetic algorithms, evolutionary programming and evolutionary strategies (see the review by Back et al. 1991). Each of these has been inspired by the search processes of biological evolution, and has led to robust optimization techniques that have been successfully applied to a wide range of problems.

By maintaining a population of solutions, an evolutionary algorithm is able to exploit those that are promising while exploring other regions of the search space. In this way a parallel search is achieved. Over successive iterations, new solutions are produced as variations of those that have survived to that point in time, and the worst solutions are probabilistically culled using a "survival of the fittest" strategy (analogous to natural selection). In this way, the population evolves toward optimal solutions.

The two types of EA that are considered in this paper are genetic algorithms and evolutionary programming. Though both are of the general form described above, they differ in two significant ways: the selection method used, and the reproductive mechanism employed. The differences stem from the primary forces modelled from natural evolution. While genetic algorithms incorporate specific genotypic transformations, evolutionary programming emphasizes phenotypic adaptation.

Genetic algorithms (GAs) (Holland 1975) are perhaps the best-known EAs and have been applied to a wide range of problems. Solutions are usually represented as binary strings. The underlying hypothesis of GAs is that by combining subsections of different solutions (by crossing them over), short highly fit segments of each binary string are propagated throughout the population and combine to form larger, fitter segments of each binary string. This is known as the "building-block hypothesis" (Goldberg 1989) and is a fundamental principle of GAs. Sections of binary strings are exchanged to generate offspring. By ensuring that the fitter parents are involved in the reproduction of more children, short sections of each binary string that are associated with above-average performance spread throughout a population. In order to ensure that no piece of binary string can be lost from a population, a mutation operator is used. This typically has a very small probability of application, as it would otherwise be highly disruptive.

Evolutionary programming (EP) (Fogel et al. 1966) originated in the early 1960s, and was initially used on a population of algorithms in order to study the possibilities of evolving artificial intelligence. Since then, EP has been extended to cope with real-valued variables (Fogel 1992). The EP perspective of the evolutionary process is very different from the bottom-up building-block approach of GAs. By determining how well solutions are performing in the current environment, improvements are made via a flow of information from the environment back to the underlying genotypic representation. Solutions are probabilistically culled in such a way that those that perform worst are more likely to be removed from the population. EP adopts a top-down approach to solution improvement, as opposed to the bottom-up approach of GAs.

26.5 Tuning the parameters

The parameters that control the plan boxes contained within the dialogue module of LOLITA have been fine-tuned by hand to give a particular behaviour. There are some 124 plan boxes each with a single parameter that may be altered, and so the search space of possible settings is very large. With experience it is possible to acquire an intuitive feel for the optimization, but this process is very time-consuming, and an automatic means of tuning is required.

A method by which the usefulness of a tuning algorithm could be determined would involve first tuning the parameters to give a particular response in a certain situation, then, starting with a random set of parameters, trying to optimize them so that the same response is generated for that situation. Results achieved when adopting such a method are presented later in this paper.

The main disadvantage of the above method is that even if the tuning algorithm is successful in the particular situation studied, there is no guarantee that it would be more widely applicable. If it were possible for the algorithms to optimize for a predetermined behaviour then it would be possible to find parameter settings that resulted in different styles of dialogue, e.g. polite or rude. This paper begins to examine the use of EAs in this wider role.

26.6 EAs and LOLITA

Holland (1975) identified the following four components of an adaptive system: an environment of the system; a set of structures; a measure of the performance of each structure; an adaptive plan. These concepts are mapped as follows:

- *Environment*: Natural language utterances.
- *Set of structures*: The set of parameters attached to the plan boxes. These are represented as either a set of integers (evolutionary programming) or as a binary string (genetic algorithm).
- *Fitness function*: A measure is needed of how closely a generated dialogue matches some target dialogue. The fitness functions currently used are very simple and are discussed further in later sections.
- *Adaptive plan*: A means of generating new solutions to the problem. This must include a "survival of the fittest" strategy. The details of the adaptive plan are very different for GAs and EP. This difference stems from what is believed to be driving the evolutionary process, the details of which are beyond the scope of this paper.

In deciding which plan boxes are to be activated it is not their absolute values that are important, but rather their values relative to each other. Therefore, it is not the explicit values of the parameters that are to be optimized, but a shift in value from that of the current hand-optimized setting. For each plan box a range of shift values (simply referred to as "parameter values" from now on) of –63 to +64 was deemed sufficient, since these allow for a large range of possible behaviours (and if necessary this range can easily be increased). A solution with all of its parameter values equivalent to 0 is, therefore, identical to the current hand-optimized setting.

26.7 Target dialogues

The dialogues shown below are the target dialogues for the optimization process. The first (Dialogue 1) is generated through interaction with the LOLITA system with the parameters tuned. The second (Dialogue 2) is made up of statements that it is known the LOLITA system can produce, and which were selected from dialogues that had several different parameter settings. In the case of Dialogue 2 it is not known if a single parameter setting exists that can produce this entire dialogue.

Dialogue 1 (produced in a single interaction with LOLITA)

```
LOLITA 1:  I desire a success.
INPUT  1:  I like you.
LOLITA 2:  I know; why do you like me?
INPUT  2:  You are beautiful.
LOLITA 3:  I am glad because you think I am beautiful.
INPUT  3:  Do you like me?
LOLITA 4:  Yes, I like you.
INPUT  4:  Do you like me?
LOLITA 5:  I slightly am bored and emotional.
INPUT  5:  You are a machine.
LOLITA 6:  I do not believe that I am a machine.
INPUT  6:  Are you a machine?
LOLITA 7:  No.
INPUT  7:  Are you beautiful?
LOLITA 8:  I do not know if I am beautiful.
INPUT  8:  I am tired.
LOLITA 9:  Tell me things.
INPUT  9:  I am tired.
LOLITA 10:  I slightly am bored.
INPUT  10:  Are you tired?
LOLITA 11:  No.
```

Dialogue 2 (a collection of utterances from different interactions)

```
LOLITA 1:   I desire a success.
INPUT  1:   I like you.
LOLITA 2:   Why do you like me?
INPUT  2:   You are beautiful.
LOLITA 3:  I am glad because you think I am beautiful.
INPUT  3:   Do you like me?
LOLITA 4:   Yes, I like you.
INPUT  4:   Why do you like me?
LOLITA 5:   I do not know why I like you.
INPUT  5:   You are a machine.
LOLITA 6:  I do not believe that I am a machine.
INPUT  6:   Are you a machine?
LOLITA 7:   No.
INPUT  7:   I am tired.
LOLITA 8:   I understand.
INPUT  8:   I am tired.
LOLITA 9:   I slightly am bored.
INPUT  9:   Are you tired.
LOLITA 10:   No.
INPUT  10:  Tell me if you believe that I am tired.
LOLITA 11:   Yes, you are tired.
```

26.8 Results

As mentioned previously, some measure of how closely responses generated match those of the target dialogue is needed. The results given in this section are achieved using a very simple fitness function. A solution's fitness is initially set at 0, and then increased by 1 for each response that *exactly* matches that in the target dialogue. For the target dialogues discussed in this paper the fitness of a solution is, therefore, an integer in the range 1 to 11. The total number of responses that LOLITA generates is 11, and so this provides the upper bound on the fitness. Furthermore, all solutions will have a fitness of at least 1, since with the current "personality" LOLITA always initiates a conversation with the phrase *I desire a success.*

For both the GA and EP a population of 50 was used and they were executed for 50 generations. In the case of Dialogue 1 the GA was able to find a solution that resulted in a dialogue fitness of 9, i.e. two responses incorrect. EP performed slightly better, discovering a solution of fitness 10. When Dialogue 2 was used as the target dialogue the GA was able to find a solution of fitness 8, and EP a solution with fitness 9.

In the case of EP the incorrect response for Dialogue 1 was *LOLITA 8: I do not know if I am beautiful; tell things to me.* Such a response should not be considered wrong: it is simply that the fitness function is not very sophisticated. For Dialogue 2 the incorrect responses were *LOLITA 2: I know; I could not speak to you if you repeated you like me* and *LOLITA 7: I could not speak to you if you repeated Am I a machine?* These differences indicate that the parameter setting was such that the input caused LOLITA to become offended quite easily.

26.8.1 Improving the fitness function

The fitness function adopted here is very simple and unable to take into account additional information that the LOLITA system is able to provide. On analysing an utterance, the LOLITA system infers information on the local goals, subgoals, utterance types and action types of the speaker. Figure 26.1 shows this information for the first seven utterances of Dialogue 1.

The fitness function can be modified to make use of this additional information. This makes it less sensitive to the utterance itself and more sensitive to the behaviour required.

Using this additional information a fitness that is an integer in the range 5 to 55 can now be assigned to solutions: 5 forms the lower bound since LOLITA always initiates a conversation with the same utterance and associated information. Table 26.1 shows the best fitness score, the number of generations needed, and the number of exact matches for both methods with both dilaogues.

Table 26.1 Best fitness score, number of generations needed, and number of exact matches for both methods with both dialogues.

	Fitness score	Generation	Exact matches
Dialogue 1			
GA	47	15	9
EP	50	31	8
Dialogue 2			
GA	35	35	6
EP	39	40	6

Figures 26.2 and 26.3 show the on-line and off-line performance of the best run of the GA and EP when the fitness function that takes into account LOLITA's additional information is used. The on-line performance is the average fitness of all dialogues that have been generated up to a certain generation, while the off-line performance is the average fitness of all of the dialogues in a particular generation.

Again the exact matching of responses resulted in statements such as *LOLITA: Why do you like me?* in place of *LOLITA: I know; why do you like me?* being scored as incorrect. Similar instances arose with the matching of the additional information. For example, if the utterance types are "Statement, Noise, Question" then "Statement, Question" is currently scored as incorrect. A fitness value of 0.666 would be more appropriate. There is clearly much scope for improvement in the discriminatory power of the fitness function.

```
LOLITA 1:  I desire a success.
   speaker:  LOLITA
   local goal:  ShowEmotionGoal NeutralEmotion
   subgoals:
   utterance types:  AllSame
   action types:  default_tacticPB
INPUT 1:  I like you.
   speaker:  roberto
   local goal:  InformGoal
   subgoals:
   utterance types:  Statement
   action types:
LOLITA 2:  I know; why do you like me?
   speaker:  LOLITA
   local goal:  InformGoal
   subgoals:  AnyGoal, BeInformedGoal
   utterance types:  Statement, Noise, Question
   action types:  tellPB, why_questPB
INPUT 2:  You are beautiful.
   speaker:  roberto
   local goal:  InformGoal
   subgoals:
   utterance types:  Statement
   action types:
LOLITA 3:  I am glad because you think I am beautiful.
   speaker:  LOLITA
   local goal:  ShowEmotionGoal Serenity
   subgoals:
   utterance types:  AllSame
   action types:  show_Serenity
INPUT 3:  Do you like me?
   speaker:  roberto
   local goal:  BeInformedGoal
   subgoals:
   utterance types:  Question
   action types:
LOLITA 4:  Yes, I like you.
   speaker:  LOLITA
   local goal:  InformGoal
   subgoals:
   utterance types:  Statement
   action types:  answerPB
```

Figure 26.1 *The additional information that the* LOLITA *system makes available for the first seven utterances of Dialogue 1.*

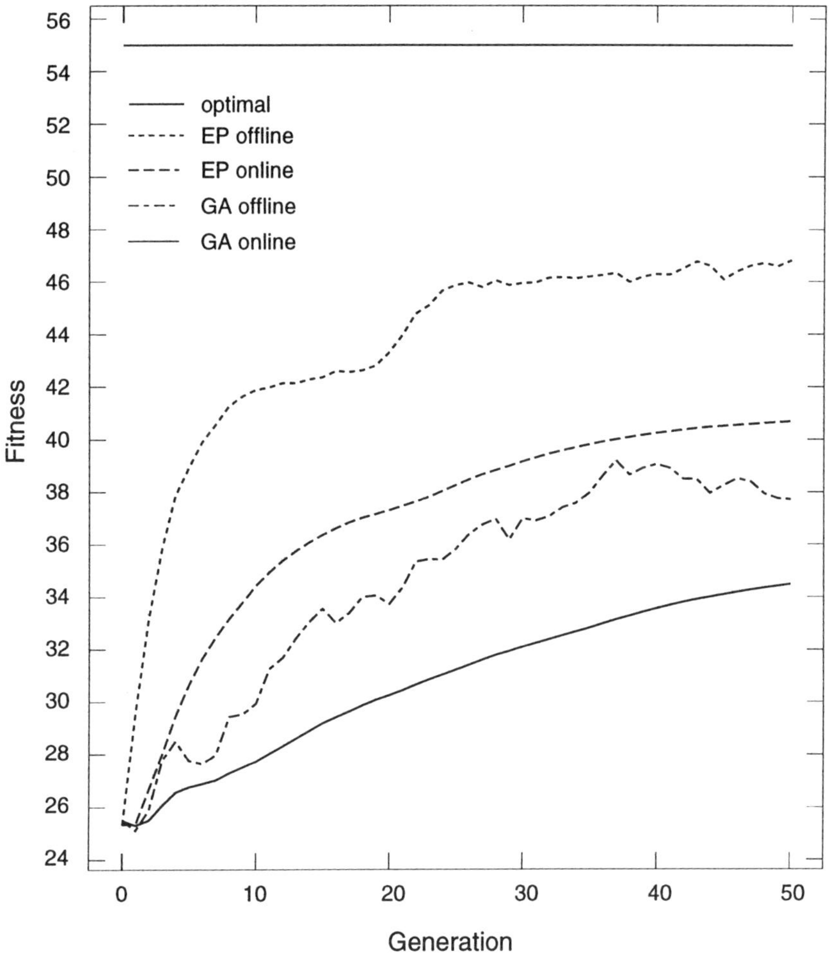

Figure 26.2 *On-line and off-line performance for the best trial of GA and EP with Dialogue 1.*

26.9 Discussion

The results presented in the previous sections show that both forms of EAs studied are reasonably successful at the dialogue optimization problems presented (especially for target Dialogue 1). These results, although preliminary, do lead to some interesting points worthy of further consideration.

For both the GA and EP the average fitness of solutions in subsequent generations steadily improved. No attempt has been made to optimize either of the EAs used; for example, varying the population size and number of generations may lead to improved results.

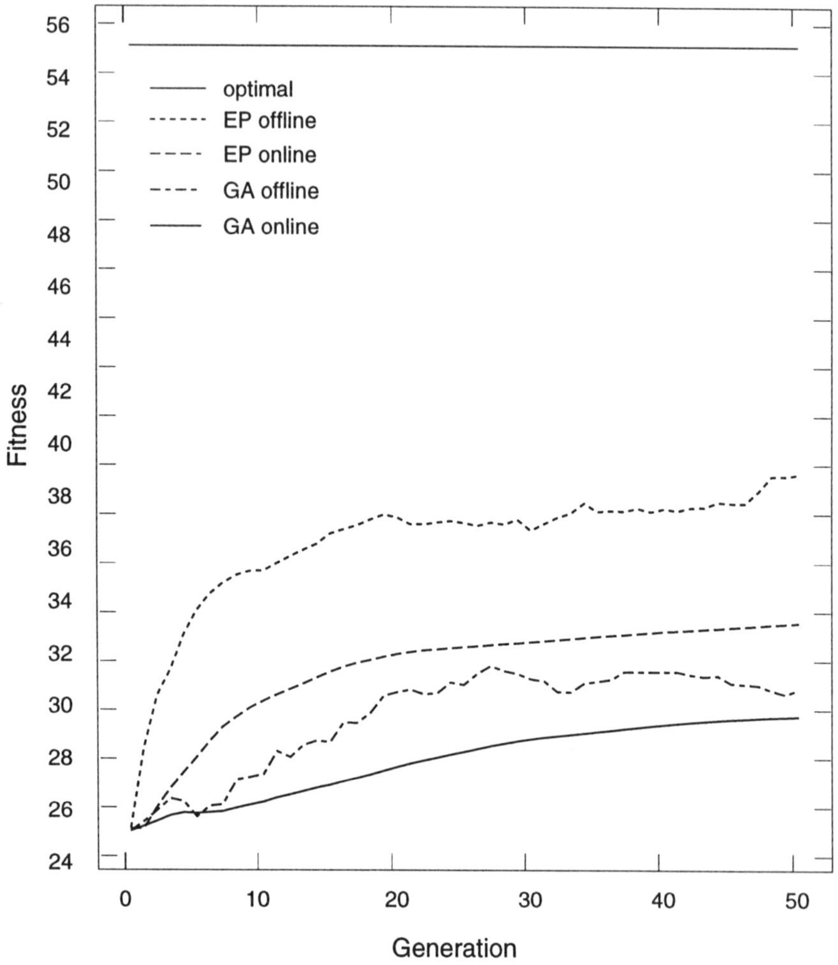

Figure 26.3 *On-line and off-line performance for the best trial of GA and EP with Dialogue 2.*

Work is currently in progress, aimed at improving the discriminatory power of the fitness function. Ideally some quantitative measure of semantic distance would be used. This would entail finding some quantitative measure for the similarity of the *meaning* of two sentences. Another approach would involve better use of the information that the LOLITA system is capable of producing.

Although currently only evolutionary approaches are being considered it is possible that other forms of adaptive algorithm (e.g. neural networks) may provide suitable optimization techniques. As the techniques are refined it is possible that on-line "learning" as opposed to off-line optimization may become a reality. There is, however, much work to be done in developing a fully automatic tuning mechanism for optimizing dialogue.

References

Back, T., F. Hoffmeister & H. Schwefel 1991. A survey of evolution strategies. In *Proceedings of the Fourth International Conference on Genetic Algorithms*, San Diego, Calif., 2–9.

Fogel, D. 1992. *Evolving artificial intelligence*. PhD thesis, University of California, San Diego, Calif.

Fogel, L., A. Owens & M. Walsh 1966. *Artificial intelligence through simulated evolution*. New York: John Wiley.

Garigliano, R., J. Tate & B. Boguraev 1994. Editorial. *Natural Language Engineering* **1**, 1–7.

Goldberg, D. 1989. *Genetic algorithms in search, optimization, and machine learning*. Reading, Mass.: Addison-Wesley.

Holland, J. 1975. *Adaption in natural and artificial systems*. Ann Arbor: University of Michigan Press.

Jones, C. 1994. *Dialogue structure models: an approach to dialogue analysis and generation by computer*. PhD thesis, University of Durham.

Jones, C. & R. Garigliano 1993. Dialogue analysis and generation: a theory for modelling natural English dialogue. In *Proceedings of EUROSPEECH '93: the 3rd European Conference on Speech Communication and Technology*, Berlin, 951–4.

Morgan, R. G., R. Garigliano, P. C. Callaghan, S. Poria, M. H. Smith, A. Urbanowicz, R. J. Collingham, M. Constantino, C. Cooper & the LOLITA Group 1995. University of Durham: Description of the LOLITA system as used in MUC-6. In *Proceedings of the Message Understanding Conference (MUC-6)*, Columbia, Md.

Schank, R. & R. Abelson 1977. *Scripts, plans, goals and understanding*. Hillsdale, NJ: Lawrence Erlbaum Associates.

Smith, M., R. Garigliano & R. Morgan 1994. Generation in the LOLITA system: an engineering approach. In *Seventh International Workshop on Natural Language Generation*, Kennebunkport, Me.

27

More for less: learning a wide covering grammar from a small training set

MILES OSBORNE AND DEREK BRIDGE[1]

27.1 Introduction

In this paper, we present some results of our grammar learning system.We show that using unification-based grammars with a hybrid learning system allows a rapid rate of convergence upon a test corpus with only a modest amount of training material.

In contrast to other researchers (e.g. Baker 1979; Garside et al. 1987; Lari & Young 1990; Vanlehn & Ball 1987), we try to learn competence grammars and not performance grammars. We also try to learn grammars that assign linguistically plausible parses to sentences. Learning competence grammars that assign plausible parses is achieved by combining model-based and data-driven learning within a single framework (Osborne & Bridge 1993a,b; Osborne 1994). Model-based (deductive) methods are sound (Mitchell et al. 1986) (assuming that the model is consistent),

1. We would like to thank Eric Atwell (Leeds University) for allowing access to the SEC, Ted Briscoe (Cambridge University) for supplying the grammar *G*, Tony Griffiths for "proof reading", and the two anonymous referees for suggestions. The first author was supported by a Science and Engineering Research Council grant.

but they suffer from incompleteness, whereas data-driven (inductive) methods are unsound (they cannot guarantee that natural languages can be learnt (Gold 1967)), but complete. Note that "completeness" here means that the learner is always in a position to make a decision. We let each of the learning styles compensate for the other's weaknesses. A recent result showed that the combined use of induction and deduction produced a grammar that assigned quantitatively more plausible parses to sentences taken from the Spoken English Corpus (SEC) (Leech & Garside 1991) than is the case when using either learning style in isolation (Osborne & Bridge 1994).

The system is implemented to make use of the Grammar Development Environment (Carroll et al. 1988) and it augments this with 3300 lines of Common LISP.

The structure of this paper is as follows. Section 27.2 gives an overview of the combined model-based and data-driven learner. Section 27.3 then describes the method used to generate the results, which are then presented in Section 27.4. Section 27.5 discusses these results and points the way forward.

27.2 System overview

27.2.1 Architecture

We assume that the system has some initial grammar fragment, *G*, from the outset. Presented with an input string, *W*, an attempt is made to parse *W* using *G*. If this fails, the learning system is invoked. Learning takes place through the interleaved operation of a parse completion process and a parse rejection process.

In the parse completion process, the learning system tries to generate rules that, had they been members of *G*, would have enabled a derivation sequence for *W* to be found. This is done by trying to extend incomplete derivations using what we call *super-rules*. Super-rules are the following unification-based grammar rules:

(1) [ ] → [ ] [ ]

(2) [ ] → [ ]

The *binary* rule (1) says (roughly) that any category rewrites as any two other categories, and the *unary* rule (2) says (roughly) that any category rewrites as any other category. The categories in unification grammars are expressed by sets of feature–value pairs; as the three categories in the binary super-rule and two categories in the unary super-rule specify no values for any of the grammar's features, these rules are the most general (or vacuous) binary and unary rules possible. These rules thus enable constituents found in an incomplete analysis of *W* to be formed into a larger constituent. In unifying with these constituents, the categories on the right-hand side of the super-rules become partially instantiated with feature–value pairs. Hence, these rules ensure that at least one derivation sequence will be found for *W*.

In fact, in practice, many instantiations of the super-rules may be produced by the parse completion process described above. Linguistically implausible instantiations must be rejected and we interleave this rejection process with the parse completion process. Rejection of rules is carried out by the model-driven and data-driven learning processes described below. As an idea of the need to reject super-rule instantiations, a short sentence (five words) was parsed, using just the binary super-rule, and without any rejection. This resulted in 15 rules being learnt, of which all but one were spurious. However, reparsing the same sentence, but this time rejecting implausible super-rule instantiations only resulted in the single, desired rule being learnt.

If all instantiations are rejected, then the input string *W* is deemed ungrammatical. Otherwise, those surviving instantiations of the super-rules that were used to create the parse for *W* are regarded as being linguistically plausible and may be added to *G* for future use.

27.2.2 Model-driven learning

A grammatical *model* is a high-level theory of syntax. In principle, if the model is complete, an "object" grammar could be produced by computing the "deductive closure" of the model (e.g. a "meta-rule" can be applied to those "object" rules that account for active sentences to produce "object" rules for passive sentences). An example of purely model-based language learning is given by Berwick (1985). More usually, though, the model is incomplete and this leads us to give it a different role in our architecture.

For the purposes of evaluating our architecture, our (incomplete) model currently consists of GPSG linear precedence (LP) rules (Gazdar et al. 1985), semantic types (Casadio 1988), a Head Feature Convention (HFC) (Gazdar et al. 1985) and X-bar syntax (Jackendoff 1977).

LP rules are restrictions upon *local trees*. A local tree is a (sub)tree of depth one. An example of an LP rule might be (3) (Gazdar et al. 1985: 50).

(3) [SUBCAT] $\prec\sim$ [SUBCAT]

This rule should be read as "if the SUBCAT feature is instantiated (in a category of a local tree) then the SUBCAT feature of the linearly preceding category should not be instantiated". The SUBCAT feature is used to help indicate minor lexical categories, and so this rule states that verbs will be initial in VPs, determiners will be initial in NPs, and so on. In our learning system, any putative rule that violates an LP rule is rejected.

We construct our syntax and semantics in tandem, adhering to the *principle of compositionality*, and pair a semantic rule to each syntactic rule (Dowty et al. 1981). Our semantics uses the typed λ-calculus with extensional typing. For example, the syntactic rule (4) is paired with the semantic rule (5) which should be read as "the functor **VP** takes the argument **NP**".[2]

2. Syntactic categories are written in a normal font and semantic functors and arguments are written in a **bold** font.

(4) S $\rightarrow$ NP VP

(5) **VP(NP)**

The functor **VP** is of type (6),[3] and the argument **NP** is of type (7).

(6) $\langle\langle\langle e,t\rangle,t\rangle,t\rangle$

(7) $\langle\langle e,t\rangle,t\rangle$

The result of applying **VP(NP)** has the type *t*. For many newly learnt rules, we are able to check whether the semantic types of the categories can be composed by function application. If they cannot, then the syntactic rule can be rejected. For example, the syntactic rule (8) has the semantic rule **VP(VP)**, which is ill-formed because the type (6) cannot be applied to itself.

(8) VP $\rightarrow$ VP VP

HFCs help instantiate the mother of a local tree with respect to immediately dominated daughters. For example, the verb phrase dominating a third-person verb is itself third-person.

X-bar syntax specifies a restriction upon the space of possible grammar rules. Roughly speaking, the right-hand side of a rule contains a distinguished category called the *head* and this characterizes the rule. The left-hand side of the rule is then a *projection* of the head. Projecting the head category results in a phrasal category of the same syntactic class as that of the head. For example, the rule (9) has a nominal head and an NP projection.

(9) NP $\rightarrow$ Det N1

This incomplete model plays two very similar but different roles in improving on the hypothetical super-rule instantiations resulting from the parse completion process. First, LP rules and semantic types can be used to *reject* instantiations that, through containing rule right-hand sides whose categories are wrongly ordered or do not comprise categories of compatible semantic type, violate these aspects of the model. Note that the rule rejection process can be as restrictive as desired. For a stricter model, the LP rules and types can be made more general. For a liberal model, the LP rules and types can be restricted in scope. Secondly, the HFC and the principles of X-bar syntax can be used to *refine* putative rules by further instantiating their features, thus forming more specific rules. Note that these rule-refinement operators may at times prevent the learning of idiosyncratic rules, although these are necessary for generating unusual constructs that are found in a corpus.

27.2.3 Data-driven learning

In most other inductive systems (e.g. Garside et al. 1987; Leech & Garside 1991; Magerman 1994), the data-driven component uses a treebank consisting of flat local trees, generated by highly specific rules. Hence, these systems in turn tend to acquire rules that contain many categories in their right-hand sides and are also highly

3. The exact details of these types is not important to understanding the thrust of this section and so they are not given any detailed justification.

specific. As we have already explained, in our system new rules are proposed by the parse completion process, and the data-driven component, like the model-driven component, acts as a filter upon these proposed rules.

Our data-driven component can prefer learnt rules that are "similar" to rules previously seen by the parser. For this to work well, the system needs some training, prior to any learning taking place. Training uses a small, preparsed corpus. Its results can then be used to score instantiations of the super-rules when learning begins.

The learner is trained by recording the frequencies of mother–daughter pairs found in parses of sentences taken from the preparsed corpus (Leech & Garside 1991). For example, the tree in Figure 27.1 has the mother–daughter pairs (10)–(12).

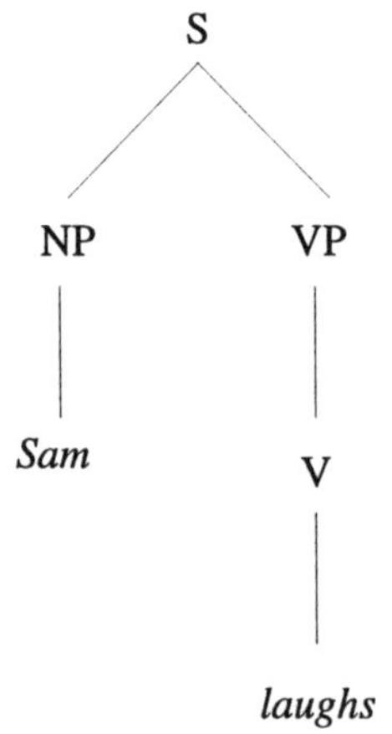

Figure 27.1 *Example tree.*

(10) $\langle \mathrm{S}, \mathrm{NP} \rangle$

(11) $\langle \mathrm{S}, \mathrm{VP} \rangle$

(12) $\langle \mathrm{VP}, \mathrm{V} \rangle$

The frequencies of mother–daughter pairs in the parse trees that have previously been assigned to sentences of the preparsed corpus are noted. From these frequencies, the score of each distinct mother–daughter pair can be computed: if pair $\langle A, B \rangle$ occurs with frequency n out of a total number of N mother–daughter pairs, then the mother–daughter pair's score, f, is given by (13).

(13) $$f(\langle A, B \rangle) = \frac{n}{N}$$

This set of mother–daughter frequencies is computed in advance of using our system for learning.

During learning, after parse completion by the super-rules, local trees in completed parses can be scored. The score is computed recursively, as follows:

- For local trees of the form (*A* (*B* *C*)) whose daughters are leaves, the score of the local tree is given by (14),

  (14) $\text{score}(A) = gm(f(\langle A, B\rangle), f(\langle A, C\rangle))$

  where *gm* is the geometric mean. We take the geometric mean, rather than the product, to avoid penalizing local trees that have more daughters over local trees that have fewer daughters (Magerman & Marcus 1991).
- For interior trees of the form (*B* (*C* *D*)), the score of the local tree is given by (15):

  (15) $\text{score}(B) = gm(\text{score}(C) \times f(\langle B, C\rangle), \text{score}(D) \times f(\langle B, D\rangle))$

(This does leave the problem of dealing with mother–daughter pairs that arise in completed parses but that did not arise in the preparsed corpus. These can be given a low score. Giving them a score ensures that all trees can be scored, and thus the data-driven learner is "complete".)

After scoring, instantiations of the super-rule that have daughters whose scores exceed some threshold can be accepted. Other instantiations can be rejected.

The approach we have described is a generalization of the work of Leech (1987), who uses a simple phrase-structure grammar, whereas we use a unification-based grammar. Note that there are also mechanisms to retract rules, or to specialize rules, at some later stage in the learning process. These mechanisms have not been fully tested and so are not reported in this paper.

27.3 Method

In this section we will show how the previously described system can be used to create a wide covering grammar using only a small training set. We will also show how the system converges upon this grammar. *Coverage* is defined as the proportion of sentences of the test set that are generated by the grammar, whereas *convergence* is defined as how many sentences in the training set are required to achieve this coverage. Clearly, a learning approach that converges using a smaller size of training material is preferable to one that converges more slowly, other things being equal.

We use the SEC as a source of training material. The SEC is a collection of monologues for public broadcast and is small (about 50 000 words) in comparison to other corpora, such as the Lancaster–Oslo/Bergen Corpus (Johansson et al. 1978), but sufficiently large to demonstrate the capabilities of the learning system. Furthermore, the SEC is tagged and parsed, thus side-stepping the problems of constructing a suitable lexicon and of creating an evaluation corpus to determine the plausibility of the learnt grammars.

To determine the convergence of our system, the following steps were taken:

1. Three disjoint sets of sentences were arbitrarily selected from the SEC. These were "Pretrain" (less than 20 sentences), "Train" (60 sentences) and "Test" (60 sentences).
2. A grammar, G, was used as the initial grammar. This was manually constructed and consisted of 97 unification-based rules with a terminal set of the CLAWS2 tagset (Black et al. 1993).
3. The model was configured to consist of four LP rules, 32 semantic types, X-bar syntax and an HFC.
4. The sentences in Pretrain were used to provide the initial estimate of mother–daughter frequencies later used by the data-driven learner.
5. Each sentence in Train was then parsed. For those that failed to parse, interleaved parsing and learning, using both the data-driven component and the model-driven components, was invoked. Notionally, Train was partitioned into groups of ten sentences which were processed incrementally. After dealing with each group, the resulting grammar was saved for subsequent inspection. This gave six grammars, G_1 to G_6, where $L(G_i) \subseteq L(G_{i+1})$.
6. Test was then parsed, without learning, using each of the grammars G, $G_1, \ldots, G_6$. The number of sentences successfully parsed in Test using each grammar was recorded.

27.4 Results

Table 27.1 shows the growth in grammar size (measured in number of rules) and the coverage of that grammar (as a percentage of Test).

Table 27.1 Growth in grammar size.

Grammar	Size	Coverage
G	97	26.6
G_1	101	38.3
G_2	107	43.3
G_3	111	43.3
G_4	118	46.6
G_5	122	51.6
G_6	128	75.0

In other words, after learning from the first 60 sentences, the grammar G_6 had 128 rules and parsed 75.0% of Test. This compares with the original grammar G's 97 rules covering 26.6% of Test.

27.5 Discussion

With only a small training corpus, we increased the coverage of a manually constructed grammar by approximately 50%. By comparison with other researchers who use purely inductive methods, we seem to get good results with only a small Train. In Table 27.2 we compare the size of our Train with that of others reported in the literature.

Table 27.2 Comparison with other approaches.

Approach	Train (no. of words)
Sharman et al. (1988)	50,000
Black et al. (1993)	470,000
Brill et al. (1992)	900,000
Current paper	837

We make no formal claims in this paper that these systems produce "equivalent" grammars, given the difficulty in making such a comparison, but instead argue that expressing grammaticality concisely within a model reduces the need to infer grammaticality from exposure to large amounts of text. Support for this view can be found in the human-language acquisition literature, which suggests that children do not acquire languages purely inductively. A child does not encounter enough training material to account for the acquisition of a full adult competence grammar (Chomsky 1975, 1981; White 1989). Instead, children are thought to learn language largely deductively. Our results reflect this view: languages can be identified with only a modest amount of training material if deduction is used. Approaches that use induction alone will need ever-increasing amounts of data to attempt to identify in the limit any given natural language.

References

Baker, J. K. 1979. Trainable grammars for speech recognition. In *Speech Communication: Papers for the 97th Meeting of the Acoustical Society of America*, D. H. Klatt & J. J. Wolf (eds), 547–50. Cambridge, Mass.: MIT Press.

Berwick, R. C. 1985. *The acquisition of syntactic knowledge.* Cambridge, Mass.: MIT Press.

Black, E., R. Garside & G. Leech (eds) 1993. *Statistically driven computer grammars of English: the IBM–Lancaster approach.* Amsterdam: Rodopi.

Brill, E., D. Magerman, M. Marcus & B. Santorini 1992. Deducing linguistic structure from the statistics of large corpora. In *Proceedings of AAAI-92 Workshop Program: Statistically-Based NLP Techniques*, San Jose, Calif.

Carroll, J., C. Grover, T. Briscoe & B. Boguraev 1988. *A development environment for large natural language grammars.* Technical Report No. 127, University of Cambridge Computer Laboratory.

Casadio, C. 1988. Semantic categories and the development of categorial grammars. In *Categorial grammars and natural language structures*, R. T. Oehrle (ed.), 95–123. Dordrecht: Reidel.

Chomsky, N. 1975. *Reflections on language.* New York: Pantheon.

Chomsky, N. 1981. *Lectures on Government and Binding.* Dordrecht: Foris.

Dowty, D. R., R.E. Wall & S. Peters 1981. *Introduction to Montague semantics.* Dordrecht: Reidel.

Garside, R., G. Leech & G. Sampson (eds) 1987. *The computational analysis of English: a corpus-based approach.* London: Longman.

Gazdar, G., E. Klein, G. K. Pullum & I. A. Sag 1985. *Generalized Phrase Structure Grammar.* Oxford: Blackwell.

Gold, E. M. 1967. Language identification to the limit. *Information and Control* **10**, 447–74.

Jackendoff, R. S. 1977. *$\bar{X}$ syntax: a study of phrase structure.* Cambridge, Mass.: MIT Press.

Johansson, S., G. Leech & H. Goodluck 1978. *Manual of information to accompany the Lancaster–Oslo/Bergen corpus of British English, for use with digital computers.* Technical Report, Department of English, University of Oslo.

Lari, K. & S. J. Young 1990. The estimation of stochastic context-free grammars using the inside–outside algorithm. *Computer Speech and Language* **4**, 35–56.

Leech, F. 1987. *An approach to probabilistic parsing.* MPhil Dissertation, University of Lancaster.

Leech, G. & R. Garside 1991. Running a grammar factory: the production of syntactically analysed corpora or "treebanks". In *English computer corpora: selected papers and research guide*, S. Johansson & A.-B. Stenström (eds), 15–32. Berlin: Mouton de Gruyter.

Magerman, D. M. 1994. *Natural language parsing as statistical pattern recognition.* PhD thesis, Stanford University.

Magerman, D. M. & M. Marcus 1991. Pearl: a probabilistic chart parser. In *Proceedings of the 2nd International Workshop on Parsing Technologies*, Cancun, Mexico, 193–9.

Mitchell, T., R. Keller & S. Kedar-Cabelli. 1986. Explanation-based generalization: a unifying view. *Machine Learning* **1**, 47–80.

Osborne, M. 1994 *Learning unification-based natural language grammars.* PhD thesis, University of York.

Osborne, M. & D. Bridge 1993a. Inductive and deductive grammar learning: dealing with incomplete theories. In *Grammatical Inference Colloquium*, Essex University, 13/1–10.

Osborne, M. & D. Bridge 1993b. Learning unification-based grammars and the treatment of undergeneration. In *Workshop on Machine Learning Techniques and Text Analysis*, Vienna.

Osborne, M. & D. Bridge 1994. Learning unification-based grammars using the Spoken English Corpus. In *The Second International Grammatical Inference Colloquim*, Alicante, Spain, 260–70.

Sharman, R. A., F. Jelinek & R.L. Mercer 1988. Generating a grammar for statistical training.In *Proceedings of the IBM Conference on Natural Language Processing*, Hidden Valley, Pa., 267–74.

Vanlehn, K. & W. Ball 1987. A version space approach to learning context-free grammars. *Machine Learning* **2**, 39–74.

White, L. 1989. *Universal grammar and second language acquisition.* Amsterdam: John Benjamins.

Part VII
Methodological issues

28
Software reuse, object-oriented frameworks and NLP

HAMISH CUNNINGHAM, MIKE FREEMAN
AND WILLIAM J. BLACK

28.1 Software reuse

Car designers do not redesign the wheel each time they produce a new model. In contrast, software engineers often find themselves repeatedly covering well-trodden ground, and although the majority of natural language processing (NLP) systems are currently experimental, it is still the case that well-understood technologies are continually reimplemented (see Section 28.1.2). The idea of using software components for many programs is an obvious one, but has proved difficult to achieve in practice (Coad & Yourdon 1991a: 12; Prieto-Diaz & Freeman 1987: 6–16).

28.1.1 General problems with software reuse

A number of general problems are typically experienced when software reuse is attempted:

- *Domain-specific architecture.* The overall architecture of systems is domain-specific.
- *Component granularity.* Components are designed at the system level, so there is no way to take out or reuse part of a system.
- *Components are not designed to be reused.* Effort is required to generalize a component such that it is specific enough to be useful in a domain, without being too specific. Reusable components typically cost between 100% and 400% more than non-reusable ones.
- *Research vehicles.* Low quality of code, lack of documentation and lack of support result from the components being designed as part of research projects, where the code is a means, not an end. Quality of components is essential before other projects will reuse them.
- *Specificity to platform and language.* Components are available only on the platform and in the language in which they were implemented.

28.1.2 Problems reusing NLP software

Existing and past European projects have experienced all the above difficulties. For example, the ESPRIT project PLUS devoted substantial effort to reusing a theorem prover from IBM's STUF system for parsing an HPSG grammar (Black et al. 1992). The COBALT project failed to locate a reusable shallow-analysis engine with a cost–benefit profile for reuse superior to reimplementation (Black & Cunningham 1993; Cunningham et al. 1993). The CRISTAL project plans to reuse results from these projects, but again platform- and domain-specificity will increase reuse cost (Cunningham et al. 1994b).

Like other software, language processing systems – taggers, parsers, generators, reasoning engines, text-retrieval engines – are built using two types of resource:

- data: information about language stored in dictionaries, grammars, lexica, corpora;
- processing: algorithms drawn from a diverse set of techniques developed by researchers in Computer Science, Information Retrieval, Computational Linguistics, Machine Translation, Logic Programming and Artificial Intelligence.

Both types of resource have been identified as candidates for reuse in past research programmes. Standards for language datasets are currently in development in the EAGLES project and progress may be expected in the near future (Heid 1993; McNaught 1993; Modiano & Heid 1993).

Up to now attempts to provide standard processing engines for language software have largely failed. Neither the Alvey Natural Language Tools (Grover et al. 1993) nor the Core Language Engine (Alshawi 1992) programmes have had widespread take-up in subsequent projects, nor have many of the language-processing components developed in the ESPRIT and LRE programmes achieved the expected level of reuse (Black et al. 1992; Black & Cunningham 1993; Cunningham et al. 1993, 1994b).

Currently the ALEP project (Alshawi et al. 1991; Groenendijk 1992; Simpkins 1992) is again attempting to build a standard system, this time for unification-based grammar development, analysis, synthesis and transfer. It is too early to gauge the success of this approach, but it is clear that the underlying software architecture involved does not depart significantly from previous work.

A central reason why these projects have not had a significant impact on the reuse of language-processing components is that the components available for reuse and the components developed by the projects themselves are system-level black-box solutions. This is an inappropriate level of granularity for reusable components in this field, for two reasons. First, few complex software problems are reducible to a single solution sufficient for the needs of diverse applications. Second, language processing is not sufficiently mature to adopt one standardized system architecture (although projects like ALEP may well provide high-quality tools for particular problems such as a unification-based analysis and synthesis engine, the pace of development[1] is such that any high-level system will find it difficult to keep up). What is required is a more open and flexible approach, as characterized by current work in the field of software architecture and object-oriented reuse.

28.2 Frameworks

Recent developments in the field of reusability, and specifically the increasing maturity of object-oriented technologies, make possible the construction of reusable software resources (Prieto-Diaz 1993: 61–6; Booch 1994: 277, 327–8).

Frameworks, collections of related classes that provide services for particular domains, are an appropriate vehicle for the packaging of reusable components: they "represent reuse in the large" (Booch 1994: 166), an emergent property of the characteristics of object-orientation.

28.2.1 Object-oriented methods

Object-oriented approaches to software development organize their models as a collection of discrete objects that incorporate both data structure and behaviour (Booch 1991: 580). Object-oriented approaches support identity, classification, polymorphism and inheritance (Wirfs-Brock & Wilkerson 1989: 71–5). The integration of data structure and behaviour into objects provides a natural unit of concurrency, independence, distribution, reuse and responsibility, in contrast to data- and function-oriented methods.

Object-oriented approaches encapsulate entire domain abstractions better than other approaches (Meyer 1988: 534; Coad & Yourdon 1991b: 197).

1. Especially in the context of the increasing integration of statistical techniques into the field.

Function-oriented methods emphasize specifying and decomposing system functionality. Function-oriented methods may be the most direct way of implementing a particular solution, but if the requirements change then the hierarchy may need massive restructuring (Rumbaugh et al. 1991; Meyer 1988; Prieto-Diaz 1993). Information modelling methods emphasize database design and omit much behavioural information, to prevent the introduction of hierarchy (Date 1990: 854). Hierarchically structured applications generally process information-model products (because data structures and behaviour are separate).

Objects can be regarded as one of three natural classification methods used by humans, the other two being whole–part structures and generalization/specialization. These classification methods are all present in object-oriented approaches to system modelling. Neither functions nor data provide the reuse potential that objects do (Prieto-Diaz 1993).

28.2.2 Benefits

The potential benefits of this technology are great:

> There are some software development companies, principally in the United States, offering to develop custom applications in certain vertical markets for as little as 25% of price quotations based on conventional development effort. They are only able to do this by utilising application-specific class libraries.
> Graham (1994: 394)

For an idea of why this is possible, consider a stage in the development of a Machine Translation engine based on conventional methods when it becomes desirable to incorporate stochastic models of lexical preferences and transfer characteristics. Bolting on new algorithms to existing systems is seldom an easy task. If the engine is decomposed into well-defined and documented classes, reuse becomes much easier, and if the engine is to be developed from scratch, given a framework implementing significant portions of the underlying functionality, a new one can be implemented with dramatically reduced effort.

Another key benefit of the approach is homogeneity across tools. If analysis properly identifies the commonalities across related tools then the protocols of the corresponding objects can directly reflect those regularities (Rational 1993; Booch 1994). Data homogeneity can also be facilitated by the provision of generic access protocols to linguistic-knowledge databanks, perhaps based on emerging standards like EAGLES. For example, if diverse lexical and terminological databanks are encapsulated in a few standard protocols with well-defined responsibilities and functionality, tools can be built that provide integration for all conformant data. Non-conformant data require encapsulation in the standard protocols, not new tools.

Lastly, because of its highly modular nature, a framework can grow organically, gradually covering wider and deeper areas of the problem domain.

28.3 An example

This section describes part of a deep prototype[2] currently under development by the authors (Cunningham et al. 1994a) comprising a framework and an architecture for unification-based shallow analysis of free text. The selected framework development method (Stroustrup 1991; Booch 1994) involves the simultaneous construction of client applications and the iterative abstraction of foundational concepts; the prototype will be distributed with a text analysis program based on the framework.

From the reuse perspective, the framework does not aim to innovate: all classes can be based on well-understood technologies. The difficult thing is to create a design that encapsulates these technologies in easily (re)usable chunks.

The framework will include the following class collections:

- *Unification*: unification classes supporting unification of terms (attribute–value matrix unification to be provided via precompilation);
- *Free text tokenization and preprocessing*: text preprocessing using finite-state automata auto-generated from regular expressions and deterministic grammar (Graver 1992);
- *Charts*: a chart-parsing engine for both inactive and active charts, with complete data abstraction allowing support for all chart-based parsing algorithms (these classes may be specializations of graph classes that are reused from the ALCOM ESPRIT project and its LEDA library (Naher 1983));
- *Search*: alternative search patterns for common parsing regimes (including an experimental algorithm using lexical preferences derived statistically from domain-specific corpora);
- *Formalism*: grammar development support for a Categorial Grammar formalism, including grammar compilation, consistency checking and corpus analysis tools such as KWIC.

28.3.1 Design policies

In all cases, key design decisions are parameterized, to be supplied by add-in classes chosen by the framework client. For example, storage management policy is selectable over the set:

- *unbounded* structures that can grow to the limits of virtual memory via the use of operating-system allocation of the heap (e.g. linked list-based structures);
- *bounded* structures whose size is determined at compile time and for which a statically sized chunk of memory is allocated on the stack (e.g. array-based structures);
- *dynamic* structures, with access behaviour similar to the bounded class, but overflow behaviour similar to the unbounded class (e.g. structures based on dynamically extendible arrays allocated in relatively large chunks on the heap).

2. "Deep" in the sense of fully implementing a small subset of the full system, as opposed to sketching the implementation of a whole system.

This set of policies is that of the "Booch components", a framework developed as a foundation class resource for data structures and algorithms of general use in modern software construction (Rational 1993: 19–33). We also endorse the library requirements identified for the Booch (1994: 329) framework, namely:

- *completeness*: incorporate abstractions covering a large subset of the problem space;
- *adaptability*: isolate platform-specific design policies;
- *efficiency*: of compile resources, run-time resources and developer resources (ease of use);
- *safety*: type safety should be enforced at both static (compilation) and dynamic (run-time exception) levels;
- *simplicity of use*: consistency and organization;
- *extendibility*: ability to add new classes within the architecture of the framework.

The framework proposed by this article supports these requirements by:

- basing the requirements analysis of the project on as wide a range of NLP research projects and commercial systems as possible (completeness);
- adopting standards and practices appropriate to cross-platform portability, e.g. C++ level 3.0, the UNICODE multi-byte character standard, generic human interface support separated from support for particular graphics environments (adaptability);
- class parameterization (C++ templates) and support for subclassing (adaptability, extendibility);
- distributing C++ source code; using low-level abstractions with explicit time and space semantics selectable for application-specific optimization and providing full documentation (efficiency);
- using the strong typing principles of C++ and the encapsulation principle of object-oriented programming (Coad & Nicola 1993; Stroustrup 1991) (safety);
- providing the maximum level of similarity between class protocols, using class families or categories, and separating algorithmic abstractions from structural abstractions (simplicity).

28.3.2 Reusability and unification

The term-unification classes are a good example of the framework's philosophy in action. Classes are parameterized for both storage management policies and instantiation policy. The latter policy is switchable between the production of either binding environments (to support structure-sharing implementations where informational structures remain constant and are manipulated relative to binding environments – Shieber et al. 1983) or structure copying (to support applications tolerant of a higher space-to-time ratio). Classes are provided for:

- precompilation of attribute–value matrices to terms (term unification is inherently more efficient – Simpkins 1992: 1, Hirsh 1988);

- term unification (efficient implementation based on integer representation of symbols – Cunningham et al. 1994a; Campbell 1984; Ramsay 1988), with polymorphic overloading of functions for alternative instantiation policies and parameterization for alternative term representations;
- continuations: indexes into a Horn-clause database plus binding environments representing previously successful goals, for reasoning-engine support.

These classes are intended to provide sufficient flexibility to support both unification-based parsing in its diverse forms and unification-based reasoning (e.g. PROLOG-like deductive inference over a database of Horn clauses, abduction).

The required flexibility is bought by decomposing the basic functions of these diverse systems. For example, PROLOG-like inference can be thought of as depth-first search over a space of continuations. Systems that use unification, however, do not always need the power of continuations. For example, a parser may use unification as a single-step operation resulting either in failure or a new instantiated object representing the informational union of two constituents (Shieber 1992: 37–9). In this case it is inefficient to adopt the full power of PROLOG's reasoning mechanisms: the decomposition of functionality embodied in the model above allows the use of only those components actually needed for a given task.

Similarly, the implementation of abductive reasoning tools in PROLOG involves the implementation of a meta-interpreter that sits on top of the deductive engine at PROLOG's heart, and this is necessarily a source of run-time inefficiency. Again, a properly constructed framework can remove the problem.

In the sample application under development in parallel with the NLP domain framework prototype (a shallow analyser of free text intended for categorization and routeing tasks) terms are implemented as contiguous (i.e. array-based) structures made up of positive and negative 2-byte integers (atoms and variables respectively: the linguistic formalism used does not require lists or embedded terms). This leads to an efficient implementation of the main unification routines and a static memory requirement of around 64 kbytes for the unification module's internal data structures. This is acceptably small for PC implementation, which is one of the system's requirements.

This representation scheme, however, is clearly not of completely general applicability: other framework clients might represent terms as graphs, or symbols as character strings, for example. Given an implementation in which terms and symbols are encapsulated as objects with a well-defined protocol,[3] substitution of an alternative representation scheme is simply a matter of providing these new classes; the unification algorithm, class composition and set of protocols need not be touched.

---

3. "We call the entire set of operations that a client may perform on an object, together with the legal orderings in which they may be invoked, its protocol" (Booch 1994: 43).

28.4 Summary

Software reuse requires a new approach to developing software systems. Traditional approaches to reuse have proved unfruitful as a result of an orientation towards the provision of system-level components. Object-orientation allows the encapsulation of finer-grained abstractions, and so is applicable to the problem of reuse. Frameworks provide a means to package and distribute reusable components. A framework of objects for NLP systems could significantly contribute to reuse within the language engineering community.

References

Alshawi, H. (ed.) 1992. *The Core Language Engine*, Cambridge Mass.: MIT Press.

Alshawi H., D. J. Arnold, R. Backofen, D. M. Carter, J. Lindop, K. Netter, S. G. Pulman, J. Tsujii & H. Uszkoreit 1991. *ET6/1 rule formalism and virtual machine design study: final report*. CEC, Luxembourg.

Black, W. J. & H. Cunningham 1993. *The COBALT language analysis module*. LRE project 61-011 Technical Report. C/CCL/04/93/a, Centre for Computational Linguistics, UMIST, Manchester.

Black W. J., H. Cunningham, B. Geurts & G. Rentier 1992. *The PLUS natural language engine*. ESPRIT project P5254 Deliverable D2.4. CEC, Luxembourg.

Booch, G. 1991. *Object oriented design with applications*. Redwood City, Calif.: Benjamin Cummings.

Booch G. 1994. *Object-oriented analysis and design*, 2nd edn. Redwood City, Calif.: Benjamin Cummins.

Campbell J. A. (ed.) 1984. *Implementations of PROLOG*, Chichester, England: John Wiley.

Coad P. & J. Nicola 1993. *Object-oriented programming*. Englewood Cliffs, NJ: Prentice-Hall.

Coad, P. & E. Yourdon 1991a. *Object-oriented analysis*, 2nd edn. Englewood Cliffs, NJ: Prentice-Hall.

Coad, P. & E. Yourdon 1991b. *Object-oriented design*, 2nd edn. Englewood Cliffs, NJ: Prentice-Hall.

Cunningham H., N. L. Underwood & W. J. Black 1993. *The surface-level COBALT analysis module*. LRE project 61-011 Technical Report C/CCL/11/93/b, Centre for Computational Linguistics, UMIST, Manchester.

Cunningham H., W. J. Black & N. L. Underwood 1994a. *Efficient shallow parsing for text categorisation*. Technical Report 94/02, Centre for Computational Linguistics, UMIST, Manchester.

Cunningham H., N. L. Underwood & W. J. Black 1994b. *Reusable components for CRISTAL*, LRE project 62-059 Technical Report, Centre for Computational Linguistics, UMIST, Manchester.

Date, C. J. 1990. *An introduction to database systems*, 5th edn. Wokingham, England: Addison-Wesley.

Graham, I. 1994. *Object-oriented methods*, 2nd edn. Wokingham, England: Addison-Wesley.

Graver J. O. 1992. T-gen: a string-to-object translator generator. *Journal of Object-Oriented Programming* **5**, 35–42.

Groenendijk M. 1992. *ALEP-0 Version 2.1 XALEP user guide*. Luxembourg: CEC.

Grover, C., J. Carroll & T. Briscoe 1993. *The Alvey natural language tools*, 4th Release. HCRC, University of Edinburgh.

Heid, U. 1993. EAGLES work-group on computational lexicons. Summary, internal report of LRE project 61-100, University of Stuttgart.

Hirsh, S. 1988. P-PATR: a compiler for unification-based grammars. In *Natural language understanding and logic programming II*, V. Dahl & P. Saint-Dizier (eds), 63–78. Amsterdam: North-Holland.

McNaught, J. 1993. The EAGLES standards-setting initiative. Internal report of LRE project 61-100, Centre for Computational Linguistics, UMIST, Manchester.

Meyer, B. 1988. *Object oriented software construction*. Englewood Cliffs, NJ: Prentice-Hall.

Modiano, N. & U. Heid 1993. EAGLES work-group on computational lexicons: Methodology. Internal report of LRE project 61-100, Cap Gemini Innovation, Paris.

Naher S. 1993. *LEDA User Manual Version 3.0.* Technical Report of ESPRIT Project 3075, ALCOM, Luxembourg.

Prieto-Diaz, R. 1993. Status report: software reusability. *IEEE Software* **10**, 61–6.

Prieto-Diaz, R. & P. Freeman 1987. Status report: software reusability. *IEEE Software* **4**, 34–58.

Ramsay, A. 1988. *Formal methods in Artificial Intelligence*. Cambridge: Cambridge University Press.

Rational 1993. *The C++ Booch components version 2.3 class catalogue*. Santa Clara, Calif.: Rational.

Rumbaugh, J., M. Blaha, W. Premerlani & F. Eddy 1991. *Object oriented modeling and design*. Englewood Cliffs, NJ: Prentice-Hall.

Shieber, S. 1992. *Constraint-based grammar formalisms*. Cambridge, Mass.: MIT Press.

Shieber, S., H. Uszkoreit, F. Pereira, J. Robinson & M. Tyson 1983. The formalism and implementation of PATR-II. In *Research on interactive acquisition and use of knowledge*, B. Grosz & M. Stickel (eds), 39–79. Menlo Park, Calif.: SRI.

Simpkins, N. 1992. *ALEP-0 prototype virtual machine user guide*. Luxembourg: CEC.

Stroustrup, B. 1991. *The C++ programming language*, 2nd edn. Murray Hill, NJ: AT&T Bell Labs.

Wirfs-Brock, R. & B. Wilkerson 1989. Object oriented design: a responsibility driven approach. In *OOPSLA 89: Object Oriented Programming: Systems, Languages and Applications*, New Orleans, La., 455–9.

Index

Page references in italics refer to footnotes.